Introduction to Medical Microbiology

Introduction to Medical Microbiology

MARCUS M. JENSEN

Professor of Microbiology, Brigham Young University

DONALD N. WRIGHT

Professor of Microbiology, Brigham Young University
and
Clinical Professor of Pathology, University of Utah

Prentice-Hall, Inc., Englewood Cliffs, New Jersey 07632

Library of Congress Cataloging in Publication Data

Jensen, Marcus M.
  Introduction to medical microbiology.

  Includes index.
  1. Medical microbiology. I. Wright, Donald N.
II. Title. [DNLM: 1. Microbiology. QW 4 J525i]
QR46.J46   1985   616'.01   84-13355
ISBN   0-13-487380-7

Editorial/production supervision:
  Zita de Schauensee
Cover design: Maureen Eide
Chapter-opening and front matter
  design: Judy Winthrop
Line illustrations: Vantage Art
Manufacturing buyer: John Hall
Art production: Charles Pelletreau
Cover photo: TAP Pharmaceuticals

Cover illustration: A scanning electron micrograph showing
invasion of lung tissue by the bacterium *Pseudomonas aeruginosa*
(see p. 339). These bacterial cells have entered the lungs from the
blood stream along with some red blood cells (concave disks).
Bacteria are adhering to lung tissue and cell division is seen in
the bacterium at the center of the photo. (Courtesy TAP
Pharmaceuticals, North Chicago, Ill.)

© 1985 by Prentice-Hall, Inc., Englewood Cliffs, New Jersey 07632

Printed in the United States of America

10 9 8 7 6 5 4 3 2

ISBN 0-13-487380-7 01

Prentice-Hall International, Inc., *London*
Prentice-Hall of Australia Pty. Limited, *Sydney*
Editora Prentice-Hall do Brasil, Ltda., *Rio de Janeiro*
Prentice-Hall Canada Inc., *Toronto*
Prentice-Hall of India Private Limited, *New Delhi*
Prentice-Hall of Japan, Inc., *Tokyo*
Prentice-Hall of Southeast Asia Pte. Ltd., *Singapore*
Whitehall Books Limited, *Wellington, New Zealand*

Contents

v

Preface

The optimal satisfaction with a textbook is largely dependent on the use of that book for its intended purpose. It is hoped this preface will help to clarify the authors' intent. This book is self-instructive and is adaptable to nonclassroom as well as classroom settings. Careful attention has been paid to readability of the material.

Introduction to Medical Microbiology has been written with the student in mind. The content is aimed not at the critical professional but at those beginning students desiring a broad approach to microbiology with emphasis on the role of microorganisms in disease processes. The text is arranged for easy access to the essential elements of medical microbiology for those students who need or desire a single course in the subject without taking prerequisite or subsequent courses. It is directed principally toward those students in nursing and other allied health areas, but can also be used in general education courses.

No attempt has been made to provide a compendium of all that is known about microorganisms. Rather, an effort has been made to provide only that information essential to an appreciation of the role of microorganisms in the disease process. The basis for this textbook is a successful course syllabus that has been used for many years in the instruction of students of nursing and other health sciences.

The early chapters are devoted to basic principles of microbiology, methods used to control microorganisms, and host-microorganism relationships relevant to a study of microbial diseases. Subsequent chapters deal specifically with disease-producing microorganisms with emphasis on the diseases they cause, modes of transmission, diagnosis, treatment, prevention, and control; that is, those concepts of greatest concern to personnel involved in patient care.

Various approaches are used in different textbooks to arrange and present the study of infectious diseases. One approach is to arrange the diseases according to the taxonomic classification of the causative microorganisms. Another approach is to discuss the diseases of an organ system, such as the respiratory tract, in one section and those of another organ system in a different section. Still another approach is to discuss diseases in groups according to their mode of transmission; that is, diseases transmitted by the airborne route in one section and those transmitted by water in another section, etc. Each of these approaches has certain advantages and disadvantages. The presentations of diseases by organ systems or by mode of transmission are useful in helping the student relate these diseases to a clinical setting or an epidemiological problem. However, these approaches are also cumbersome in that a single disease may involve more than one organ system or may be transmitted by more than one route, and therefore the same disease must be discussed in several different sections. In this text, the various diseases will be discussed according to the taxonomic categories of the causative microorganisms, as it is felt a better organized and more concise coverage of the subject can be accomplished with this approach.

Provo, Utah   Marcus M. Jensen

                                                                   Donald N. Wright

Historical Developments in Medical Microbiology

1

Infectious diseases have been the greatest pestilences in human history and only in the past 75 to 100 years have many of our major infectious diseases been brought under control. In years past severe outbreaks of infectious diseases periodically swept across nations or through cities to ravage inhabitants. Classic examples of these epidemic scourges are smallpox, typhus, cholera, and plague. Outbreaks of smallpox, which periodically struck cities, would often kill from 10 to 90% of the inhabitants while the great plague pandemic of the Middle Ages killed an estimated one-fourth of the inhabitants of Europe. The disease of tuberculosis, which develops slowly in the body and rarely causes explosive outbreaks, has always been with us; until the present century approximately 30% of the world's inhabitants who reached adulthood died of tuberculosis before reaching old age. Childhood infectious diseases have always been present as well; before 1900 about one of every two children died, primarily due to these diseases, before reaching 10 years of age.

Today the number of persons dying from infectious diseases in developed countries is only a small portion of what it was in earlier times. Developments that led to the control of many devastating microbial diseases of humans represent some of the great triumphs of modern technology. Yet many infectious diseases are still not effectively controlled; moreover, as social and physical living conditions change, new patterns of these diseases develop. Often these new patterns result from new medical procedures that, while benefiting patients in some ways, render them more susceptible to certain types of infections in other ways. A person working in health care today must be aware of conditions that cause these changing patterns of infectious diseases and must then be able to adapt procedures to minimize or control such infections.

Serious infectious diseases are still widespread in underdeveloped countries, particularly those caused by parasites and those transmitted because of unsanitary conditions.

The discoveries that led to an increased understanding and control of infectious diseases involved many people over many years. By the latter half of the nineteenth century the contagious nature and mode of transmission of many diseases had been demonstrated. This information, coupled with an increased ability to study microorganisms, led to the formation of the germ theory of disease and ushered in the *golden age of microbiology.* This period of discovery spanned the years from about 1875 to 1900, during which time the foundations of the science of microbiology were established.

Developments that preceded and established the basis for the germ theory of disease came from three independent branches of research—that is, observations on the contagious nature of disease, vaccination, and basic research on the nature of microorganisms. Out of the central concept of the germ theory of disease arose various subdisciplines that specialize in the study of different types of microbial agents as well as the methods used to treat and control infectious diseases. Some historical highlights of medical microbiology are outlined in Figure 1-1 and are discussed next.

EVENTS PRECEDING THE GERM THEORY

Contagion

The idea that certain diseases could be passed from person to person by contact existed in many ancient cultures. The most notable examples of awareness of contagion are Biblical references to the disposal of human wastes and regulations to avoid contact with lepers. The ancient Greek civilization was more aware of this concept than many later cultures. Aristotle reportedly instructed Alexander the Great to have his armies boil their drinking water and bury their dung. Yet many later cultures seemed unaware of the contagious nature of diseases. One dominant philosophy before the nineteenth century held that diseases resulted from contaminations of earthly influences, planetary conjunctions, or supernatural forces. The name *influenza* stems from the Middle Ages when it was thought that certain positions of the stars "influenced" the onset of this disease. Yet despite such philosophies some scientists correctly observed the contagious nature of infectious diseases. One such interpretation was recorded in a book entitled *De Contagione et Contagiosis Morbis* (Contagion and Contagious Diseases) written in 1547 by an Italian physician, *Girolamo Fracastoro.* Fracastoro theorized that tiny imperceptible particles ("seeds of disease") spread from person to person. He postulated three forms of contagion: (a) by direct contact, (b) by fomites (a term first introduced by Fracastoro in referring to contaminated inanimate objects), and (c) at a distance—that is, by air or water. Unfortunately, his concepts were several hundred years ahead of their time and generally did not become part of the medical philosophy of his day.

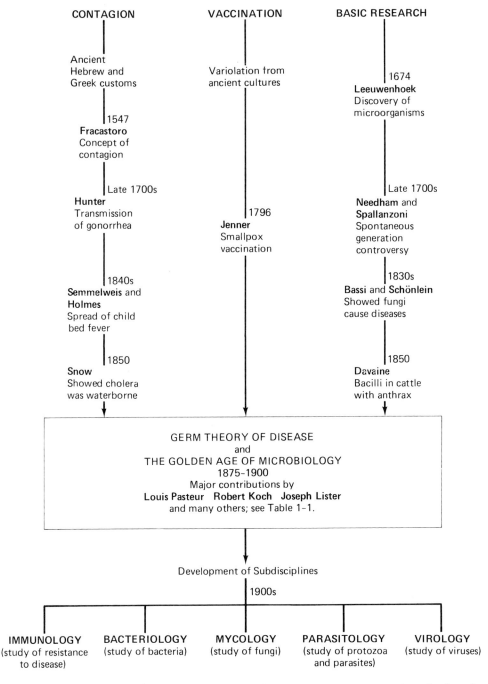

Figure 1-1 Historical highlights in medical microbiology, showing three independent branches of research coming together in the latter part of the nineteenth century to formulate the germ theory of disease and usher in the "Golden Age of Microbiology." In the twentieth century, subdisciplines of medical microbiology developed.

Rather convincing work was done in the 1700s by *Micheli, Tillet,* and *Prevost* on the transmission of plant diseases and the prevention of transmission by the use of chemical agents. This work, however, had little apparent impact on those concerned with diseases of humans or animals. In the latter half of the eighteenth century the experiments of the noted British surgeon *John Hunter* helped emphasize the concept of contagious diseases. Yet he also inadvertently and somewhat tragically confused the entire concept. In an attempt to prove the contagious nature of gonorrhea, he purposely inoculated the skin of his arm with pus from a person with gonorrhea. His concept was proven when he developed a pussy gonorrheal lesion at the site of inoculation. Unfortunately, the experiment was confused because the patient from whom the pus was taken had syphilis as well. This disease was also successfully transmitted to the unfortunate Dr. Hunter and resulted in his untimely death. Because of this error, for years afterward many persons believed gonorrhea and syphilis were different manifestations of the same disease.

During the first 30 years of the nineteenth century some chemical antimicrobials, mostly chlorine compounds and primarily for odor control, came into use in some medical facilities. Several applications, however, also involved treating infected wounds, purifying water, and disinfecting hands. Notable observations were made between 1830 and 1860 on the mode of spread of childbed or puerperal fever, measles, and cholera. During the 1830s and 1840s independent observations were made on the transmission of a serious disease called childbed fever by the noted American physician-poet *Oliver Wendell Holmes* and a young Hungarian physician, *Ignas Semmelweis.* They proposed methods for controlling this disease by having physicians wash their hands regularly with chloride solutions. Semmelweis trained in the obstetrical service of the general hospital of Vienna and while there became greatly concerned about the high death rate from childbed fever in women who gave birth in that hospital. By careful observation (Figure 1-2), he detected certain patterns of this disease. Patients examined shortly after the physician had autopsied a cadaver frequently contracted childbed fever. He theorized that "cadaveric particles" carried by the physician from the cadaver to the patient were responsible for the disease. Semmelweis instructed those working under him to wash their hands thoroughly with chlorinated water after having worked with a cadaver or a diseased patient. Consequently, the mortality rate from childbed fever on his service was greatly reduced. Unfortunately, his observations and similar ones by Holmes were not readily accepted by many of the medical profession of their time. Semmelweis was more abused than honored for trying to introduce "radical new concepts of little value."

In 1846 *Panum,* a 26-year-old Danish physician, was sent by his government to investigate an outbreak of measles in the Faroe Islands. After interviewing thousands of patients, he determined that measles was contracted by contact with a person who already had measles and that the disease did not arise spontaneously as some authorities thought. He also determined the incubation time for the disease and clearly observed that those who had had the disease were immune when reexposed. His work presented a clear and accurate picture of the epidemiology of measles.

I. Abtheilung.

Klinik für Aerzte.

1841	Geburten 3036,	Todte	237,	Percent-Antheil	7.80
1842	» 3287,	»	518,	»	»	15.75
1843	» 3060,	»	274,	»	»	8.95
1844	» 3157,	»	260,	»	»	8.23
1845	» 3492,	»	241,	»	»	6.90
1846	» 4010,	»	459,	»	»	11.44
	» 20042,	»	1989,	»	»	9.92

II. Abtheilung.

Klinik für Hebammen.

1841	Geburten 2442,	Todte	86,	Percent-Antheil	3.52
1842	» 2659,	»	202,	»	»	7.59
1843	» 2739,	»	164,	»	»	5.98
1844	» 2956,	»	68,	»	»	2.80
1845	» 3241,	»	66,	»	»	2.03
1846	» 3754,	»	105,	»	»	2.79
	» 27791,	»	691,	»	»	3.38

Figure 1-2 A table from the research of Semmelweis showing a higher death rate (9.92%) from childbed fever in women giving birth in the clinic attended by physicians (Klinik für Aerzte) compared to a death rate of 3.38% in the clinic attended by midwives (Klinik für Hebammen). Translations: *Geburten* = births; *Todte* = deaths; *Abtheilung* = division.

Important observations were made on the communicable nature of cholera through a detailed study by *John Snow*. In 1854 he showed that persons using water from the Broad Street pump in London were much more likely to contract cholera than those obtaining their water from other pumps (Figure 1-3). He further showed evidence of fecal contamination at the Broad Street pump and correctly deduced that this contamination was responsible for the outbreaks of cholera.

Immunization

Since antiquity people had observed that those surviving one attack of certain diseases were immune to a second attack. Most notable were observations on smallpox (also called variola). It was further noted that both a major and a minor form of smallpox occurred and recovery from one conferred immunity against both forms.

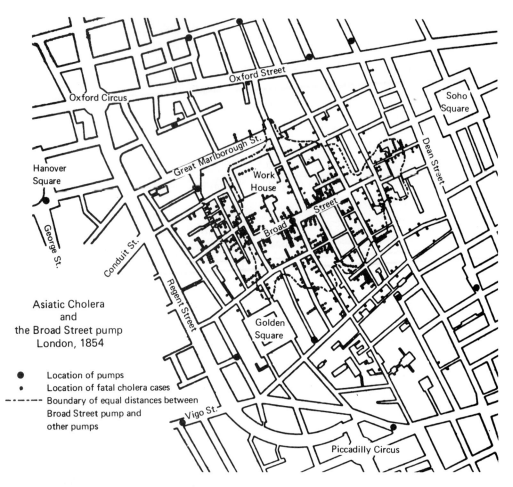

Figure 1-3 A map of the Broad Street London showing the clustering of outbreaks of cholera among persons using water from the Broad Street pump. From the study of John Snow in 1854. (Modified from J. P. Fox, C. E. Hall, L. R. Elveback: *Epidemiology Man and Disease*, Figure 10-10, p. 227. Copyright © 1970 by Macmillan Publishing Company)

Death rates from the minor form were considerably less than the risk of naturally acquiring and dying of the major form. Therefore in some countries before the nineteenth century, primarily in Asia, Africa, and, to some extent, North America, a procedure called variolation was practiced. This procedure entailed purposely exposing persons to the minor form of smallpox. The English physician *Edward Jenner,* who was aware of the practice of variolation, carried the concept a step further. Jenner observed that milkmaids, who often contracted a mild disease called cowpox, rarely came down with smallpox. Therefore in about 1796 he deliberately inoculated persons with materials taken from cowpox lesions (Figure 1-4). This process came to be known as vaccination, a term based on the Latin word for cow (*vacca*). In spite of some early opposition, the practice of vaccination against smallpox eventually became widely adapted and started a procedure that in time led to the complete eradication of this disease.

All the foregoing studies on the contagious nature of some diseases and vaccinations were accomplished through empirical observations and without correlation with discoveries that were being made in the new science of microbiology.

Discovery of Microorganisms and Early Basic Research

The discovery of microorganisms in 1674 came not from research by scholars and scientists of that day but from the astute observations of a layman. *Antony van Leeuwenhoek* of Delft, Holland, was not well educated in the classical manner of this day, but he had become very skilled in his hobby of grinding glass lenses and making simple one-lens microscopes (Figure 1-5). These microscopes gave magnifications of

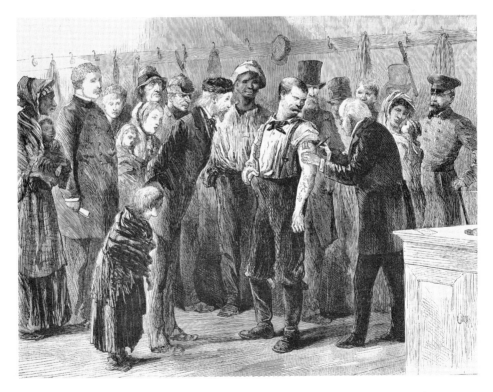

Figure 1-4 Early smallpox vaccination procedure in which cowpox material was introduced into the skin. (The Bettmann Archive)

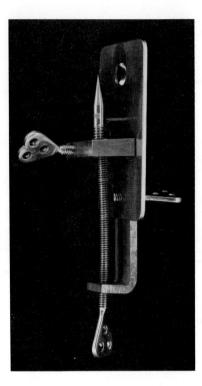

Figure 1-5 A replica of the type of single-lens microscope used by Leeuwenhoek. The object was placed on the pointed tip and brought into focus by turning the screws. (From Thomas D. Brock, *Biology of Microorganisms*, Third Edition, Figure 1.2, p. 3. Copyright © 1979 by Thomas D. Brock. Reprinted by permission of Prentice-Hall, Inc.)

up to 300 times and through a special method of illumination, which he kept a secret but was probably a form of dark-field lighting, he was able to observe the fine structure of many materials. While observing pond water in 1674, he was amazed to see many very small creatures, apparently algae or protozoa. He called these creatures *animalcules.* This discovery greatly intrigued Leeuwenhoek, who spent most of his spare time over the next 50 years making observations of microorganisms that he found in various materials. Encouraged by friends, he communicated his discoveries to the Royal Society of London. Leeuwenhoek wrote his first letter to the Royal Society somewhat apologetically, for it was in his own simple Dutch dialect and not in the scholarly Latin then customary in scientific writing. Yet using this simple language, he was able to accurately describe his important discovery (Figure 1-6). Impressed with Leeuwenhoek's discovery, the Royal Society encouraged him to continue his observations and correspondence. Between 1673 and the time of his death in 1733 Leeuwenhoek sent over 150 letters to the Royal Society. In his simple, colorful way Leeuwenhoek accurately described protozoa, fungi, algae, and bacteria. He was honored by being made an honorary member of the Royal Society, the preeminent society for scientific research of his time. Today he is recognized as the "Father of Microbiology." Neither Leeuwenhoek nor his contemporaries made any connection between these recently discovered "animalcules" and diseases, however.

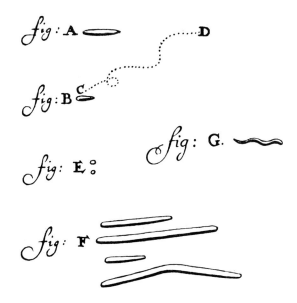

LEEUWENHOEK'S FIGURES OF BACTERIA FROM THE HUMAN MOUTH
(Letter 39, 17 Sept. 1683)
Enlarged (× 1½) from the engravings published in *Arc. Nat. Det.*, 1695.

Fig. A, a motile *Bacillus*.
Fig. B, *Selenomonas sputigena*. C . . . . D, the path of its motion.
Fig. E, Micrococci.
Fig. F, *Leptothrix buccalis*.
Fig. G, A spirochæte—probably " *Spirochaeta buccalis*," the largest form found
in this situation.

Figure 1-6 Reproductions of microorganisms drawn by Leeuwenhoek in one of his letters to the Royal Society. (From C. Dobell, *Anthony and His Little Animals*. New York: Dover Publications, 1960)

Studies of microorganisms were limited during the first 150 years after their discovery and were considered little more than biological curiosities. Because of technical difficulties, most biologists of that era found it unprofitable to study microorganisms. The Swedish naturalist *Linnaeus,* in an attempt to include microorganisms in his scientific classification of plants and animals in 1758, referred to them as the class "chaos." This name perhaps best described the contemporary state of knowledge regarding microorganisms in the eighteenth century.

The systematic laboratory investigation of microorganisms accelerated in the latter half of the eighteenth century. During this time microorganisms became the central subject of a controversy concerning spontaneous generation (life arising from nonliving matter). Studies by *Redi* a century earlier had laid to rest such theories as the idea that flies arose spontaneously from decomposing meat. In 1784, however, *John Needham,* after conducting a series of experiments with bacteria in which bacterial growth appeared in broth that had been boiled, concluded that only spontaneous generation could explain his results. Clearly Needham's findings were a result of resistant bacterial spores and poor aseptic techniques. In any case, Needham's theory received wide support as well as notoriety. *Spallanzani* challenged it and conducted an extensive series of experiments to show that microorganisms arose only from other microorganisms of the same type. The controversy between Spallanzani and Needham continued for many years and increased scientific interest in microorganisms. The spontaneous generation theory smoldered on for an additional 100 years until finally disproved by *Pasteur* and *Tyndall.*

By the mid-1800s investigators started to recognize the possible role of microorganisms as causative agents of disease. In 1836 *Bassi* showed that fungi were the cause of a disease in silkworms; a few years later *Schönlein* demonstrated the association of fungi with a human skin disease called favus. *Hansen* discovered bacilli in cells from leprosy patients in 1847. In 1850 *Davaine* carried out preliminary studies in which he observed large bacilli in the blood of cattle with anthrax; he suggested that these organisms might be the cause of this disease. Then in 1865 *Villemin* experimentally transmitted tuberculosis to animals. The full impact of these studies was not initially recognized; they were, however, a prelude to the formulation of the germ theory of disease and an introduction to the *golden age of microbiology* during the latter part of the nineteenth century.

GERM THEORY OF DISEASE AND GOLDEN AGE OF MICROBIOLOGY

The central figures in establishing microbiology as a science were the French scientist *Louis Pasteur* and the German physician *Robert Koch.*

Pasteur (Figure 1-7) first gained recognition as a chemist when he successfully separated left- and right-handed crystals of tartaric acid. Then in the 1850s his studies turned to the process of fermentation and he concluded that microorganisms were responsible for this process. In a short series of studies published in 1860 and 1861 Pasteur helped disprove the lingering theory of the spontaneous generation of microorganisms. Because of his knowledge of fermentation, Pasteur was asked to help solve the problem of the so-called wine disease. In this study he scientifically determined that undesirable wine was produced by the presence of undesirable microorganisms. To resolve this problem, he applied mild heat to the grape juice in order to destroy the unwanted microorganisms, a process now called *pasteurization* (Figure 1-8). Pasteur was next requested to cure a silkworm disease that was gradually destroying the French silk industry. After many trials and setbacks and five years of effort, Pasteur demonstrated that a protozoan caused this disease and he introduced

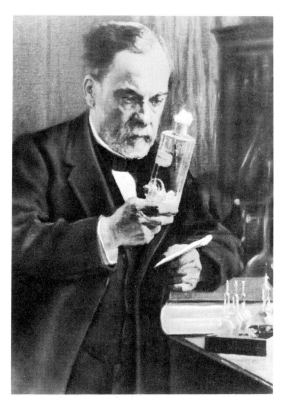

Figure 1-7 A painting of Louis Pasteur by Edelfeld. (The Bettmann Archive)

methods to limit its spread. Then by 1876 Pasteur turned to the study of the contagious diseases of vertebrates. Carrying out extensive experiments with anthrax and chicken cholera, Pasteur helped establish the causative role of specific bacteria for these diseases. Among his greatest contributions were the development of vaccines for their control. Later in the mid-1880s Pasteur developed a successful treatment for persons exposed to rabies.

Koch was fascinated with research on microorganisms early in his medical career. Working under makeshift conditions in the 1870s (Figure 1-9), he developed systematic methods for studying microorganisms. His first studies, reported in 1876, clearly demonstrated the role of a specific bacterium as the causative agent of anthrax. By 1880 Koch was receiving increased support for his work and could spend his full efforts in research. He continued to improve the methods used to study microbial diseases, with some of his most important work centering on tuberculosis. Before his death in 1910 Koch became a central force for microbiological research and, with his associates, made many notable contributions to medical microbiology.

Great research institutes developed around both Pasteur and Koch and became the major centers for microbiological research during the latter part of the nineteenth century.

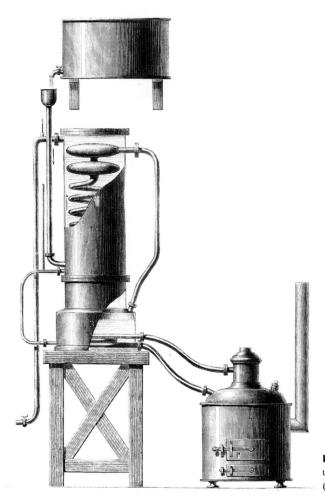

Figure 1-8 An early type of apparatus
used for the pasteurization of wine.
(Institut Pasteur, Paris)

While both Pasteur and Koch carried out important work in France and Germany, significant developments were being made in Great Britain by the surgeon *Joseph Lister*. Lister was familiar with the studies of Pasteur on fermentation and putrifaction and in 1865 he reasoned that microorganisms could be causing the putrifaction or pus formation (suppuration) associated with wounds. He further reasoned that dressing the wound with some material capable of killing these germs might help prevent the suppuration. Noting that carbolic acid (phenol) was effective in preventing sewage odors, Lister chose to use this substance as his antiseptic agent. This choice was fortunate and Lister had great success in preventing wound infections. He extended his methods to surgeries by soaking ligatures in disinfectants and by performing operations under a spray of phenol (Figure 1-10). Lister's methods were readily accepted and by the end of the nineteenth century aseptic surgery had become a standard procedure.

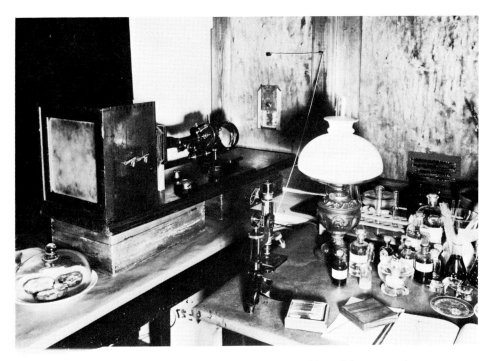

Figure 1-9   A room in Koch's house that was converted into a laboratory and was used during his early studies in microbiology. (The Bettmann Archive)

Numerous other discoveries were made by other scientists during this *golden age of microbiology* (see Table 1-1). By 1900 microbiology was a well-established science and the relationship between microbes and many diseases had been clearly determined. Even more important, methods for treating and controlling some diseases were developed during this time. In the early 1900s numerous contributions broadened our knowledge of microbiology. Out of this early knowledge came the various subdisciplines of medical microbiology shown in Figure 1-1.

CHEMOTHERAPY

Knowing that living biological agents were responsible for disease in humans led naturally to an investigation of the means to use in infection control. Extensive studies were carried out in the early 1900s in Germany by *Paul Ehrlich* to find chemicals that would specifically destroy microorganisms in infected tissues. His success was limited, but he firmly established the concept of using chemicals to treat infectious diseases (chemotherapy).

Later developments in chemotherapy in the 1930s revolutionized our ability to treat bacterial diseases. From England in 1928 *Alexander Fleming* had reported his chance discovery of strong antibacterial properties produced by the secretions of the

TABLE 1-1 SOME IMPORTANT DISCOVERIES MADE IN MEDICAL MICROBIOLOGY DURING THE "GOLDEN AGE OF MICROBIOLOGY," 1875–1900

Year	Discoverer	Discovery
1877	R. Koch	Proved that anthrax is caused by a bacterium.
1877	F. Cohn	Demonstrated bacterial spores.
1878	J. Lister	First grew bacteria in pure culture.
1879	A. Neisser	Discovered the cause of gonorrhea.
1880s	L. Pasteur	Developed vaccines and treatment for rabies.
1881	A. Ogston	Discovered staphylococci cause wound infection.
1882	R. Koch	Discovered the cause of tuberculosis.
1883	T. Klebs	Discovered the cause of diphtheria.
1884	A. Nicolaier	Discovered the cause of tetanus.
1884	R. Koch	Discovered the cause of cholera.
1884	G. Gaffky	Discovered the cause of typhoid fever.
1884	E. Metchnikoff	First observed phagocytosis by white blood cells.
1887	D. Bruce	Discovered the cause of Malta fever.
1890	E. von Behring and S. Kitasato	Discovered bacterial toxins and how to develop antitoxins.
1892	W. Welch and G. Nuttal	Discovered the cause of gas gangrene.
1892	D. Ivanovski	First demonstration of a virus.
1894	A. Yersin	Discovered the cause of plague.
1897	E. Van Ermengen	Discovered the cause of botulism food poisoning.
1898	K. Shiga	Discovered the cause of dysentery.
1900	W. Reed	Showed yellow fever was transmitted by mosquitoes and was caused by a virus.

mold *Penicillium* (Figure 1-11). This substance he called penicillin. By 1938 *Florey* and *Chain* had purified this material and demonstrated its usefulness in treating bacterial infections. Stimulated by the advent of World War II, scientists soon found methods for the mass production of penicillin and this antimicrobial agent became available to the world.

The development of another important chemotherapeutic agent during this era involved several groups of scientists. In the early 1930s *Domagk*, a German pathologist, found that a chemical called prontosil had significant chemotherapeutic effects on some bacterial infections. Then in 1935 the *Trefouels*, a husband and wife team working in France, discovered that the antibacterial activity of prontosil was due to the sulfanilamide segment of the molecule. This finding rapidly led to the development of various "sulfa" compounds that became useful chemotherapeutic agents.

Penicillin and sulfa drugs were the first highly effective compounds developed for treating specific bacterial diseases. Over the past 40 years untold millions of patients have been treated by using these two agents. Moreover, these chemicals were continually improved over the years and since 1940 many additional chemotherapeutic agents have been developed.

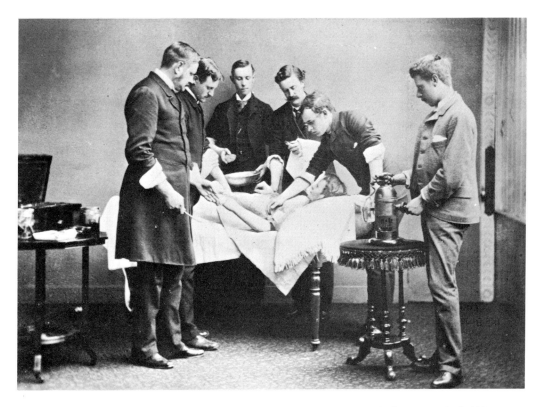

Figure 1-10 An operation in Edinburgh, about 1870, using the carbolic spray method of Lister. Masks, gloves, caps, and gowns were not yet being used. (The Bettmann Archive)

MOLECULAR BIOLOGY

Many advances in all areas of microbiology occurred since the 1940s. The most impressive contributions, however, are those that led to a preliminary understanding of how molecules work together inside a living cell—a field of study now referred to as *molecular biology.* Microorganisms and, in particular, viruses were extensively used in these studies because of their relative structural simplicity. Using bacterial cells, *Avery, MacLeod,* and *McCarty,* working in New York, first reported the genetic role of DNA in 1944. Then in 1953 *Watson* and *Crick,* working in England, discovered the structure of DNA. Following these early discoveries, various scientists have demonstrated how DNA functions as the genetic storehouse of information and how this information is used to direct the various cellular activities. As a result of this information, it is now hoped that scientists will be able to develop new methods for treating many human diseases.

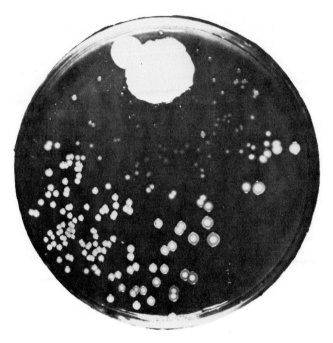

Figure 1-11 A photograph of Alexander Fleming's original plate showing the growth of the mold *Penicillium notatum* and its inhibitory action on bacterial growth. (The Bettmann Archive)

SUMMARY

1. Microbiology is a rather recent scientific discipline that has grown rapidly during the past 100 years. Originally the primary concern and interest regarding the microorganism centered around its ability to produce serious, often fatal disease. Later the microorganism proved a great tool in the study of life and much that we know regarding genetics, biochemistry, cellular physiology, and molecular biology was derived through careful study of these life forms.

2. Microbiology took a great leap forward with the general acceptance of the germ theory of disease. This awakening led to a period known as the Golden Age of Microbiology during which most infectious disease agents now known were discovered.

3. Concurrent with the discovery of infectious agents developed a parallel science based on a study of resistance to infection. This discipline, immunology, today ranks as one of the most challenging and exciting fields of scientific discovery. Later on the development of antimicrobial therapy, centered in the antibiotics, brought a new success to the world of the microbiologist.

The Scope of Microbiology

2

The cell is the basic unit of all living systems and each one contains the unique components of life. Life forms exist either as multicellular forms or as single cells. The multicellular forms, such as plants and animals, consist of millions of cells of diverse types that function together and depend on each other. Microorganisms are single-cell forms of life; each cell is an individual and is able to carry out the biological functions necessary to perpetuate itself. Because most single-celled life forms can be seen only with the aid of a microscope, they are called *microorganisms* and are the subjects of microbiology. The total number of individual microorganisms is staggering and far exceeds the number of all other forms of life combined. Microorganisms have adapted to grow in many and diverse environmental niches (Table 2-1). Within the digestive tract of humans or other animals, for example, as many as 10^{10} microorganisms may be present in one gram of fecal material while a gram of fertile topsoil may contain more than 10^9 microorganisms. Yet other environments may be relatively free of microorganisms; for example, outside air may contain less than one microorganism per liter or a clean surface exposed to sunlight may contain no viable microorganisms.

The environments in which microorganisms have adapted to grow are diverse and, in some cases, extreme. Certain microorganisms grow in hot springs at temperatures close to the boiling point, for instance, whereas others are able to grow on snow banks. Microorganisms may have a profound effect on their surroundings and are responsible for many essential biological phenomena in nature that are necessary to maintain balanced life systems on the earth. By and large, the overall effect of microorganisms on other life forms is beneficial; without microorganisms other life forms

TABLE 2-1   COMMON HABITATS WHERE BACTERIA
ARE PRESENT

Habitat	Approximate number of bacteria
Garden soil (surface)	9.7×10^6/g
Garden soil (30 cm deep)	5.7×10^5/g
Lakewater (shallow)	10^4/ml
Lakewater (deep)	10^2/ml
Seawater	1.1×10^3/ml
Human skin	10^6/sq cm
Human mouth	10^7/ml
Human intestine	4×10^{10}/g
Milk	10^3 to 10^6/ml
Cheese	10^8/g
Sunlit surface	few
Air	few

on this planet would probably be unable to survive. Although this textbook deals primarily with microorganisms that cause diseases in humans, it is also important for readers to be aware of the beneficial role of microorganisms. This chapter briefly mentions some of the nonmedical applications of microbiology and introduces various groups of microorganisms. In describing microorganisms, it is necessary to use units of measurement unfamiliar to most beginning students of microbiology. As with all scientific measurements, these units are part of the metric system and are included in Table 2-2.

BASIC CELL TYPES

Two basic cell types exist; they are called *eucaryotic* and *procaryotic* cells. Basically eucaryotic cells are larger and more complex than the procaryotic cells and possess a membrane-enclosed nucleus; eucaryotic means a true nucleus (*eu* = true; *karyon* = nucleus). All plants, animals, fungi, protozoa, and algae consist of eucaryotic cells. Procaryotic cells have no nuclear membrane or true nucleus (*pro* = early). Only the

TABLE 2-2   THE UNITS OF MEASUREMENT USED IN MICROBIOLOGY

Unit of measurement	Abbreviation	Equivalent
Meter	m	39.37 inches
Centimeter	cm	1/100th of a meter (10^{-2}m)
Millimeter	mm	1/1000th of a meter (10^{-3}m)
Micrometer[a]	μm	1/1000th of a millimeter (10^{-6}m)
Nanometer[b]	nm	1/1000th of a micrometer (10^{-9}m)
Angstrom	Å	1/10th of a nanometer (10^{-10}m)

[a]Formerly called a micron.
[b]Formerly called a millimicron.

microorganisms classed as bacteria and the cyanobacteria are procaryotic cells. The eucaryotic microbes are sometimes called *eucaryotes* and the procaryotic microbes *procaryotes*. The morphology of these cell types is discussed in greater detail in Chapter 3. The differences between eucaryotic and procaryotic cells are of more than academic interest to the medical microbiologist. Much of the rationale in the treatment of many microbial infections capitalizes on these differences, a concept that will be expanded in subsequent chapters.

CLASSIFICATION

Classification of microorganisms, and all other forms of life, is an endeavor to arrange the various life forms into related groups. *Taxonomy* is the term used when referring to the science of classification. All classification schemes start out with major divisions (kingdoms) and move down through a series of progressively smaller and less inclusive categories. The smallest category (species) is one in which all members are alike in all or most major characteristics. The various taxonomic categories are defined in Table 2-3. A dual name (binary nomenclature) is given to each species and uses both the genus and species name. The scientific names are given in Latin or are Latinized and are descriptive or honorary. The species *Pasteurella multocida,* for example, has a genus name to honor Louis Pasteur, who discovered this bacterium, and the species name *multocida* because it is able to infect the cells of many different animal hosts. Another example is the bacterium *Neisseria gonorrhoeae,* the causative agent of gonorrhea, that was discovered by Albert Neisser. When used repeatedly in the same report, the genus name is only written out the first time; on repeated uses the genus name is abbreviated with only the first letter—that is, *N. gonorrhoeae.* The genus name is always capitalized and the species name is lower case; both names are either underlined or italicized. Often a common name may be used in general references to a given bacterium. For example, *N. gonorrhoeae* may be called the gonococcus.

An "International Code of Nomenclature of Bacteria" has been adopted by microbiologists to achieve uniform naming of microorganisms in all parts of the world. Classification schemes and names are periodically changed as new information becomes available. Occasionally changes are proposed that are not accepted by

TABLE 2-3 THE TAXONOMIC CATEGORIES OF LIVING ORGANISMS

Kingdom (major division)
    Phylum (groups of related classes)
        Class (groups of related orders)
            Order (groups of related families)
                Family (groups of related genera)
                    Genus (groups of related species)
                        Species (living organisms that are alike)

TABLE 2-4 TAXONOMIC KINGDOMS

Kingdom	Members
Animalia	Multicellular animals
Plantae	Multicellular plants
Fungi	Molds, yeast, and mushrooms
Protista	Protozoa and microscopic algae
Procaryotae	All procaryotic microbes

all microbiologists. A periodically updated publication called "Bergey's Manual of Determinative Bacteriology" serves as the standard reference source for the classification and naming of bacteria.

Early classification schemes divided all forms of life into either the plant or the animal kingdom. As early as 1866 Haeckel, a German biologist, recognized that microorganisms could not readily be classified into either the traditional plant or animal kingdom because they shared properties of both kingdoms. He proposed the addition of a third kingdom called Protista (first life), which would contain the single-celled microorganisms. Proposals have been made to divide microorganisms into the following three kingdoms (Table 2-4):

1. Kingdom Procaryotae (also called Monera in one scheme), which contains the procaryotes—that is, the cyanobacteria, which are photosynthetic microbes (formerly classified as blue green algae)—and the bacteria (including the rickettsiae and chlamydiae)
2. Kingdom Protista, which consists of the protozoa and the microscopic algae
3. Kingdom Fungi, which consists of the molds and yeast.

Viruses, unique types of subcellular microbiological agents, do not fit well into this classification scheme, but are often listed as a separate category close to the bacteria for convenience.

MAJOR GROUPS OF MICROORGANISMS

The purpose here is to give a brief overall view of the characteristics of the major groups of microorganisms, with an emphasis on nonmedical areas. The medical aspects will be covered in later chapters.

Fungi

A large group of nonphotosynthetic, plantlike eucaryotes, fungi include such diverse organisms as yeast, molds, and mushrooms (Figure 2-1). Yeast are globular-shaped cells about 10 to 30 μm in diameter that multiply by budding. They are best known

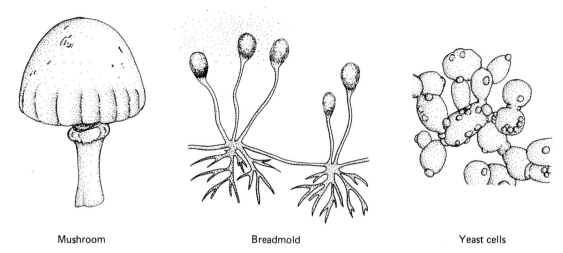

Mushroom   Breadmold   Yeast cells

Figure 2-1 Three different types of fungi. The mushroom is close to natural size. The bread mold and yeast are greatly enlarged.

for their use as a leavening agent for bakery goods and for their ability to produce alcohol.

Molds are organisms that consist of masses of branchlike filaments called *hyphae* and are most frequently recognized by their fuzzy growth on various foods and other organic matter. Reproduction in fungi usually results from the formation of large numbers of seedlike structures called *spores*. Mushrooms, although not microscopic in size, are actually complex arrangements of single, independently functioning cells that have the appearance of multicellular structures. The fungi are widely distributed in nature and readily grow in dark, damp places where organic matter is found. Only a relatively small number of molds and yeast is able to cause diseases in humans (see Chapter 29). Large numbers can cause diseases in plants and lower animals, however. These diseases have a significant impact on reducing the world's food supply.

The most notable function of fungi is their ability to decompose organic matter. They secrete powerful enzymes that dissolve organic food sources. When moisture is present and other environmental factors are not extreme, fungi continually attempt to grow on a wide variety of organic substances. Organic matter in contact with the soil is rapidly decomposed by fungi as part of the natural, essential recycling process in nature. Such products as foods, paper, lumber, fabrics, paint, and rubber can all be decomposed by fungi. This process may be beneficial or detrimental, depending on circumstances; that is, the decomposition of dead plants in the soil is beneficial whereas the decomposition of lumber stored for building is detrimental. Societies spend a great deal of time and effort to treat and store materials so that they will not be damaged by fungal growth; yet even so large quantities of foods and other materials are lost each year due to the action of fungi. On the other hand, some by-prod-

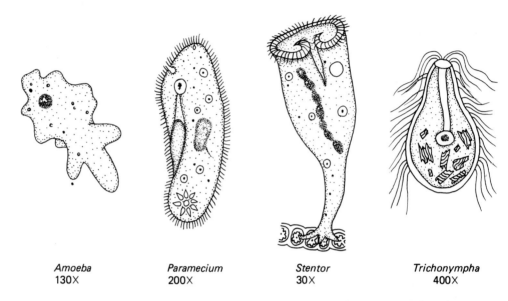

| Amoeba | Paramecium | Stentor | Trichonympha |
| 130× | 200× | 30× | 400× |

Figure 2-2   Four different types of protozoa with degrees of enlargement indicated.

ucts of fungal growth have commercial value and large-scale industrial fermentation processes produce such fungal products as penicillin, alcohols, cheeses, and solvents.

Protozoa

The protozoa are a group of microorganisms that are animallike in their structure and function. They are eucaryotic cells and possess many intracellular components that are characteristic of higher forms of life. Most protozoa have some form of active locomotion and they vary considerably in their size and shape (Figure 2-2). The smallest protozoa are only a few micrometers in diameter whereas others may be seen with the unaided eye. Protozoa are able to ingest food particles by folding their outer membrane around the food and then pinching off the membrane to form an intracellular vacule. Protozoa inhabit most bodies of water, are found in soil, and live in the digestive tract of many higher forms of life. Because of their relatively large size and motility, protozoa are easily seen by the microscopic examination of water from such sources as stagnant ponds. Protozoa have a moderate influence on the quality of water and on the various biological cycles in nature. While a great majority of the protozoa do not cause diseases in higher forms of life, those that do are responsible for some of the most serious, such as malaria and African sleeping sickness.

Algae

Algae (singular alga) are a large morphologically and physiologically diverse group of eucaryotic micro- and macroscopic organisms (Figure 2-3). All contain chlorophyll, which allows them to carry out the process of photosynthesis. This process results in

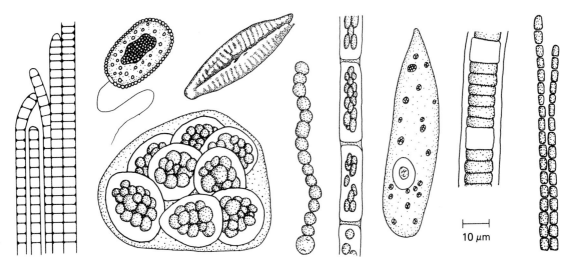

Figure 2-3 Different species of algae and cyanobacteria reproduced to scale (see 10 μm bar).

the production of energy-containing compounds and oxygen. Many algae occur as single cells, ranging in size from less than 1 μm to upward of 60 μm in diameter. They may be shaped as spheres, rods, or spindles. Others occur in multicellular colonies that are often visible to the naked eye and take on a wide variety of shapes. Some, such as seaweeds, appear much like multicellular plants. The presence of chlorophyll gives diverse pigmentations to the algal cells and this characteristic is used in their classification. Along with their scientific names, they are also referred to as yellow-green, green, red, or brown algae. Thousands of different species exist and are found in most moist environments. Many algae are free living in waters; others grow in soils or on the surfaces of plants and rocks, and similar environments. The wide diversity of algae is reflected by the fact that some grow on ice or snow whereas others are able to grow in hot springs. The only health problem commonly associated with algae is the production of toxins, which may be consumed by aquatic animals, such as shellfish. When algae levels are high, during the summer months, enough toxins may be retained in the shellfish to cause illness when eaten by humans.

Because algae are involved in many biological cycles and are important contributors to the overall balance in nature, they play important roles in the well-being of humans and most other forms of life. They aid in soil fertility by adding organic matter and some species are able to fix atmospheric nitrogen. Some are harvested from the sea and used directly as human or animal food. Agar, a solidifying agent used in microbial culture media or as a thickening agent in various foods, is extracted from seaweeds. Currently a great deal of interest is being shown in the mass culture of algae as a source of food. Large numbers of algae are found in oceans, seas, lakes, ponds, and streams. Small free-floating algae make up a part of the life forms referred to as *plankton*. Plankton are at the beginning of the food chain in aquatic environments and are often consumed by small aquatic animals (zooplankton), which, in turn, are eaten by small fish, which are eaten by larger fish, and so on. Some larger aquatic animals, such as the blue whale, eat algae directly. Essentially all sea and freshwater animals depend on the presence of algae for food. Algae are found in most bodies of water and in depths of 45 to 180 meters. The amount of organic matter resulting from the photosynthesis occurring in algae in aquatic environments exceeds the amount of materials produced from all plants on terrestrial surfaces.

Bacteria

Bacteria are procaryotes and are smaller and less complex than the eucaryotic cells. Normally bacteria have rigid cell walls and are shaped as spheres, rods, or helices (Figure 2-4). Bacteria are found in virtually every environmental habitat and some types have adapted to grow on minimal nutrients or under extreme environmental conditions. Some, for example, are able to grow on inorganic compounds, others in hot springs, in cold storage food, or on the bottom of the ocean under extreme pressure; still others grow in areas completely devoid of oxygen. Most bacteria multiply by the cell dividing into two daughter cells (binary fission). Under proper conditions growth may be very rapid with cell division occurring as often as every 12 to 15 minutes. The rapid growth of bacteria may lead to profound changes in the surrounding environment. Although many important infectious diseases of humans are caused by bacteria, most are not able to cause disease. Many bacteria produce beneficial environmental changes, such as the decomposition of waste products, aiding in soil fertility, or production of useful chemicals.

Two groups of small bacteria, between 0.3 and 0.5 μm in diameter, called rickettsiae and chlamydiae are able to multiply only inside living eucaryotic cells. Because of this small size and dependency on living host cells (characteristics that are also shared by viruses), the rickettsiae and chlamydiae have in the past been grouped next to or with the viruses. It is now well established that the rickettsiae and chlamydiae have definite cellular structures and are best considered small obligately parasitic

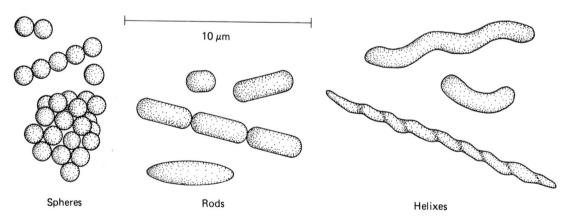

10 μm

Spheres   Rods   Helixes

Figure 2-4 Bacterial cells showing representatives of the three basic cell shapes.

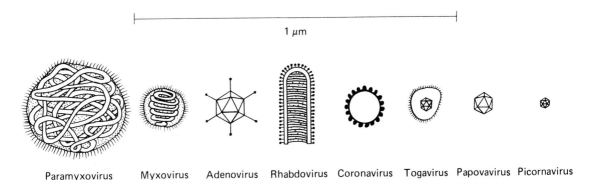

Figure 2-5   The shapes and relative sizes of various types of viruses that infect animals.

bacteria. Because of their dependency on living host cells, they have no direct influence on the outside environment. Nevertheless, these microbes can cause some important human diseases.

Viruses

Viruses are a unique type of biological agent. All other organisms described previously are complete cells with the capabilities of carrying out metabolic activities and other functions of life. Viruses, however, are not complete cells and have no independent metabolic activity. Viruses might best be described as independent genes encased in a protein coat. Each virus has a single molecule of nucleic acid; this molecule contains genetic information (see Chapter 5). The virus is covered with a coat that consists of a geometric arrangement of protein molecules. When a virus enters a living cell, the viral genes are released and the information contained in them may be expressed in the host cell. The information on the viral genes may redirect the cell to make virus particles and eventually the cell may be destroyed or altered. The only effects produced by viruses are on the host cells; when found outside host cells, viruses are simply a collection of molecules with no apparent life functions. Most viruses have definite geometric forms, the most common being spherical; some of the others are rod, brick, bullet, or tadpole shaped (Figures 2-5 and 31-2). They range in size from about 25 to 300 nm in diameter. Almost every form of life has specific viruses that are able to infect its cells. Viruses have no effects on nonliving substances. Still, their effect on living cells can be destructive and many common diseases of humans are caused by viruses.

NONMEDICAL APPLICATIONS OF MICROBIOLOGY

Most of the material in this textbook will deal with medical microbiology; yet microorganisms are used or play an important role in various other areas. This section briefly discusses several nonmedical applications of microbiology.

Soil

Most microbes occur in the upper one-half meter of soil and one gram of fertile farm soil may contain as many as 4 to 5 billion microorganisms. These large numbers of microorganisms are actively involved in the decomposition of organic matter. This process is a vital phase in the natural recycling of the elements needed for living systems. The photosynthetic algae add organic matter to the soil by their growth and death. Some bacteria and algae are able to convert (fix) atmospheric nitrogen into a form that can be used by plants. Acids produced by microbes aid in dissolving rocks, an important step in the formation of soil. Overall microorganisms are a major factor in the development of fertile soil.

Water

Microorganisms are found in all bodies of fresh- and saltwater. The numbers and types vary greatly, just as the conditions of the water vary. Some microbes are natural inhabitants of water whereas others are transient, having entered from sewage, land runoff, or other external sources. As in soil, microorganisms are vital links in the recycling of nutrients in the aquatic food chain. Much of the world's food supply is made possible by the activities of these aquatic microbes. Maintaining the proper biological balance of these aquatic systems is one of the great challenges of present-day technology and is essential for the continued survival of most life forms on this planet. The important role of algae in the aquatic food chain was mentioned earlier. An overabundance of algal growth, however, may be detrimental to a body of water; this situation may occur when concentrations of nutrients are high and the water is warm. A massive growth of algae is called a *bloom* (Figure 2-6). Such blooms may kill fish and make the water unsuitable for recreational activities. All lakes are slowly filling with sediments and microbial debris contributes significantly to this process. Excess nutrients in the water may accelerate the rate of filling, mainly by the increased growth of algae.

Water may serve as an important vehicle for the transmission of disease-producing microorganisms. The proper treatment of water for human consumption and the treatment of sewage are of vital importance in maintaining a healthy environment. Decomposition of organic matter by microorganisms is an important step in the treatment of sewage.

Dairy

Milk provides an excellent medium for the rapid growth of many types of microorganisms and great care is needed during the collection and processing of milk in order to minimize microbial contamination. In general, the quality of milk is directly related to the numbers and types of microorganisms it contains and so the dairy industry spends a lot of time and money in controlling microorganisms. Pasteurization, which is the application of mild heat, destroys disease-producing and many non-

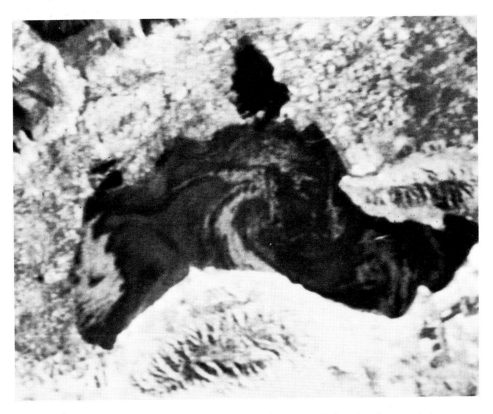

Figure 2-6 A shallow freshwater lake, about 35 kilometers in length and surrounded by mountains, photographed from a space satellite during the summer. The swirls and areas of contrast show massive blooms of algae. (NASA)

disease-producing bacteria commonly found in milk. When this procedure is combined with storage at low temperatures, the storage time of milk is greatly increased.

Certain microorganisms, under controlled conditions, induce desirable changes in milk (Figure 2-7). Such dairy items as yogurt, sour cream, and buttermilk result from the fermentation of milk products through the addition of selected acid-producing bacteria. Cheeses are produced by the controlled growth of selected microorganisms on curdled milk, a process called ripening. Different cheeses are produced by the action of different microorganisms.

Food

Like dairy products, most foods provide excellent media for the growth of many types of microorganisms. Generally microbial growth in food is undesirable and produces changes in texture and flavor commonly called spoilage. Yet the action of microorganisms may sometimes be desirable, as in the production of pickles and sauerkraut.

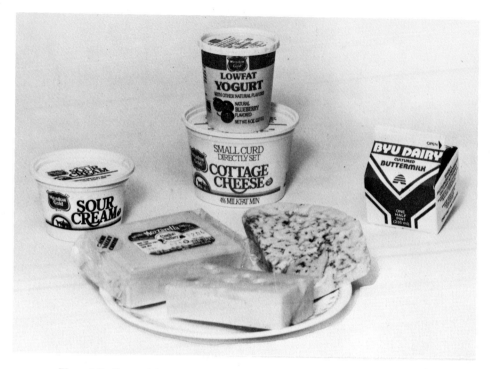

Figure 2-7 Some of the dairy products that are produced by the action of microorganisms on milk components.

As noted, food industries make great efforts to prevent detrimental changes to food by microorganisms. Much of what is done in food processing is directed toward the control of such microbial spoilage. Such processes as drying, smoking, salting, freezing, refrigerating, heat processing (canning), and the use of chemical preservatives are the major methods in preventing or slowing the spoilage of foods. Because of the everincreasing costs of foods and the limited supplies of certain foods in many countries, reducing spoilage waste is increasingly important and offers a challenge to food microbiologists. Some estimates indicate that as much as 25% of the world's food supply is lost to spoilage by microorganisms or by infestation by insects or rodents.

Microbes may be used to a limited extent as a direct food source, such as yeast as a food supplement. The potential for microorganism use as a food source is great and active research projects are currently underway to develop methods of using the rapid-growth capabilities of microorganisms as a means of producing food substances. When compared to other forms of life, microorganisms are much more efficient producers of proteins. A rapidly growing culture of microorganisms under controlled conditions, for instance, is able to produce as much protein in one day as a meat-producing animal can produce in several weeks. Furthermore, microbes can do so in a small space and often by using waste products or inexpensive organic materials as their food source. This area of research offers a possible means of ensuring a proper food supply for the world's increasing population. Currently the appeal of microorganisms as a basic food for humans is limited. The term *single-cell protein* is used when referring to this type of product to make it sound more appealing. Although most humans are not yet ready to trade their roast beef for "bacterial-protein patties," single-cell protein may become an important food supplement for meat-producing animals that are, in turn, processed for human consumption.

Industrial Uses

Many by-products of microbial growth are useful and the field of industrial microbiology uses the action of microorganisms to produce these products. In some cases, the useful product can be produced only by microorganisms; in others, the microbial process is the most economical means of production. To be economically feasible, the raw material should be relatively inexpensive and readily available while the end product must be of greater value. These conditions are fulfilled in many processes and today industrial microbial processes are the basis of large commercial industries. Some products produced by microorganisms include solvents, organic acids, alcohols, including alcoholic beverages, enzymes, and antibiotics.

The increasing costs and scarcity of petroleum and natural gas have renewed interest in microbial fermentations that can convert plant materials into methane gas and alcohols. These products can then be used for heating or in internal combustion engines. Because plant materials are renewable, these processes could greatly reduce our dependence on nonreplenishable petroleum products.

Biological Tools

Microorganisms are widely used as biological models for scientists who wish to study fundamental principles of living systems. When working with bacteria, it is possible to start with a single cell, which will then replicate rapidly so that within a day trillions of identical cells can be produced. This population of identical cells is much easier to study than a population of mixed cells that might be obtained from animal or plant tissues. Much of what we know about the biological activities of cells has evolved through studies of bacterial cells reproduced in this manner.

It has now become possible to pass some genes from other forms of life into bacteria and from one type of bacterium to another. This process, referred to as genetic engineering or *recombinant DNA*, is allowing microorganisms to be used in unique ways. One of the first practical developments of genetic engineering was to place the human insulin gene into a bacterium. As this bacterium divided, the insulin gene divided and was passed to each daughter cell. Within a short time trillions of bacteria, each producing human insulin, were available. Consequently, inexpensive human insulin can be produced for the treatment of diabetics. Many other applications of this new technology now being developed will allow common microbial cells to provide new and beneficial products for mankind.

SUMMARY

1. Microorganisms hold a legitimate place in the world of living things. Although unique in many attributes, these single cells exemplify all the characteristics normally associated with biological systems.

2. The microworld of biology can be divided into several logical major groups. These groups are classified and named according to the systems used for larger life forms. The smallest and simplest forms are the viruses. More complex and larger are the procaryotic bacteria and three groups of eucaryotic organisms (fungi, protozoa, and algae) often included within the designation "micro-organism."

3. Microorganisms are ubiquitous in their habitat. They are found throughout the world, in, on, and around every conceivable environment. They play a major role in maintaining ecological balance and are often used in procedures that are beneficial to human beings.

Cellular Anatomy

3

All cells share some fundamental characteristics in their structural components and biochemical functions. These similarities permit scientists to extrapolate information obtained from the study of one type of cell to other cells and much of what we know about the biochemical reactions in the complex eucaryotic animal cells was first discovered through studies of the simpler procaryotic cells. Still, there are many differences between cell types, particularly when comparing procaryotic with eucaryotic cells. A knowledge of these differences is essential in understanding why some chemical agents can be used to treat particular diseases successfully. Chemicals like penicillin that specifically interfere with the function of components found in procaryotic cells but that are not present in eucaryotic cells have proven effective chemotherapeutic agents. The concept of chemotherapy is covered in Chapter 9. The following discussion deals with the major cellular components of procaryotic cells and gives a brief description of the major components of eucaryotic cells.

PROCARYOTIC CELLS

Because most procaryotic cells of importance in medical microbiology are bacteria, this section is limited to a discussion of bacterial anatomy.

Sizes and Shapes

Bacteria are the smallest independently living cells, with most ranging from 0.25 to 8.0 μm in diameter or length. Some are slightly larger. The thousands of different

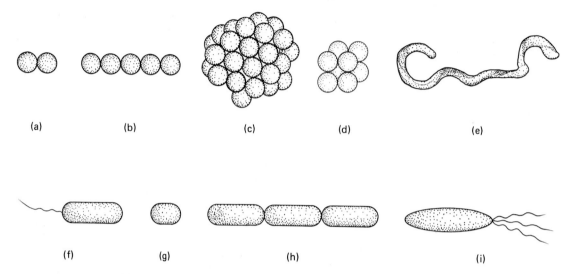

Figure 3-1 Some of the general shapes and arrangements of bacteria: (a) diplococci, (b) streptococci, (c) staphylococci, (d) sarcinae, (e) spirillum, (f) bacillus with monotrichous flagellum,
(g) coccobacillus, (h) streptobacillus, and (i) bacillus with lophotrichous flagella.

species occur in one of three general shapes: (a) spherical, (b) rod or cylindrical, and
(c) curved or helical (Figure 3-1).

Spherical bacteria are called *cocci* (singular coccus) and each species exhibits
one of the characteristic arrangements of cells shown in Figure 3-1. The cylindrical-
shaped bacteria are called *bacilli* (singular bacillus) or rods; most occur as single cells
and not in arrangements like the cocci. Under certain growth conditions some bacilli
also occur in pairs or chains. Certain bacilli characteristically lie side by side in pali-
sadelike arrangements and others may occur in Y or branching-shaped arrangements.
Some bacilli are short, stubby rods between 0.5 and 1 μm in length with a diameter
only slightly less than the length. Such cells, especially if they have rounded corners,
have an elliptical shape and appear to be as much coccal shaped as rod shaped; the
term *coccobacillary* is sometimes used to describe this shape. Many bacilli have definite rod shapes with some species being significantly larger than others.

Some helical bacteria are called *spirilla* (singular spirillum) whereas others are
grouped into the *spirochetes* and usually occur as individual cells. Chains of these
organisms may occur, however. Many variations exist between species as to length
and number and amplitude of spirals.

Components of Procaryotic Cells

Many components found in bacterial cells are shown in Figure 3-2.

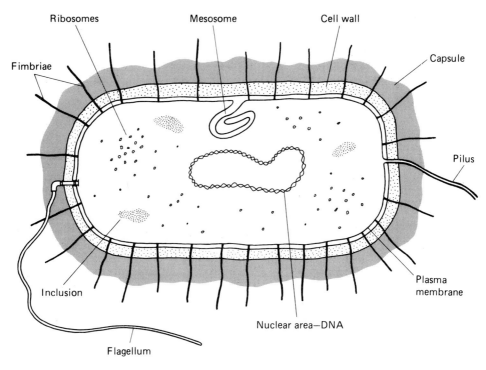

Figure 3-2   A schematic diagram of a composite procaryotic bacterial cell.

Cell wall

The bacterial cell wall is a unique and important structure. No comparable structure is found in any animal cell and the chemical structure differs from the cell walls found in higher plants. The cell wall is rigid and gives shape to the cell. Because bacterial cells are directly exposed to the external environment, the cell wall provides a necessary protection for the cell. Bacteria usually live in fluids that contain relatively low concentrations of ions (atoms with + or − charges) whereas the inside of the cell (cytoplasm) contains high concentrations of ions. Water is drawn to the area of high ionic concentration and thus tends to flow into the cell. This situation creates a pressure inside the cell (osmotic pressure). Because the internal osmotic pressure of bacterial cells is relatively high, these cells would swell and burst if it were not for the support of the rigid cell wall. The cell wall is also necessary for cell division. Cell walls are porous and allow the free passage of fluids and small molecules.

Two types of cell walls are found among the different species of bacteria and divide bacteria into one of two staining types called either *gram positive* or *gram negative*. The gram stain, a cell-staining procedure developed by Dr. Christian Gram, is used to differentiate the two types of cell walls. Briefly, when subjected to the gram stain, the gram-positive cell walls retain a crystal violet-iodine complex whereas the gram-negative cell walls do not. The gram stain is discussed in more detail in Chapter 6.

A structure common to both gram-positive and gram-negative cell walls is a large, insoluble chemical structure called *peptidoglycan* (sometimes called murine or mucopeptide). Peptidoglycan forms a coarse, layered, rigid meshwork that surrounds the cytoplasm and maintains the shape of the cell. A layer of peptidoglycan consists of two types of alternately joined molecules called *N-acetylglucosamine* and *N-acetylmuramic acids* that form long chains. A cell wall may have many such layers. The layers are joined together by short chains of four amino acids (tetrapeptides) that connect above and below with *N*-acetylmuramic acid and also connect with other short side chains of amino acids that cross-connect the long chains of the peptidoglycan structure (Figure 3-3). The peptidoglycan structure is found only in cell walls of bacteria.

The cell walls of gram-positive bacteria consist of many layers of peptidoglycan that may form 85 to 90% of this structure. Gram-positive cell walls may also contain polysaccharides (complex sugars) and teichoic acids (complex molecules composed of sugar, amino acids, and lipids).

The gram-negative cell wall is more complex than the gram-positive wall. It contains a thin, rigid, inner peptidoglycan component, not more than two layers thick, that constitutes only 5 to 20% of the total cell wall materials. Outside this peptidoglycan layer is an *outer membrane* composed of lipoprotein (large molecules of

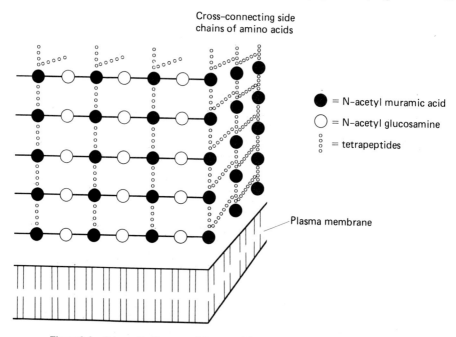

Cross–connecting side chains of amino acids

● = N–acetyl muramic acid

○ = N–acetyl glucosamine

⋮ = tetrapeptides

Plasma membrane

Figure 3-3   Schematic diagram of gram-positive cell wall with multiple layers of peptidoglycan.

lipid and protein complexes) and lipopolysaccharide (large molecules of lipid and sugar complexes) molecules associated with a typical double-layer, phospholipid-type membrane (see cytoplasmic membrane). The arrangement of these various components in the gram-negative cell wall is shown in Figure 3-4. The outer membrane forms the major part of the gram-negative cell wall.

The type of cell wall possessed by a bacterium may influence the types of clinical signs and symptoms seen in an infection caused by that bacterium. The lipopolysaccharide components of gram-negative cell walls, for instance, have toxic effects on infected animal hosts and cause such signs of disease as fever, diarrhea, and shock. These lipopolysaccharides are called *endotoxins* (Chapter 14) and play an important role in the disease-producing capabilities of gram-negative bacteria.

The type of cell wall may also determine the response of bacterium to certain antibiotics. The classic example is penicillin, which selectively interferes with the formation of the amino acid cross-linkages of the peptidoglycan meshwork when new cell wall is being formed during cell division. Without the cross-linkages, the cell wall is weak and ruptures; this condition results in the death of the bacterium in most environments. Because the major component of gram-positive cell walls is peptidoglycan, most gram-positive bacteria are highly susceptible to penicillin. On the other hand, the peptidoglycan layer forms only a small portion of the gram-negative cell wall and is covered with the thick outer membrane. The outer membrane hinders penicillin from reaching the peptidoglycan; even with some damage to the peptidoglycan layer, the other components may hold the cell wall together. Therefore penicillin is not effective in treating infections caused by many gram-negative bacteria. Because animal cells have no peptidoglycan, they are unaffected by penicillin.

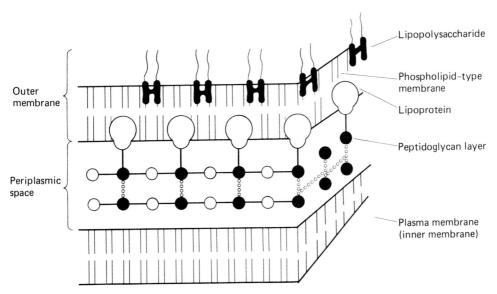

Figure 3-4   Schematic diagram of gram-negative cell wall.

Capsule

Some bacteria produce a slimy or gel-type material that adheres to the outside of the cell wall. It forms a layer around the cell that is called a *capsule* (Figure 3-5). Most capsular materials are polysaccharides. The capsule may offer a protective covering to help prolong the survival of some bacteria. In large amounts this material is termed a *glycocalix* and may be important in providing a natural-growth environment for the cells. The capsule may slow the rate at which white blood cells are able to ingest (phagocytize) the bacteria that have invaded the tissues of an animal. The capsule gives the bacteria a greater opportunity for survival and thus a better chance to cause disease. The disease-producing capabilities of some bacteria are directly related to the presence of a capsule.

Flagella

Flagella (singular flagellum) are long, hairlike appendages, composed of the protein flagellin, that extend out from some bacterial species. They are present on many species of bacilli, on some spirilla, but on very few species of cocci. Flagella are attached to the cytoplasmic membrane by a small hook at the end of the structure and are able to rotate rapidly. Some flagella have been measured at over 2000 rpm. This movement propels the bacterium through fluids. Some bacteria are able to move 30 times the length of their cell in one second; such directional movement of bacteria requires a large amount of available energy. The term *trichous*, which means hairlike, is used when referring to the arrangements of flagella on bacterial cells (Figure 3-1). Certain bacteria have only a single flagellum and are called *monotrichous*; some have tufts of flagella and are called *lophotrichous*; still others have flagella protruding from all areas of the cell and are called *peritrichous*.

Fimbriae and pili

The structure of the fimbriae (Latin-fingers) and pili (Latin-hairs) is similar in some ways to flagella, but these structures are not associated with motility. Fimbriae and pili are short, hairlike structures that project out from the cell wall. They are present

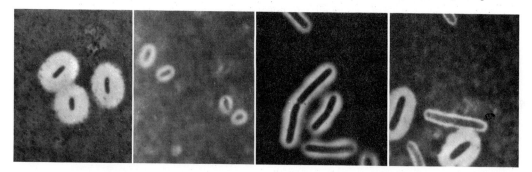

Figure 3-5 Various sized capsules present on different species of the genus *Bacteroides*; magnified 1000 to 1200×. (J. L. Babb and C. S. Cummins, *Inf. Imm. 19*:1088–1091, Figure 1, with permission from ASM)

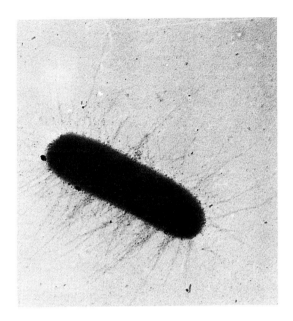

Figure 3-6 Numerous hairlike fimbriae projecting out from the cell wall of the bacterium *Escherichia coli.* (Courtesy Dr. K. V. Nagaraja)

on some bacterial species but not on others. Fimbriae are quite numerous over the entire surface of a bacterium and function as attachment sites between the bacterium and other surfaces (Figure 3-6). The ability of some bacteria to attach to and infect certain tissues is partly a function of their fimbriae. Pili are generally longer than fimbriae and only one or a few may be present on the surface of a bacterium. Pili seem to function as hollow tubes through which genetic materials may pass. Certain viruses that infect bacteria (bacteriophages) specifically attach to pili and inject their nucleic acid into the bacterial cell through the pilus. Some pili may be involved in a mating process (conjugation) in which they form a tube between two bacterial cells through which DNA may pass. The terms fimbriae and pili were used interchangeably in the past; however, the preceding definitions are now recommended to distinguish between the two functional types of short, hairlike appendages.

Cytoplasmic membrane

The cytoplasmic membrane, also called the protoplasmic or the plasma membrane, is a thin, fragile membrane located just inside the cell wall; it completely surrounds the internal cellular components. This membrane forms a functional barrier between the inside of the cell and the external environment. Numerous essential biological functions are carried out by the activities of these membranes. Bacterial cytoplasmic membranes are involved in the synthesis of cell wall materials, excretion of enzymes (exoenzymes) essential to the nutrition of the cell, determination of selective permeability and transport of nutrient and waste products into and out of the cell, and essential energy-producing chemical reactions.

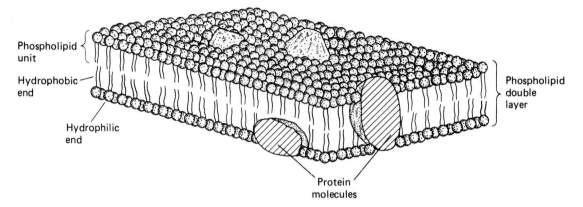

Phospholipid unit

Hydrophobic end

Hydrophilic end

Phospholipid double layer

Protein molecules

Figure 3-7   Cross section of a cytoplasmic membrane composed of two layers of phospholipid units with their hydrophilic ends pointing to the outside and their hydrophobic ends pointing to the center of the membrane. Protein molecules are "floating" in the "fluidlike" phospholipid membrane.

The cytoplasmic membrane is only 7 to 10 nm in thickness and consists primarily of phospholipids and proteins. The phospholipid molecules have one end that is soluble in water (hydrophilic) and another end that is insoluble (hydrophobic); this situation causes these molecules to form a typical double-layer unit membrane with the hydrophilic ends pointing out and the hydrophobic ends pointing in (Figure 3-7).

Many bacteria contain an invaginated and highly convoluted section of cytoplasmic membrane called *mesosome*. Certain mesosomes are thought to be involved with the formation of new cross walls that form when the cell divides.

The structure of the cytoplasmic membrane is similar in both procaryotic and eucaryotic cells. The functional integrity of this membrane is essential for the survival of the cell and any process or chemical that disrupts its structure or function causes the death of the cell. Several chemicals that function as disinfectants (Chapter 8) have an effect on this membrane.

Cytoplasm

All components inside the cytoplasmic membrane are collectively referred to as *cytoplasm*. Much of the cytoplasm is made up of proteins, nucleic acids, carbohydrates, and lesser amounts of other substances suspended in fluid. Certain anatomically distinct structures found in the cytoplasm are discussed next.

Ribosomes

Ribosomes consist of protein and ribonucleic acid (RNA) and enormous numbers are found in each cell; they are involved in the important function of protein synthesis. Ribosomes are about 20 nm in diameter and are made up of two unequal-sized lobular subunits, a 30 S- and a 50 S-sized component (Figure 3-8). The two subunits are separated when not involved with protein synthesis. When directly involved in protein synthesis, they are arranged in aggregates called *polyribosomes* (see Chapter 5).

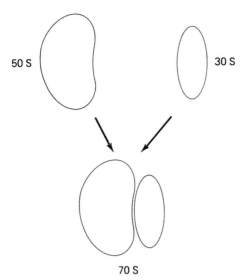

Figure 3-8 The two components of ribosomes that combine to form a 70 S unit when attached to *m*RNA during protein synthesis.

It is possible to separate such particulate components as ribosomes from other organelles by the technique of ultracentrifugation. Under high gravitational forces exerted by this procedure particles separate into layers, based on their density. The bacterial ribosomes have a density value of 70 S; the S refers to Svedberg units or the sedimentation constant. The 70 S size of the procaryotic ribosomes is slightly smaller than the 80 S size of ribosomes of eucaryotic cells and this difference is associated with a basic difference in the ability of the antibiotic streptomycin to combine with ribosomes. Streptomycin is able to combine and interfere with the function of 70 S ribosomes but not with 80 S ribosomes. Consequently, streptomycin can be used as an antibiotic that can selectively interfere with procaryotic cells.

Nuclear region

The nuclear region is that part of the cytoplasm where the DNA molecule is located. Each bacterium possesses a large circular DNA molecule with a molecular weight of about 3×10^9 that contains the genetic information needed by the bacterium. This "chromosome" appears to be attached at one point to the bacterial cell membrane. The absence of a membrane surrounding the nucleus is one of the main characteristics used to distinguish procaryotic cells from eucaryotic cells.

Cytoplasmic inclusions

Granules or globules are observed in many bacteria and are collectively referred to as *inclusions*. Many inclusions are aggregates of lipid, sulfur, carbohydrates, or a form of phosphate called volutin that can be stored by the cells as reserve food and energy supplies. The area of the cell that they occupy varies with the growth rate and nutritional state of the cell. Inclusions are not surrounded by membranes but are often made visible by special stains.

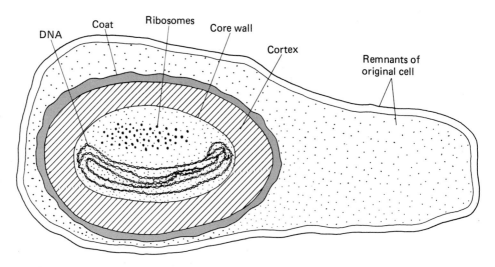

DNA Coat Ribosomes Core wall Cortex Remnants of original cell

Figure 3-9 Major components of a bacterial endospore.

Endospores

Three genera of gram-positive bacilli, *Bacillus*, *Clostridium*, and *Sporosarcina* (Chapter 20), are able to form a unique structure called an *endospore* or simply a *spore* (Figure 3-9). These spores are formed inside the bacterial cell, hence the prefix *endo*. The term *vegetative* is used to refer to the actively growing, nonspore stage of a bacterium. Under optimal conditions of growth the vegetative bacteria multiply without the formation of spores; that is, the spore is not a necessary step in replication. When growth conditions become unfavorable, however, such as a limitation in nitrogen or an energy source, the formation of endospores is stimulated. One spore develops per cell and forms a dormant, resistant stage for the cell. The spore is formed by a sequence of changes called *sporulation*. This process involves the development of a cytoplasmic membrane around the DNA molecule, followed by the formation of a layer called a *cortex*, a spore coat of protein; finally, water is removed to dehydrate and mature the spore. The mature spore is highly resistant to destruction by heat or chemicals and may remain dormant for long periods. Some spores have germinated—that is, developed back into the vegetative stage—after lying dormant for many years. The bacterial spore is the most stable form of life; consequently, special efforts must be made to destroy them in order to achieve sterile conditions.

EUCARYOTIC CELLS

Eucaryotic cells are larger and much more complex than procaryotic cells (Table 3-1). Many diverse eucaryotic cells exist, ranging from yeast cells (microorganisms with some similarities to the procaryotic bacteria) to highly specialized cells found in multicellular animals. The major components found in eucaryotic cells of animals are shown in Figure 3-10.

TABLE 3-1 COMPARISON OF PROCARYOTIC AND EUCARYOTIC CELLS

Characteristic	Procaryotic cells	Eucaryotic cells
Internal membrane-bound organelles	Absent	Numerous; e.g., golgi, mitochondria, chloroplasts, lysosomes
Nucleus	Not membrane bound	Membrane bound
Flagella	Submicroscopic	Complex microscopic
Ribosomes	Small (70 S)	Large (80 S)
Cell wall	Complex peptidoglycan	Simple-polysaccharide
Mitotic structures	Absent	Present
Chromosomes	Singular-circular, no histone	Multiple with histones
Membrane structures	Mesosome	Endoplasmic reticulum
Endospores	Present	Absent
Membranes	Lack steroids	Contain steroids

Cell walls

Of the eucaryotic cells, only fungi, algae, and plant cells have cell walls. Chemically these walls are much simpler than the cell walls of bacteria. Most eucaryotic cell walls are composed of cellulose or other carbohydrates. The formation of these walls is not affected by penicillin.

Flagella and cilia

Some eucaryotes have flagella or cilia as organs of locomotion. The eucaryotic flagella are more complex than those present on procaryotic cells but perform much the same functions. Cilia are structurally similar to the flagella except they are much shorter and large numbers are usually arranged over the entire surface of the cell. Cilia are found only on some protozoa and some specialized animal cells, such as the ciliated epithelial cells of the respiratory tract.

Cytoplasmic membrane

This membrane is structurally similar in both procaryotic and eucaryotic cells. The cytoplasmic membrane is the outer limiting membrane of most protozoa and all animal cells and it invaginates and convolutes extensively through the interior of the cell to form a structure known as the *endoplasmic reticulum*. The membrane forming the endoplasmic reticulum appears to be continuous with the nuclear membrane. Various membrane-bound vacuoles and organelles are located throughout the interior of eucaryotic cells.

Vacuoles

Vacuoles are membrane-bound areas within the cytoplasm of some cells. They are associated with food storage, digestion, osmotic regulation, and excretion of waste products. Their number and sizes may change with the physiological state of the cell.

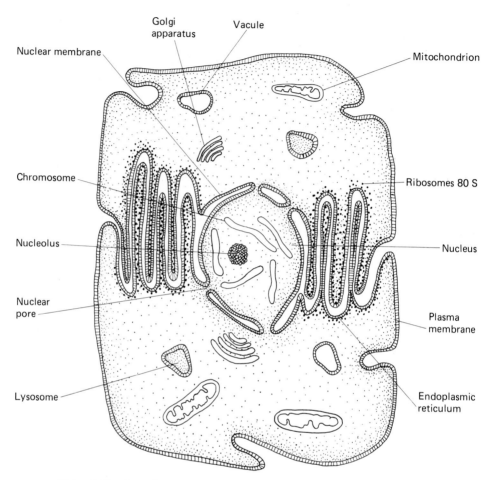

Figure 3-10 General eucaryotic cell diagram showing the major cellular components.

Lysosomes

Lysosomes are membrane-bound bodies that contain digestive enzymes and are found in such cells as the white blood cells that ingest (phagocytize) foreign particles. The lysosomes fuse with other vacuoles containing foreign particles to produce a vacuole called a phagolysosome in which digestion occurs (see Chapter 11).

Ribosomes

The function of the eucaryotic ribosomes is the same as the procaryotic ribosomes. The eucaryotic ribosomes are located along the endoplasmic reticulum and are the sites of protein synthesis. These ribosomes have a size of 80 S, which is larger than the procaryotic ribosomes.

Nucleus

The nucleus of eucaryotic cells is a prominent membrane-bound structure that contains the genetic material of the cell. A smaller structure inside the nucleus is the nucleolus, a structure associated with the synthesis of ribonucleic acid. Two membranes enclose the nucleus. The outer membrane is continuous, at least in part, with the endoplasmic reticulum. Round pores or holes pass through both membranes and allow the passage of large molecules between the nucleus and the cytoplasm.

Other organelles

Other major structures found in eucaryotic cells are *mitochondria, golgi bodies*, and *chloroplasts*. Mitochondria are rod-shaped structures about 1×3 μm in size and are associated with energy storage and transfer. Golgi bodies are aggregates of membranes and seem to be associated with the transport of enzymes out of the cell. Chloroplasts are prominent chlorophyll-containing structures found in eucaryotic cells that carry out photosynthesis. The sizes and shapes of chloroplasts vary among the different types of cells.

SUMMARY

1. Bacteria are procaryotic cells with limited shape variation and unique cell wall structures. The composition of the cell wall is a determinant in the staining characteristics of the bacteria, dividing them between gram-positive and gram-negative species.

2. Bacteria possess a number of organelles related to cellular function. Among them, flagella, fimbriae, capsules, and endospores are the most noticeable. Other organelles are similar in shape and function to those observed in eucaryotic cells. An organelle of singular importance in eucaryotic cells, the mitochondria, is not found in procaryotic forms, although a compensating mesosomal structure can often be observed.

Cellular Functions

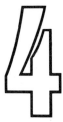

Any chemical change or reaction that occurs within a cell is called *metabolism*. These reactions are involved with the breakdown of food materials for the release of energy, a process called *catabolism*, and with the production of new cellular components, a process called *biosynthesis* or *anabolism*, which requires energy. Catabolism and biosynthesis are usually coupled together such that the energy released from one reaction can be used by the other. The rate of metabolic activity in an actively growing bacterial cell is phenomenal. Some bacteria are able to go through several generations in less than one hour. This rapid synthesis of new cellular material requires the breakdown of relatively large amounts of nutrient with its associated release of energy, plus the biosynthesis of enough new material to double the cell mass for each generation. In order to facilitate this rapid growth, the small size of bacterial cells provides for a large surface area relative to cell mass, which, in turn, allows for a rapid interaction between the intra- and extracellular environments.

This chapter briefly outlines the steps involved in the release and transfer of energy as well as the production of new building blocks needed for cell growth. The structure and functions of enzymes and other proteins are also discussed. The intention is to present a conceptual overall view of cellular metabolism and, by necessity, omits many details of this complex subject. Appendix A, however, is included for those desiring a more in-depth presentation of this subject.

ENERGY METABOLISM

Figure 4-1 presents a simplified outline of the reactions involved in energy metabolism and the biosynthesis of cellular materials. The original source of energy used in a vast majority of biological systems is the sun. Radiant energy from the sun is converted through the process of photosynthesis into a form of chemical energy that can be used by the living organisms that require organic matter as their source of energy. Green plants growing on land and algae in water are the major forms of life that carry out the essential process of photosynthesis.

During the process of photosynthesis the atoms contained in carbon dioxide (CO_2) are rearranged, a process that results in the formation of molecules containing long chains of carbon atoms connected to hydrogen and oxygen atoms. The ratio of atoms in these molecules is one carbon atom and one oxygen atom to two hydrogen atoms (CH_2O)—that is, one carbon atom plus water; these molecules are called *carbohydrates*. Along with the formation of carbohydrates, molecules of free oxygen (O_2) are also formed as part of the photosynthetic reaction, the entire reaction being

$$CO_2 + H_2O \longrightarrow CH_2O + O_2$$

Radiant energy from the sun is needed to connect the molecules together during the synthesis of the carbohydrate molecules; this energy is stored as chemical energy in the bonds between the atoms. The carbohydrate molecules are said to be *reduced* and were formed by the removal of oxygen and the addition of extra hydrogen atoms to carbon dioxide. Energy is required to form a reduced compound and much of this energy is retained in the compound. In turn, this stored energy can be released at a later time when oxygen is again added to the molecule or when hydrogen atoms are removed, a process called *oxidation* (Figure 4-2).

Various sizes of carbohydrate molecules are formed by photosynthetic plants and algae. The most common molecules are the simple sugars, called *monosaccharides*, usually containing five or six carbon atoms. Two monosaccharides may combine to form a *disaccharide*; many monosaccharides connected together form *polysaccharides*. Starch and cellulose are the major polysaccharides produced by plants and algae.

The stored energy in the chemical bonds of carbohydrates and other molecules, such as proteins and lipids, is made available to the cell through a complex series of metabolic reactions. The main source of energy for most cells is a six-carbon sugar called *glucose*. Many glucose molecules may be incorporated into larger polysaccharides; before they can be used by the cell, glucose must be separated from the larger carbohydrate molecule. This splitting is accomplished in microbial cells by digestive enzymes that are released from the cells into the extracellular environment. In gram-negative bacteria these extracellular digestive enzymes are often concentrated in the space between the peptidoglycan layer and the outer membrane of the cell wall where the larger molecules can be broken down efficiently. The glucose molecules

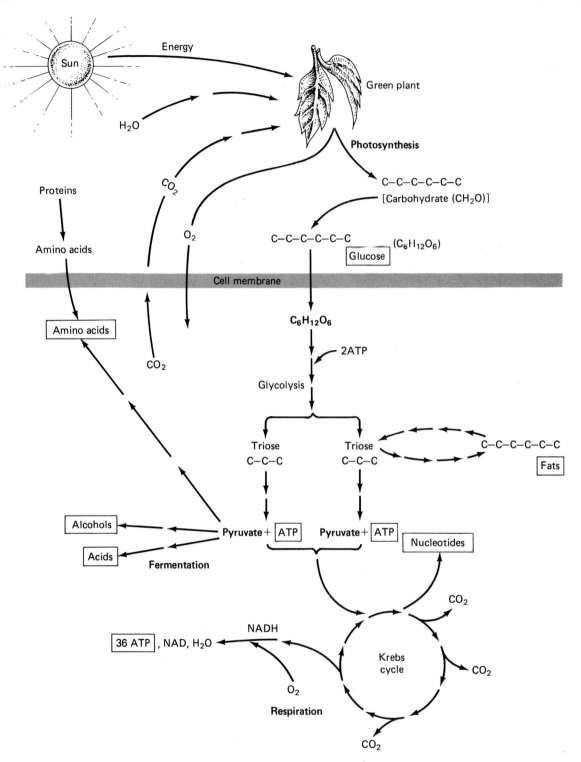

Figure 4-1 A simplified schematic diagram illustrating the source of cellular energy and the biosynthesis of cellular materials. The reactions above the cell membrane are representative of

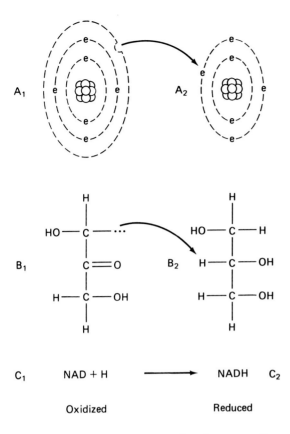

A_1 A_2

B_1 B_2

C_1 NAD + H   ⟶   NADH C_2

Oxidized   Reduced

Figure 4-2 Oxidation-reduction reactions involve the transfer of electrons. Losing an electron (A_1) results in oxidation while adding an electron results in chemical reduction (A_2). In metabolism, hydrogen is often transferred with the electron, thus losing hydrogen (B_1, C_1) results in oxidized molecules while gaining hydrogen produces reduced molecules (B_2, C_2).

contained in starch molecules are easily split from the larger molecule whereas the sugars that make up cellulose are more difficult to separate. Various microbes, however, are endowed with a wide array of enzymes that are able to break down some of the most complex and resistant carbohydrates, such as cellulose. Most digestion of the cellulose that is formed by plants is done by microorganisms. Thus carnivorous animals are unable to digest many plant cellulose carbohydrates whereas herbivorous animals, such as cattle, sheep, and rabbits, are able to feed on plants because of the kinds of microorganisms that live in their alimentary tract. These microorganisms are able to break down cellulose into small molecules that can be handled by the digestive fluids of the animal. Glucose molecules readily pass across the bacterial cytoplasmic membrane; once inside the cell, they enter into a series of reactions that slowly extract the energy contained in their chemical bonds (see Appendix A).

The first series of reactions in the process of glucose catabolism, called *glycolysis*, begins with several changes occurring in the structure of the glucose molecule, followed by the splitting of these six-carbon sugars into two molecules containing three carbon atoms each (Figure 4-3). These three carbon compounds are further altered to form a compound called *pyruvic acid*. The energy obtained by these metabolic processes is briefly stored in molecules called *adenosine triphosphate* (ATP)

photosynthesis (requiring water, carbon dioxide, and light energy for the synthesis of carbohydrate and the release of oxygen). The metabolic reactions occurring in bacterial and animal cells which require chemical energy such as glucose are shown below the cell membrane. These reactions produce the necessary ATP and cellular components for growth while releasing both carbon dioxide and water as end products.

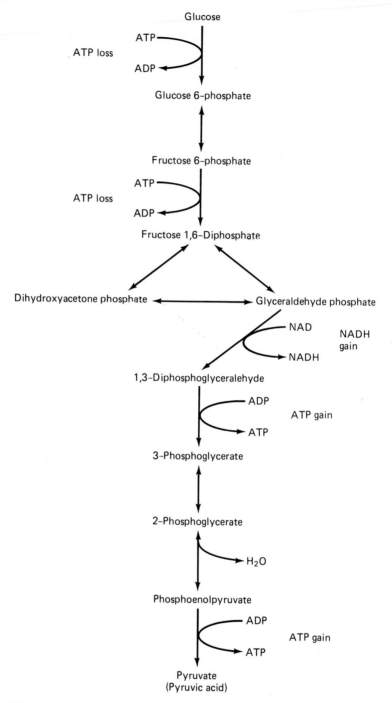

Figure 4-3 Simplified schematic of the glycolytic pathway. Note that two ATP molecules are required to activate this pathway, while ATP is produced in converting glyceraldehyde phosphate to pyruvate. This process results in a net increase of two ATP molecules because the six carbon glucose molecules are converted into two three-carbon glyceraldehyde phosphate molecules.

(Figure 4-4). ATP contains three phosphate groups, two of which are connected by high-energy bonds that are readily available for various cellular functions. When energy is released, the ATP molecule loses a phosphate group and is changed to an adenosine diphosphate (ADP) molecule. The ADP molecule can be changed back into an ATP molecule when energy becomes available from the oxidation of other compounds (Figure 4-5). In the reactions that change glucose to pyruvic acid two ATP molecules are used to prime the reaction; then two ATP units are generated for each of the two pyruvic acid molecules formed. Thus the net yield at this point is two ATP molecules because four were generated and two were used to prime the reaction. The reactions of glycolysis do not use oxygen and if oxygen is not available (anaerobic metabolism), pyruvic acid may subsequently be converted into such products as alcohol and organic acids. These metabolic reactions that proceed without oxygen are called *fermentation* (Figure 4-1). A net gain of only two ATP molecules is produced in the conversion of one molecule of glucose to alcohol. At this phase most of the energy is still contained in the alcohol molecule. Only certain types of microorganisms are able to produce alcohols or some other products of fermentation. Many such compounds have commercial value and controlled fermentation is carried out on a mass scale in many industrial processes. Because most of the energy originally present in glucose is still found in the alcohol molecules and because it is easily released by combustion with oxygen, much effort is now being directed toward increasing production of alcohol to be used as a supplemental fuel for combustion engines.

Many microorganisms use oxygen (aerobic metabolism) and are able to oxidize pyruvic acid completely to CO_2 and H_2O with the transfer of the released energy to ADP molecules forming ATP. When reactions use oxygen, the process is called *respiration*. This process proceeds when pyruvic acid enters into a series of reactions called the *tricarboxylic acid* (TCA) or *Krebs cycle*. In the Krebs cycle the carbohydrates are further oxidized and released hydrogen is transferred to an appropriate carrier molecule, such as nicotinamide adenine dinucleotide (NAD). The reduced NAD (carrying the hydrogen atom, NADH) enters an electron transport system in which the hydrogen atom is transferred to an oxygen atom, thereby resulting in the ultimate formation of water (Figure 4-6). Thus the chemical energy contained in pyruvic acid is slowly released through a stepwise series of reactions involving the passage of electrons from the carbohydrate to oxygen and resulting in the formation of water and the release of CO_2. In all, for every glucose molecule metabolized by the cell, 38 ATP molecules are generated by this process. Using the two ATP molecules to initiate the glycolytic reaction, a net total of 36 available ATP molecules are generated. Therefore, most of the energy available to the majority of cells results from respiration. The CO_2 that is formed as a by-product of respiration is released from the cell into the atmosphere where it is again able to enter into the reactions of photosynthesis and be converted back into an energy-containing carbohydrate. On the other hand, the oxygen given off as a by-product of photosynthesis is used in the respiration reactions of the cell, thus forming one of the important chemical cycles involved in the balance of living systems.

ATP

(a)

ADP

(b)

AMP

(c)

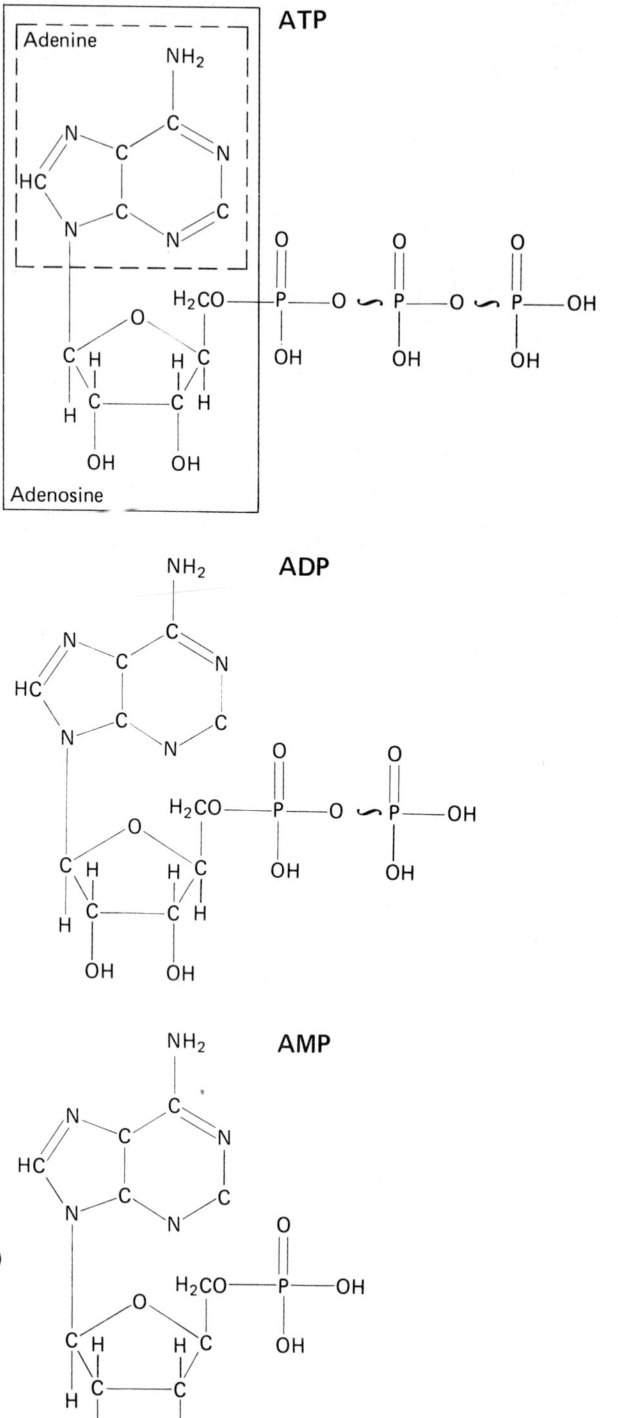

Figure 4-4 Adenosine tri (a), di (b), and mono (c) phosphate showing the position of the high energy (∿) phosphate bonds.

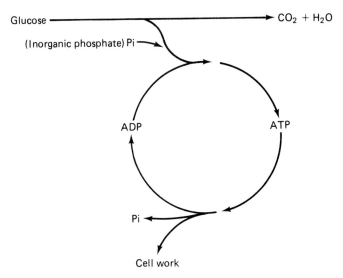

Figure 4-5 The ATP-ADP cycle. Energy obtained through the oxidation of glucose is used to form ATP. This energy is then released by ATP to carry out energy-requiring cellular processes. The resultant ADP is then available to be used in the formation of a new ATP molecule.

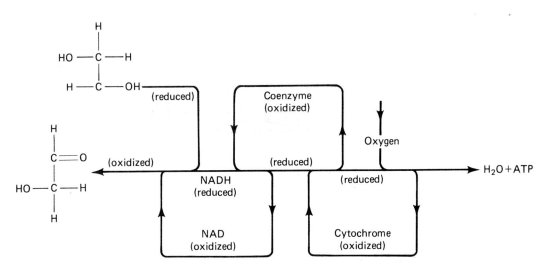

Figure 4-6 A schematic diagram representing the transfer of hydrogen from the oxidation of carbohydrate to NAD and from NADH to the electron transport system which ultimately uses two hydrogen atoms to reduce an atom of oxygen to a molecule of water. These reactions result in a concurrent production of ATP (see appendix A for details).

TABLE 4-1 THE MAJOR CATEGORIES OF MONOMERS
AND THE POLYMER FORMED FROM THEM

Monomers	Polymers
Amino acids	Proteins (polypeptides)
Simple sugars	Carbohydrates (polysaccharides)
Fatty acids, monoglyceride	Lipids
Nucleotide bases	Nucleic acids

BIOSYNTHESIS

In addition to providing energy through the catabolic reactions just discussed, the metabolic activities of the cell are also engaged in producing building blocks needed for the formation of new cellular components. This process is called *biosynthesis* or *anabolism* and requires energy obtained from the ATP molecules. All living cells consist of a large number of complex organic molecules called *polymers*. Polymers are so called because they are produced by connecting large numbers of smaller molecules called *monomers*. Only about 150 different types of precursor monomers are needed to form the thousands of different polymers found in a living cell. Many monomers are produced through the various metabolic pathways within the cell whereas others come directly from nutrients and are carried into the cell through the cytoplasmic membrane (Figure 4-1). Most polymers, also referred to as macromolecules, are of the following four general types: (a) polysaccharides, (b) proteins, (c) nucleic acids, and (d) lipid complexes. Polysaccharides are polymers of simple sugars and were discussed earlier in this chapter. Proteins are polymers that consist of monomers called amino acids. The myriads of protein macromolecules are formed from 20 different types of amino acids. The structure and functions of proteins are discussed later. Nucleic acids are polymers composed of chains of monomers called nucleotide bases. Their structure and functions are discussed in the following chapter. The lipid complexes vary in composition, with fatty acids, alcohols, sugars, and amino acids as precursor monomers. Some monomer–polymer relationships are shown in Table 4-1.

STRUCTURE AND FUNCTIONS OF PROTEINS

Proteins function both as important structural components of the cell and as enzymes that regulate the chemical reactions of cells. By controlling the types of proteins produced, all other characteristics of the cell are also controlled. To help understand this relationship, some knowledge of the structure and enzymatic functions of proteins is needed.

The 20 amino acid monomers that constitute the polymeric protein molecules are analogous to letters of the alphabet whereas the protein molecules are analogous to words of the printed language. The amino acids are connected end to end, forming long chains, and each protein molecule, in order to be formed properly, must contain a specific sequence and number of amino acids, just as correctly spelled words must have a proper sequence and number of letters (Figure 4-7). Yet a protein molecule contains many more amino acids, usually several hundred, than the number of letters in a word.

Amino acids are so called because they contain an amine group (NH_2) at one

end and a carboxylic acid group (O—OH) at the other end of the molecule. The arrangement of atoms in between the amine and the carboxylic acid groups is different for each amino acid. The structures of two amino acid molecules are shown in Figure 4-7. When the amino acids are brought together under specific conditions, a reaction occurs between the amine group of one amino acid and the carboxyl group of the other. In this reaction a water molecule is split off.

The bond that forms between amino acids is called a *peptide* bond and a macromolecule containing many amino acids is called a *polypeptide*. A complete protein molecule may consist of one or several polypeptides. The sequence of amino acids in the protein is called the *primary structure* of the polypeptide. As the polypeptide forms, it coils into a spiral or helical arrangement called the *secondary structure*. Next, the helix folds on itself and forms chemical bonds between different segments of the molecule. The result is called the *tertiary structure* and gives the protein molecule a specific three-dimensional shape (Figure 4-7). The primary structure of the polypeptide determines the secondary and tertiary configuration. In addition, some protein molecules are formed by connecting several polypeptides. Such an arrangement is called a *quaternary structure*. Any amino acid can be connected to any other amino acid; moreover, because of the large numbers of amino acids in a protein, an almost unlimited number of different types of protein molecules can be formed from the 20 amino acids.

An important function of some proteins is to serve as enzymes. All enzymes are proteins; however, not all proteins are enzymes. Enzymes are the *catalysts* of living systems. A catalyst is a substance that reduces the energy needed to start a chemical reaction and that may increase the rate of the reaction but is not used up in the reaction itself (Figure 4-8). Most chemical reactions that occur in living systems will not proceed without the proper enzymatic catalyst. So without enzymes, life functions as we know them would stop. Enzymes are very specific and almost every reaction of the thousands that occur in a cell requires a distinct and specific enzyme. Thus a simple bacterial cell must be able to synthesize hundreds of different types of protein molecules just to supply the needed enzymes. The specificity of an enzyme is a result of the three-dimensional configuration of the protein molecule. This shape allows the enzyme to react temporarily with and properly orient the compounds involved in chemical reaction so that the energy required to start the reaction is reduced (Figure 4-9). After the reaction occurs, the enzyme disassociates and is free to repeat the process. Most enzymes are able to catalyze thousands of reactions per second.

Some enzymes direct the synthesis of complex molecules from simple precursor subcomponents; others may change the arrangement of the atom within a molecule;

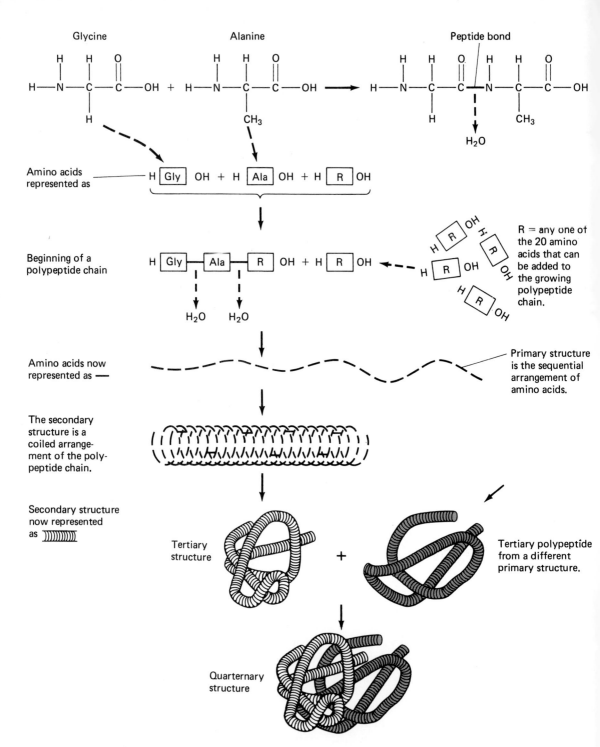

Figure 4-7 Formation of protein molecules from amino acid monomers. Formation and structure of primary, secondary, tertiary, and quaternary structure are shown.

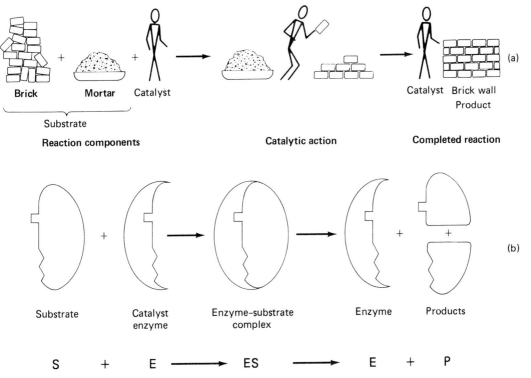

Figure 4-8 A catalyst enters a chemical reaction, facilitates the reaction by increasing the interaction between substrate molecules, then leaves the reaction unchanged. (a) This can be exemplified by a bricklayer, who uses brick and mortar (substrates) and combines them into a finished product. (b) An enzyme is a biological catalyst. It facilitates a chemical reaction, makes it go, and is left unchanged by the reaction.

still others may break down complex compounds into simpler molecules. The chemical that is acted on by an enzyme is called a *substrate*. Enzymes are usually named by adding the suffix *-ase* to the name of the substrate or reaction catalyzed. An enzyme that breaks down proteins would be called a protease, for instance, whereas one that catalyzes the reaction to form a DNA macromolecule would be called a DNA-polymerase. A list of some enzymes and their functions is given in Table 4-2.

What a cell can and cannot do depends on the type of enzymes it possesses. The great diversity of activities of various microorganisms is a function of the types of enzymes they possess. If all the necessary enzymes are formed, the cell will function properly. If an essential enzyme is not properly formed, the cell may die. If an enzyme that catalyzes a minor reaction is missing, the cell may survive but take on different characteristics. Similarly, if a cell acquires the ability to produce a new enzyme, the cell may acquire a new characteristic. Therefore controlling the synthesis of protein molecules means that all other reactions of the cell are controlled. Fundamentally, then, the genetic control of a cell or an organism is a control of protein synthesis. The

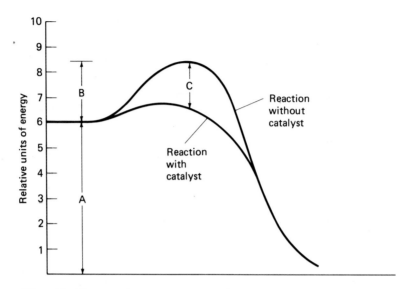

Figure 4-9 How a catalyst works. Catalysts such as an enzyme reduce the energy of activation, B, needed to initiate a chemical reaction. The energy available in the substrate is represented by A. The amount of energy conserved by the catalyst is represented by C.

discovery of how a cell can store and transfer to offspring the information necessary to line up the amino acids into the proper sequences in order to form the proper enzymes has been one of the great scientific achievements of the past 30 years. This topic will be discussed in the next chapter.

TABLE 4-2 ENZYMES AND ENZYMATIC FUNCTIONS

Enzyme class	Examples	Functions
Hydrolase	Amidase, esterase, phosphatase	Breaking of chemical bonds by the addition of water
Isomerase	Mutase, epimerase	Molecular rearrangement producing one isomer from another
Ligase	DNA synthetase	Linking of simple molecules into complex polymers
Lyase	Deaminase, decarboxylase	Nonhydrolytic cleavage of chemical bonds
Oxidoreductase	Dehydrogenase, peroxidase	Catalyzes oxidation and reduction reactions
Transferase	Transaminase, transmethylase	Transfer of atoms or molecules from one compound to another

SUMMARY

1. Energy for life is primarily a product of the sun. This energy is organized into chemical systems by means of photosynthesis, which occurs in autotrophic life forms. Heterotrophic organisms obtain their needed energy by using autotrophs or the metabolic products of autotrophs.

2. Heterotrophic bacteria primarily use carbohydrate as an energy source. The carbohydrate is gradually oxidized through a stepwise rearrangement of the molecule. This energy, obtained in a systematic fashion, is captured in ATP, which is then used by the cell to perform energy-requiring operations, such as cell synthesis.

3. Cellular metabolism is regulated by the availability of enzymes. These proteins ensure the proper, systematic interaction of those molecules necessary to build new cell material. Other enzymes provide orderly catabolic processes that result in a continuous supply of energy to carry out cell processes.

Control of Cellular Functions

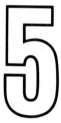

Cell genes are information-carrying molecules that contain all the information needed to direct the proper functions of the cell. When a cell divides, a full complement of the genetic information (genes) must be passed to each daughter cell. As the individual chemical reactions of the cell are catalyzed by specific enzymes, which are proteins, the information-carrying molecules of the genes must be able to direct the synthesis of the proper proteins.

It is now well established that the chemical *deoxyribonucleic acid* (DNA) is the information-carrying molecule of the gene. One of the greatest achievements in science was the discovery that DNA is the genetic material of the cell, what its structure is, how equal complements are passed to each daughter cell, the means of information storage, and how this information directs the formation of protein molecules. The following pages present the chronological developments in this series of discoveries.

DNA AS THE GENETIC MOLECULE

By the 1930s it was recognized that the information-carrying molecules of the cell were in the nucleus. Chemical analysis of the nucleus, however, showed that large amounts of both protein and DNA were present. At that time the structure of protein molecules was much better understood than the structure of DNA. DNA was known to consist of only four different monomeric components called nucleotide bases. On the other hand, the protein molecules were known to be formed by the 20 amino acids. So scientists of the 1930s had a choice between the "4-letter alphabet" of DNA and the "20-letter alphabet" of proteins for the genetic information molecule. They logically assumed that protein molecules would contain the genetic information. A series of important experiments conducted in the 1930s and 1940s by Avery, MacLeod, and McCarty, however, demonstrated that DNA is the genetic material of the cell. Using the pneumococcus bacterium, they performed a series of experiments that led to the discovery that genetic traits could be passed from one cell to another with pure extracts of DNA, a process now called *transformation* (Figure 5-1).

Structure of DNA

Once it was determined that DNA was the information-carrying molecule, various groups of scientists tried to determine how a substance containing only four monomeric nucleotide bases could contain the massive amount of information needed to be stored in the genes of the cell. Each nucleotide base was known to contain a phosphate group connected to the five-carbon sugar deoxyribose, which, in turn, was connected to a purine or pyrimidine base. Two pyrimidine bases, called *cytosine* and *thymine*, and two purine bases, called *adenine* and *guanine*, are contained in the nucleotide bases; their structures are shown in Figure 5-2.

The structure of DNA was demonstrated in 1953 when Watson and Crick, working in England, were able to construct a model of the molecule showing how the nucleotide bases fit together. Their model showed that the molecule was constructed of two long chains of nucleotides intertwined in a double helix (spiral). The deoxyribose sugar and the phosphate formed the backbone of the molecule and the purine and pyrimidine bases pointed toward the center and were connected in a specific pairing arrangement to hold the two chains together (Figure 5-3). The specific arrangement was that thymine could pair only with adenine and cytosine only with guanine. This is called *complementary pairing* and is one of the essential features that allow a DNA molecule to replicate into two identical molecules prior to cell division. Each new cell formed by division receives one of the two identical DNA molecules (chromosomes).

The Watson-Crick model demonstrated how the DNA molecule could divide. That is, when the bonds that connect the complementary nucleotides are broken (this would be done by a specific enzyme), new nucleotides can be brought in and connected at their complementary site on each DNA chain. The phosphate groups connect to the adjacent deoxyribose sugar to form the backbone of the newly forming chain of each DNA molecule. The separation of the original nucleic acid chain and the addition of new nucleotide bases continue along the entire molecule, resulting in the formation of two identical molecules (Figure 5-4). Each molecule contains one chain from the old molecule and one newly synthesized chain. Although this model showed that the complementary nucleotide pairing between the two chains of the double helix is rigidly specific, the linear arrangement of the nucleotides along the chains could be variable.

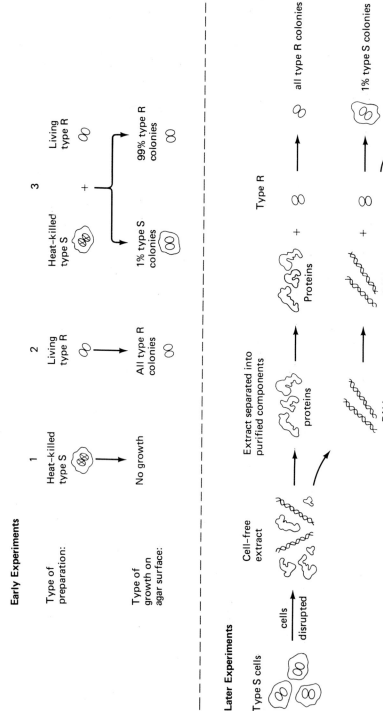

Figure 5-1 The transforming experiments of Avery and coworkers. Two strains of pneumo-cocci were used. One was a strain with a capsule that produced smooth colonies (type S); the other strain had no capsule and produced rough colonies (type R). The early experiments showed that when killed type S cells were mixed with live type R cells about 1% of the living R cells acquired genetic material from the type S cells and were transformed into type S cells. The later experiments demonstrated that the transformation was produced by purified preparations of DNA extracted from type S cells.

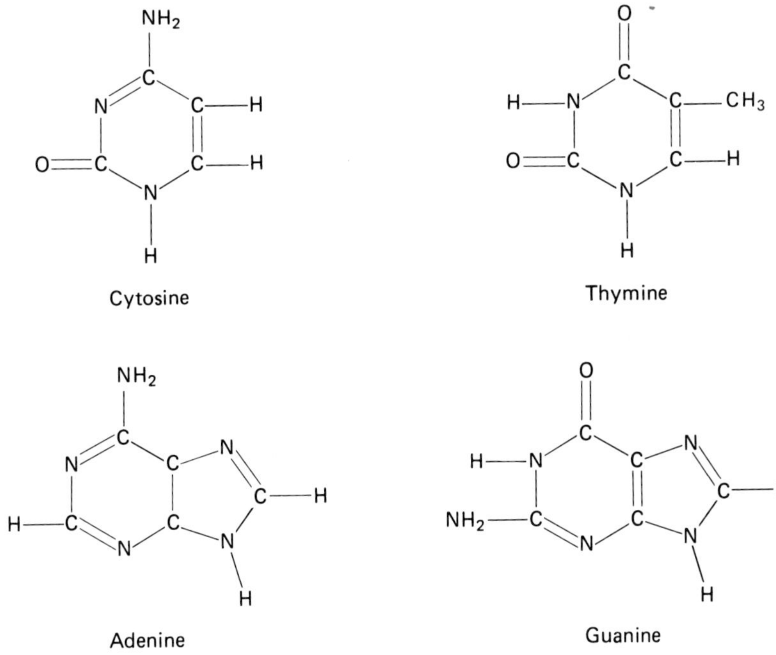

Figure 5-2　The structures of the two single-ring pyrimidine bases called cytosine and thymine, and the two double-ring purine bases called adenine and guanine.

Following the work of Watson and Crick, the challenge was to determine how the genetic information was encoded in the molecule. Obviously the information had to be encoded in the linear sequence of nucleotides along the chains of the DNA molecule. It was necessary to determine how a linear sequence of four nucleotide bases could direct the alignment of 20 amino acids into sequences that could lead to the formation of a wide variety of proteins. That is, how could the 4-letter nucleotide alphabet correspond to the 20-letter amino acid alphabet? Using one nucleotide as a letter of the genetic alphabet would obviously not be sufficient to correspond to the 20 amino acids. The next alternative was to use two neighboring nucleotides as a letter, which would give only 16 possible combinations. The next alternative was three nucleotides in sequence for each letter, which would give a total of 64 possible combinations of nucleotide bases. This base arrangement is called a *triplet code*. Toward the end of the 1950s sufficient experimental information had accumulated to show that the triplet code was the one used by DNA. Each sequence of three nucleotides forms a letter of the genetic code called a *codon* (Figure 5-5). The determination of the genetic code—that is, discovering which codon corresponded to which amino acid—took an additional 10 years and was completed in the late 1960s. Because there are 64 codons and only 20 amino acids, some amino acids were found to correspond to more than one codon. Three codons, however, did not correspond to any amino acid and were shown to function as punctuation marks in the genetic alphabet. These punctuation

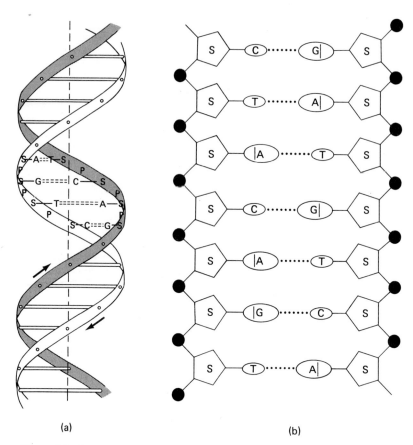

(a)

(b)

Figure 5-3 Structure of DNA molecule. (a) The molecule is made up of two polynucleotide chains. The backbone of the chains is composed of alternate sugars (S) and phosphate (P) units. The two chains are coiled in a double helix and connected by chemical bonds between the complementary bases (A:T, G:C). (b) A diagram of a section of DNA molecule uncoiled showing the alternate sugar (S) phosphate (●) backbones and the cross-connecting purine and pyrimidine bases.

marks determine when the messages for specific polypeptides start and end. The segment of bases in the DNA molecule that codes for one polypeptide is called a *cistron*. The DNA of a bacterial cell is a single molecule (about 1 mm in length) that contains approximately 10 million pairs of nucleotides, more than enough to code for the several thousand different proteins produced by the bacterial cell. That is, three nucleotide bases form one codon that corresponds to one amino acid; assuming that an average protein contains 300 amino acids, then 900 nucleotides would be needed in a single cistron to code for that protein.

During the late 1950s important research under the direction of Lwoff, Jacob, and Monod in France demonstrated how the genetic information of DNA is able to

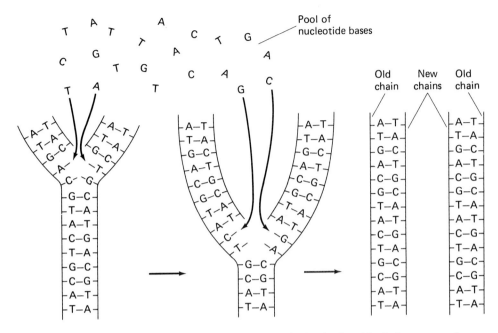

Figure 5-4 The mode of replication of a DNA molecule showing how identical sequences of nucleotide bases are maintained in each replicated molecule.

direct the synthesis of proteins. This process requires a second type of nucleic acid called *ribonucleic acid* (RNA). RNA differs from DNA in that it contains ribose sugar in place of deoxyribose sugar, uses a uracil base instead of the thymine base, and is usually single stranded.

Protein Synthesis

The process of getting the genetic information contained in the linear sequence of nucleotides along the DNA molecule into a linear sequence of amino acids in a protein molecule requires two phases, *transcription* and *translation*.

Transcription

The process of transcription involves the passage of genetic information from the DNA molecule into an RNA molecule called *messenger RNA* (*m*RNA). Transcription is controlled by specific enzymes and starts at the beginning of a cistron. A momentary separation of the strands of the DNA molecule occurs and an RNA nucleotide is brought into the appropriate complementary position on one chain of the DNA molecule. Thus if the base on the DNA molecule is thymine, a ribose containing adenine nucleotide will attach to it. When the enzyme moves to the next position on the DNA molecule, another RNA nucleotide is brought into a complementary position and is

Singlet code				
A				
G				
C				
U				

Doublet code			
AA	AG	AC	AU
GA	GG	GC	GU
CA	CG	CC	CU
UA	UG	UC	UU

Triplet code			
AAA	AAG	AAC	AAU
AGA	AGG	AGC	AGU
ACA	ACG	ACC	ACU
AUA	AUG	AUC	AUU
GAA	GAG	GAC	GAU
GGA	GGG	GGC	GGU
GCA	GCG	GCC	GCU
GUA	GUG	GUC	GUU
CAA	CAG	CAC	CAU
CGA	CGG	CGC	CGU
CCA	CCG	CCC	CCU
CUA	CUG	CUC	CUU
UAA	UAG	UAC	UAU
UGA	UGG	UGC	UGU
UCA	UCG	UCC	UCU
UUA	UUG	UUC	UUU

Figure 5-5 The possible number of letters (codons) in the genetic alphabet based on singlet, doublet, and triplet arrangements of nucleotide bases. These examples use the *m*RNA molecule. The triplet code is the one that functions in the genetic alphabet.

then connected to the adjacent RNA nucleotide through a ribose sugar-phosphate linkage. As the enzyme passes each nucleotide along the DNA molecule, the complementary RNA nucleotide is brought into place and connected to the growing *m*RNA chain. When the enzyme has passed over the last DNA nucleotide in the cistron or message, the RNA is separated from the DNA and the complementary DNA nucleotides rejoin to form the double helical orientation of the original DNA molecule. Thus the original message of the DNA molecule is both duplicated in the *m*RNA and preserved in the DNA. The process of transcription is shown in Figure 5-6.

Translation

In eucaryotic cells the *m*RNA passes from the nucleus into the cytoplasm, where translation (Figure 5-7) occurs. In procaryotic cells translation can begin as soon as the *m*RNA begins to form, for no nuclear membrane separates the DNA from the protein-synthesizing components (Figure 5-8). The formation of protein from the *m*RNA message is called *translation* because it changes the genetic information from the nucleotide "alphabet" into the amino acid "alphabet" of proteins. Translation requires the involvement of ribosomes and a form of RNA called *transfer RNA* (*t*RNA). The ribosome attaches to one end of the newly formed *m*RNA and then

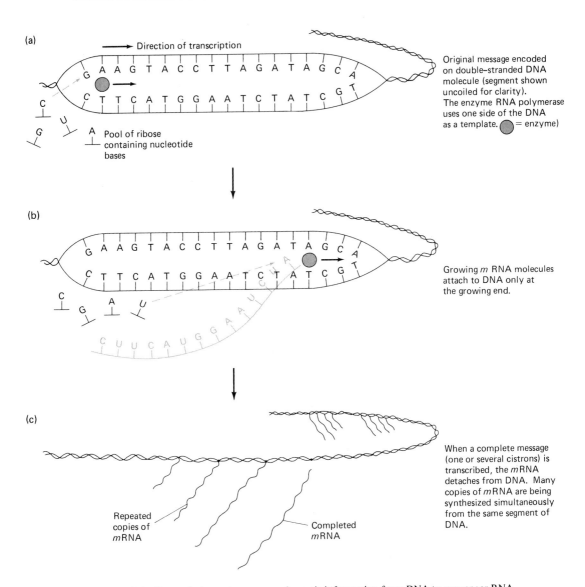

Figure 5-6 Transcription—the passage of genetic information from DNA to messenger RNA.

moves along this molecule. Other ribosomes follow in sequence along the *m*RNA like beads on a string. Usually five or six ribosomes will be strung along a *m*RNA molecule; this complex of ribosomes is called a *polyribosome*. As a ribosome moves along the *m*RNA, it directs the process of translation. Transfer RNAs are relatively short chains of nucleotides that contain a specific triplet of three nucleotides at one section of the molecule called an *anticodon*. A site exists on an end of the *t*RNA molecule

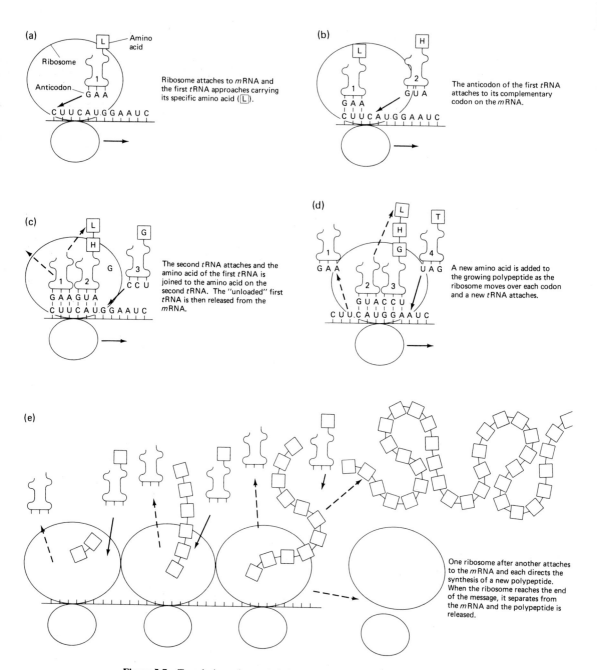

(a)

Ribosome attaches to *m*RNA and the first *t*RNA approaches carrying its specific amino acid ([L]).

(b)

The anticodon of the first *t*RNA attaches to its complementary codon on the *m*RNA.

(c)

The second *t*RNA attaches and the amino acid of the first *t*RNA is joined to the amino acid on the second *t*RNA. The "unloaded" first *t*RNA is then released from the *m*RNA.

(d)

A new amino acid is added to the growing polypeptide as the ribosome moves over each codon and a new *t*RNA attaches.

(e)

One ribosome after another attaches to the *m*RNA and each directs the synthesis of a new polypeptide. When the ribosome reaches the end of the message, it separates from the *m*RNA and the polypeptide is released.

Figure 5-7 Translation of genetic information from a nucleotide sequence to an amino acid sequence.

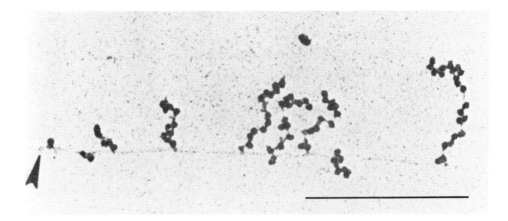

Figure 5-8 Active genes of a rapidly growing bacterium (*E. coli*). As soon as an *m*RNA molecule begins to be transcribed from DNA (presumed initiation site at arrow), ribosomes begin to attach. As the length of the *m*RNA increases, more ribosomes attach forming longer polyribosomes. In procaryotic cells, where the DNA is not separated from the ribosomes by a nuclear membrane, translation may begin before the complete *m*RNA is formed and while it is still attached to the DNA. (Bar = 0.5 μm.) (From Hamkalo and Miller, "Electronmicroscopy of Genetic Material," Figure 6a, p. 379. Reproduced, with permission, from *Annual Review of Biochemistry*, Volume 42. © 1973 by Annual Reviews, Inc.)

apart from the anticodon that will combine with only one kind of the 20 different amino acids. The connection between the *t*RNA and amino acid is energized with energy received from ATP molecules. When the ribosome passes over a codon of the *m*RNA, a *t*RNA with the complementary anticodon is connected to the *m*RNA codon and carries with it a specific amino acid. This amino acid is the one corresponding to the codon of the *m*RNA and thus also corresponds to the complementary code on the DNA molecule. The first amino acid is held in position on the ribosome by the *t*RNA while the next amino acid is brought into position by its *t*RNA and the two amino acids are then attached by means of a peptide bond. The first amino acid and its *t*RNA separate and the "unloaded" *t*RNA moves from the ribosome.

The ribosome continues to move along the *m*RNA and, as it passes over each codon, the complementary *t*RNA comes into position and connects the specified amino acid onto the growing polypeptide chain. On reaching the end of the *m*RNA, the ribosome leaves the polyribosome complex and the completed polypeptide is released. As ribosomes move along the same *m*RNA, one after the other, each forms an identical polypeptide. Consequently, thousands of proteins can be rapidly formed from a single *m*RNA molecule. The *m*RNA molecule functions only for a limited period and is then broken down by the cell's enzymes. New copies of the *m*RNA, however, are transcribed from the DNA as needed.

The same genetic code is used by all living systems, with the flow of genetic information going from double-stranded DNA to single-stranded *m*RNA to polypeptide. The only exceptions are with some viruses, which use the same code but use nucleic acid molecules other than double-stranded DNA for the storage of their genetic information (see Chapter 31).

ALTERATIONS IN GENETIC INFORMATION OF THE CELL

The properties expressed by a microorganism in a given environment are a result of the genetic information contained in the DNA and are modified by environmental conditions. The genetic information—that is, the sequence of nucleotide bases in DNA—in a cell is referred to as the *genotype* of the cell. Nevertheless, when observing cellular properties or functions, it is not the genotype that is seen but the expression of the genes. This observable property of the cell is called its *phenotype* and may be influenced by environmental conditions. When changes occur in the genotype of a cell, new messages are formed and a new phenotype may be produced.

The genotype of a microbial cell can be altered in two general ways. First, the sequence of nucleotide bases in the existing DNA molecule can be altered, a process called *mutation*. The second means of altering the genotype of a cell is by the addition or deletion of segments of DNA.

Mutations

Mutations may result from several types of changes that can occur in the sequence of nucleotides in a gene. First, one type of nucleotide may substitute for another type during replication of the DNA molecule; this is called *point mutation* (Figure 5-9). Other mutations may result from the addition or loss of one or more nucleotides in a gene; these result in a shift of the reading frame for the DNA and are called *frameshift mutations* (Figure 5-10). Point mutation causes the change of a single codon and hence the incorporation of one different amino acid into the corresponding protein; this may or may not cause a change in the phenotypic expression of the cell. Frameshift mutation results in an entirely new sequence of amino acids in the corresponding protein; this protein is usually nonfunctional, which may cause a pronounced phenotypic change in the cell.

Normally mutations occur during cell replication at a frequency of 1:100,000 to 1:10 billion for any given phenotypic characteristic. Certain agents, called *mutagens,* may increase the rate at which mutations occur. A rather lengthy list of mutagens can be compiled and includes such agents as x rays, ultraviolet light, nitrous acid, acridine dyes, alkylating agents, and nucleotide-type bases that are slightly different from the normal nucleotides in DNA. The agents that increase the mutation rate of bacterial cells are also known to increase the occurrence of cancer in humans and animals.

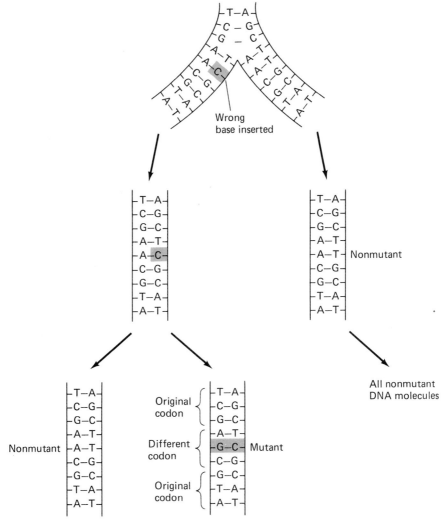

Figure 5-9   A point mutation produced by the wrong insertion of the base cystosine in the place of a thymine base. This results in one different codon in the mutant DNA molecule and one different amino acid in the resulting polypeptide.

Transfer of Genes

In addition to the large circular DNA molecule (bacterial chromosome) that contains the essential genetic information for a bacterial cell, many bacteria contain smaller, circular DNA molecules called *plasmids*. Plasmids exist and reproduce independently of the main chromosome and are not essential for the normal growth of the bacte-

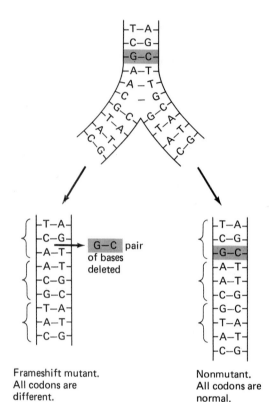

Frameshift mutant. All codons are different.

Nonmutant. All codons are normal.

Figure 5-10 A frameshift mutation in which a pair of bases were deleted. This results in a new sequence of codons starting at the position of the deletion.

rium. Yet the genes contained in plasmids are able to impart added characteristics to a cell.

Genes from both plasmids and bacterial chromosomes can be transferred from one cell to another. Three different mechanisms—*transformation, conjugation,* and *transduction*—are used in the transfer of DNA from a donor cell to a recipient cell.

Transformation

The process of transformation is the transfer of cell-free fragments of chromosomal DNA or plasmids from one cell to another. This process was referred to earlier in the experiments with pneumococci that demonstrated the genetic role of DNA (Figure 5-1). Transformation with chromosomal DNA can occur in nature only between closely related bacteria and has been demonstrated in only a few species. The DNA fragment enters the recipient cell by passing through the cell wall and plasma membrane. When donor chromosomal DNA enters a cell, it becomes positioned alongside homologous (same type) genes of the recipient cell. Enzymes cut out (excise) the homologous genes in the DNA of the recipient cell and the donor chromosomal fragment is integrated into the recipient cell's DNA in place of the excised DNA segment. This integration of donor DNA into the recipient DNA is called *recombination*. If the integrated DNA contains genetic information not previously possessed by the recipient cell, the transformation process will cause a genotypic change by adding new information and deleting the information on the excised DNA segment. Plasmids need not recombine with the chromosomal DNA and thus do not delete any information from the recipient cell, but they do add new genetic information.

Conjugation

Conjugation is the transfer of genes between bacteria that are in physical contact with one another (Figure 5-11). The contact is made by pili produced by the donor cell. The donor cell, sometimes called the male or positive cell, contains a plasmid that is readily passed to the recipient cell, also called the female or negative cell. The plasmid contains genetic information for the formation of pili, plus other characteristics. After receiving the plasmid, the recipient is converted into a donor cell with pili and plasmids.

In most cases of conjugation none of the chromosomal DNA is passed. But in a few cases the plasmid integrates into the chromosome of the donor cell, thereby making the chromosome "mobile"—that is, able to be passed to the recipient cell. Under these conditions the circular chromosome breaks and is transferred as a linear molecule into the recipient cell. Usually before all the donor chromosome can be transferred, the cells separate and the recipient receives only part of the donor DNA. This transferred DNA becomes integrated into the recipient cell DNA and imparts new genetic characteristics to the recipient cell.

In yet other cases, the plasmid that has integrated into the donor cell chromosome can reverse the process and once again become a free plasmid in the cytoplasm. When the plasmid separates, however, it often carries with it segments of the donor cell chromosome, which then become part of the plasmid. When passed to a recipient

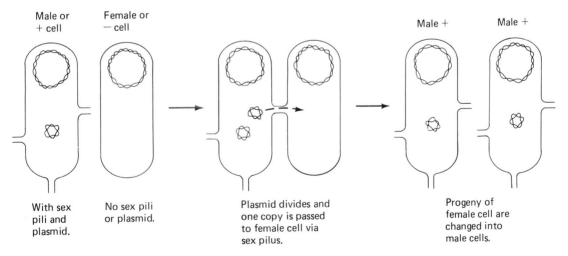

Male or + cell	Female or − cell		Male +	Male +

With sex pili and plasmid.

No sex pili or plasmid.

Plasmid divides and one copy is passed to female cell via sex pilus.

Progeny of female cell are changed into male cells.

Figure 5-11 A mechanism of conjugation in which genetic traits producing the male characteristics are passed with a plasmid to a female cell through a pilus.

cell, this plasmid also carries with it the genetic information picked up from the donor cell chromosome.

Transduction

Transduction is a process in which a bacterial virus (bacteriophage or phage) carries bacterial DNA from a donor to a recipient cell (Figure 5-12). A phage infects by injecting nucleic acid into a bacterial cell. The phage nucleic acid directs the bacterial cell to synthesize new phage nucleic acid and protein coats that are then assembled into new phage particles. When several hundred new phages have been assembled, the bacterial cell bursts and releases the phages into the surrounding medium. During the multiplication and infection cycle of the phage it is possible for some of the bacterial genes to be passed from one cell to another by several mechanisms. One type of transduction results when a phage infects a bacterial cell and causes the bacterial chromosome to fragment into many pieces. As new phage particles are assembled, a fragment of bacterial DNA or a plasmid may accidentally become packaged inside the protein coat of the phage. When this phage later infects a new cell, the DNA inside the phage is introduced into the new cell. If a fragment is carried to the new cell, it must recombine with the DNA of the recipient cell before it can be expressed. If a plasmid is transported to the recipient cell by the phage, its genetic messages can be expressed without the need to integrate into the DNA of the recipient cell.

The DNA of some types of phage integrates into the DNA of the host cell, a condition called *lysogeny,* and replicates along with the bacterial DNA during cell division. Periodically the phage DNA dissociates from the bacterial DNA and may carry a section of adjacent host cell DNA with it. When new phage DNA molecules are synthesized, the section of attached bacterial DNA is also synthesized and is packaged, along with the phage DNA, inside the protein coat of the phage. When these phages infect and integrate their DNA into the recipient cell, the attached segment of bacterial DNA is also integrated and will induce new genetic traits in the recipient cells.

The Significance of Mutations and Gene Transfer

Most mutations that occur in microorganisms result in changes that are detrimental to the optimal performance of the mutant. These mutants are usually eliminated, for they are less able to survive or compete with normal microbes. Occasionally, however, a mutation or gene transfer occurs that gives a microbe an advantage in a given environment. Such a new genotype may then be able to outcompete and replace most normal microbes in that particular environment or they may be able to grow in an environment where normal microbes are unable to grow. New genotypes that have an advantage or have adapted to a new environment may regularly develop in microbial populations where cell division occurs rapidly.

Mutations may be beneficial or detrimental to human needs. The most troublesome and frequent changes associated with medical microbiology are resistant strains of microbes that develop against antimicrobial agents. Antibiotic resistance can be

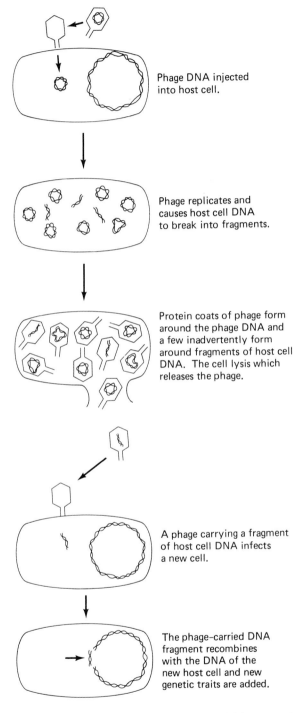

Phage DNA injected into host cell.

Phage replicates and causes host cell DNA to break into fragments.

Protein coats of phage form around the phage DNA and a few inadvertently form around fragments of host cell DNA. The cell lysis which releases the phage.

A phage carrying a fragment of host cell DNA infects a new cell.

The phage-carried DNA fragment recombines with the DNA of the new host cell and new genetic traits are added.

Figure 5-12 Generalized transduction in which bacterial genes are transferred from one cell to another by a phage.

acquired through both mutations and gene transfers. Some genes associated with plasmids or acquired by transduction impart disease-producing capabilities to some microorganisms.

Selected mutants and microbes with recombined genes are sometimes of great use. Certain mutants have been selected as highly efficient producers of products of commercial value. The original *Penicillium* mold used for the antibiotic penicillin, for instance, produced relatively small amounts of the antibiotic. By treating this mold with such mutagens as x ray and ultraviolet light, it was possible to induce a mutant that produced a 1000 times greater yield of penicillin. Such a mutant allowed penicillin to be produced much more efficiently. Some mutants of disease-producing bacteria that have lost most of their disease-causing capabilities have been effectively used as living vaccines.

Because mutagens of bacteria also tend to cause cancer in humans, many chemicals are tested each year to determine if they are able to increase the mutation rate in bacteria. These tests take only a few days and are relatively inexpensive. Only those chemicals that are mutagenic for bacteria are then further tested by slower and expensive methods using experimental animals. Thus by using bacteria in the screening tests, the number of chemicals tested in the animal system is greatly reduced and overall many more chemicals can be tested.

GENETIC ENGINEERING

Manipulated gene transfer to microorganisms by means of plasmids is currently of great interest. This technology, called *genetic engineering* or *recombinant DNA*, has the potential of developing microorganisms that are able to produce many useful products that are difficult or impossible to produce by other methods. With this technology it is possible not only to transfer genes from one type of bacterium to another but also to transfer genes from any other form of life to microorganisms. A method used in recombinant DNA is shown in Figure 5-13. Recombinant DNA is formed by first isolating and purifying plasmids of a given bacterium (*E. coli* is most often used). DNA from some other organism (referred to as foreign DNA or gene) that contains a specific gene is also isolated and purified. Both the plasmid and the foreign DNA are treated separately with a special type of enzyme called a *restriction endonuclease*. The endonuclease breaks both the plasmid and foreign DNA where identical sequences of nucleotides are located. This break is such that a short segment of single-stranded DNA is left at the ends of the broken DNA molecules. Using this procedure, the nucleotide sequences on the single strands at the ends of both DNA molecules become complementary. Such complementary single strands are called "sticky" ends, for they specifically combine with the single-stranded ends of any other DNA molecule that has been treated with the same endonuclease. When the endonuclease-treated plasmids and foreign genes are mixed together in the presence of another enzyme, called *DNA ligase*, their "sticky" ends join together and the foreign gene becomes integrated into the plasmid. The recombined plasmid can then be placed back

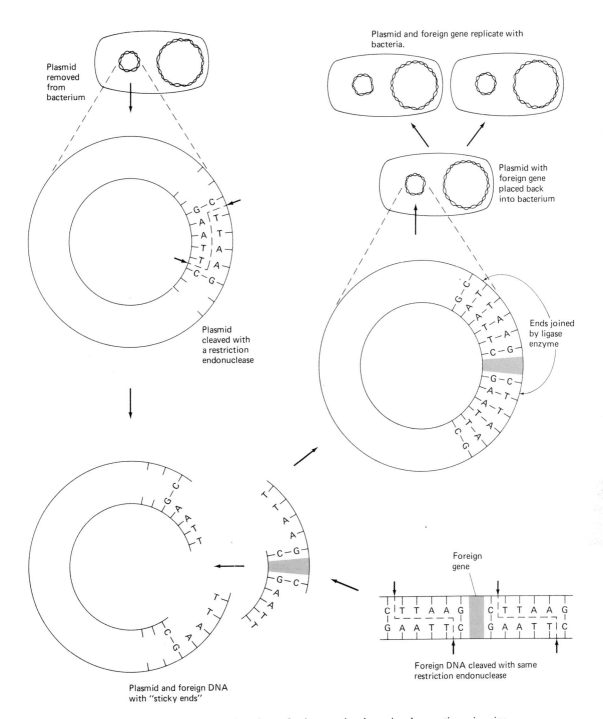

Figure 5-13 A method used to place a foreign gene in a bacterium by genetic engineering.

TABLE 5-1 SOME POSSIBLE PRODUCTS AND POTENTIAL APPLICATIONS OF GENETIC ENGINEERING

Products	Applications
Enzymes that metabolize petroleum	Clean up oil spills
Insulin	Treatment of diabetics
Human-growth hormones	Treatment of growth disorders
Animal-growth hormones	Stimulate growth for increased meat production
Interferons	Treatment of viral infections and possibly cancer
Pheremones (insect hormones)	Insect control
Endophrines	Pain killers
Antigens	Preparation of vaccines not easily produced by regular methods
Antibiotics	Improved or less expensive antibiotics
Methane or alcohol	More efficient formation of these products from cellulose waste
Nitrogen fixation	Increased soil fertility

into a bacterium. As this bacterium divides, the plasmid, including the integrated foreign gene, also divides. All the progeny bacteria will thus contain the foreign gene and will be able to produce the protein coded on this gene. Because of the rapid growth of microorganisms, large amounts of "foreign" proteins can be produced by genetically engineered microbes.

Several applications of genetic engineering are listed in Table 5-1. Some early applications of genetic engineering included the development of bacteria that could produce human insulin (Figure 5-14) and human-growth hormones. These products have now become available in relatively inexpensive forms for the treatment of diabetics and children with growth defects. Prior to these developments insulin was obtained from animals and human-growth hormone was obtained from human cadavers and was in very limited supply.

Many new vaccines, particularly against viral diseases, that could not be produced economically by conventional methods are now being developed through genetic engineering. Large amounts of an antiviral and possible anticancer agent called *interferon* (p. 409) are being produced by this new technology; it may soon be possible to treat many diseases that were not previously treatable.

Recombinant DNA technology is being applied in many other areas, such as food and energy production, in order to use the rapid growth of microorganisms to increase production and reduce the costs of many products associated with these industries. Genetic engineering is, in fact, creating a new technological revolution.

SUMMARY

1. The chemical structure of deoxyribonucleic acid and its functional operation form the basis for the principles of inheritance and control of cell activity. Through the process of replication, genetic continuity is maintained while the

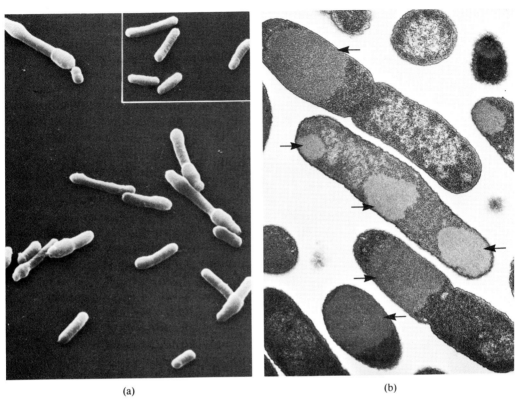

(a)   (b)

Figure 5-14 (a) Scanning electron micrograph of the bacterium *E. coli* that has been genetically engineered to produce components of human insulin. The prominent bulges are caused by the accumulation of insulin inside the bacterial cells; insert shows normal *E. coli* which lack the bulges. (b) Transmission electron micrograph of the insulin producing *E. coli* showing prominent inclusion bodies (arrows) resulting from the accumulation of bacterial-produced human insulin. (Figure 2 and 3 from "Cytoplasmic Inclusion Bodies in *Escherichia coli* Producing Biosynthetic Human Insulin Proteins," D. C. Williams et al., *Science* 215: 687–689. Copyright 1982 by The American Association for the Advancement of Science. Courtesy D. C. Williams, Eli Lilly and Co.)

processes of transcription to RNA and translation to protein account for the maintenance of cell control. Heritable change in the DNA nucleotide sequence is called mutation and results in an altered protein synthesis.

2. Bacterial genetic exchange occurs through the processes of conjugation, transduction, and transformation. These processes are analogous to sexual reproduction in higher life forms.

Growth and Nutrition of Microorganisms

6

The materials and procedures necessary for the laboratory cultivation of microorganisms developed over many years and are still developing. Our understanding of bacterial growth and nutrition is critical to the methods used in isolating and identifying disease agents in the clinical laboratory. This chapter focuses on a working understanding of the growth of bacteria and helps to define processes routinely used in diagnostic microbiology.

NUTRITIONAL REQUIREMENTS OF BACTERIA

Bacteria were first carefully studied in association with infectious diseases. It was early recognized that these microorganisms would not grow on simple substances but required a complex diet, frequently consisting of mammalian body fluids. Such nutrients are needed to supply a source of energy and provide the necessary components for cell growth. All disease-producing bacteria—all fungi, protozoa, and animal cells—require organic chemical compounds as a source of carbon and energy; such cells are called *heterotrophs*. The methods used by these cells to obtain energy from organic compounds, primarily glucose, were discussed in Chapter 4.

Certain bacteria, not of direct medical importance, use CO_2 as their source of carbon; such microbes are called *autotrophs*. Some autotrophs obtain their energy from the oxidation of inorganic compounds, such as ammonium, nitrates, sulfur, and hydrogen, and are called *chemoautotrophs*. Other autotrophs, such as algae and some bacteria, contain chlorophyll and are able to obtain energy from light through the process of photosynthesis; these microbes are called *phototrophs* or, more precisely, *photoautotrophs.*

The most common chemical elements needed by bacterial cells are carbon, hydrogen, oxygen, nitrogen, sulfur, phosphorus, potassium, magnesium, calcium, iron, and sodium. In addition, elements like zinc, molybdenum, copper, and manganese are needed in small amounts and are referred to as *trace elements.* Heterotrophic microbes obtain their carbon from organic compounds, such as sugars, proteins, and lipids. Hydrogen is usually obtained from water and oxygen from any source—water, for instance—where it is found in a dissolved state. Nitrogen, sulfur, and phosphorus can be obtained from either organic or inorganic sources. Most of the other needed elements are obtained from soluble inorganic compounds. Some bacteria, especially several of the disease-producing species, require special growth factors, such as vitamins and amino acids, which explains their need for blood or other animal body fluids.

CULTURE MEDIA

A culture medium used for the growth of a given bacterium must contain all the essential nutrients and the proper concentration of salts and ions and must have the proper pH for optimum bacterial growth to occur. Moisture is always essential, for the various ingredients must be in a soluble form or in a form that can be solubilized to facilitate diffusion into the cell.

It may be necessary in some studies of bacteria to use a chemically defined medium, called a *synthetic medium,* in which all essential nutrients are supplied as pure chemicals. Such synthetic media are often difficult to produce for heterotrophic bacteria. Therefore, for these organisms, *complex media* are used in which all ingredients are not precisely defined. Complex media are often mixtures of organic products from plants, animals, or yeasts, along with appropriate salts, and usually contain the nutrients necessary for the growth of a wide range of bacteria. Products like extracts of malted barley, muscle or other animal tissue, or baker's yeast are frequently used. Acid or enzyme digests of meats, casein, or soybean protein are also used. These products contain most nutrients, both organic and inorganic, that are needed even by the most fastidious microorganisms.

Today almost all culture media formulations are produced by commercial companies and supplied to laboratories as dehydrated products (Figure 6-1). To prepare media at the consumer's laboratory, a specified amount of a dehydrated medium is added to a given volume of distilled water. The medium is then sterilized in an autoclave (see Chapter 8) and dispensed in sterile test tubes or other appropriate containers (Figure 6-2). Currently many clinical laboratories purchase their culture media already reconstituted and dispensed in appropriate sterile containers.

Culture media are prepared in both liquid (*broth*) and solid forms. The broth

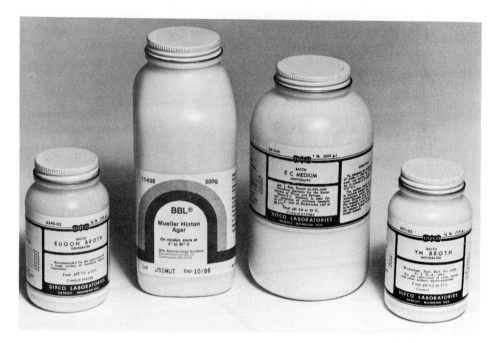

Figure 6-1 Some examples of commercially prepared dehydrated culture media. Components and instructions for preparation and use are given on the labels.

media are made simply by dissolving nutrients in water. Solid media are made by adding a solidifying agent to a broth medium. We are indebted to the laboratory of Robert Koch for the discovery of an appropriate solidifying agent for growth of bacteria. As noted, many of today's bacteriological techniques were developed in the Koch laboratory. Koch recognized that bacteria would effectively reproduce in broth, but if two or more kinds of bacteria were introduced into a broth medium, the resultant growth was a mixed culture. It was extremely difficult to study the properties of any bacterial species as long as it was mixed with other microorganisms. Earlier studies had shown that when placed on a solid medium, such as bread, solidified egg albumen, or the surface of a freshly cut potato, bacteria would grow into a colony consisting of only one kind of bacterial species. The problem for Koch, however, was that such solid surfaces lacked the necessary nutrients to grow disease-producing bacteria, or produced colonies that could not be easily distinguished from the background surface, or several different kinds of bacteria produced colonies that were indistinguishable from each other. These problems greatly limited the scientific study of disease-producing microorganisms.

Faced with this problem, Koch tried adding gelatin to clear broth media in order to obtain a solid surface on which to grow microorganisms from infectious processes.

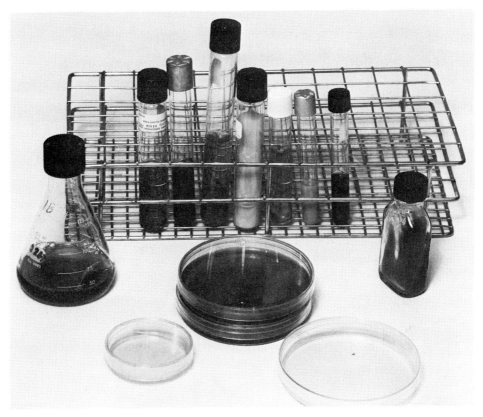

Figure 6-2 Sterilized culture media dispensed into various containers. Petri dishes containing solid agar media are in the foreground. Test tubes and flasks may contain either solid or liquid medium.

Although this approach enabled Koch to provide the necessary nutritional support for the organisms under study, and growth of various species could be distinguished by their colonial differences, it failed to provide an appropriate solution to the problem. Some bacteria digested the gelatin and at optimal bacterial growth temperatures (37°C) gelatin was no longer solid. Therefore cultures of bacteria in such a system were often equivalent to cultivation in broth.

A solution to the problem came through an observation made by Hesse, one of Koch's assistants. His wife, Frau Hesse, was aware that in Indonesia a seaweed extract was boiled with fruit juices to provide a jellylike product. Hesse concluded that if such material could be added to the nutrient broths used to grow bacteria, it might be a satisfactory solidifying agent. The seaweed extract, called *agar*, proved an ideal product to solidify culture media. Agar is inert for most bacteria and thus does not

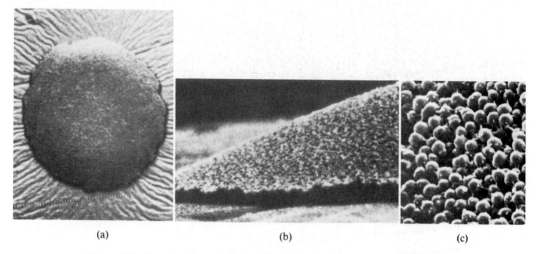

(a)   (b)   (c)

Figure 6-3   Scanning electron micrographs of colonies of gonococci shown at increasing magnifications. (a) viewed from above at 240× magnification, (b) viewed from the side at 1200× magnification and (c) 6000× magnification showing individual cells. (T. Elmros, P. Hörstedt, and B. Winblad, *Inf. Imm.* *12*:630–637, Figures 1c, 2c, and 3d, with permission from ASM)

change the nutritional qualities of the media. It also has the useful property of melting at a temperature just below the boiling point; yet once melted, it will remain in the liquid state until it is cooled to about 44°C. Consequently, the solid medium can be incubated at relatively high temperatures if necessary for the growth of bacteria while the liquid phase can be cooled to a temperature that will not damage heat-sensitive nutrients, chemicals, or live microorganisms that might need to be mixed in the me-

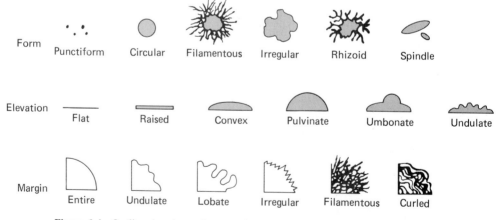

Figure 6-4   Outline drawings of some of the characteristics of various isolated bacterial colonies.

dium before it solidifies. The main advantage of solid media is that they provide a surface on which bacteria can be deposited and grown without mixing with other bacteria. Solid media are widely used for isolating, characterizing, and counting bacteria.

When a bacterial cell is deposited on the solid surface of an agar medium, the cell rapidly divides and its progeny pile up into a mass of identical cells. This mass of cells is called a *colony* (Figure 6-3) and is usually visible to the naked eye by 24 hours. The characteristics of colonies vary among bacterial species and are useful aids in helping to identify a particular species. The colonies may vary in size, texture, contour, margin, and color (Figure 6-4).

Pure Cultures

Microorganisms of various types are found growing together in natural environments. In order to study and characterize a particular microorganism, it must first be separated and grown free of other microorganisms; this is called a *pure culture*. The development and maintenance of pure cultures are important basic procedures in microbiology and are extensively used in the laboratory diagnosis of infectious diseases.

The most common method of isolating pure cultures is called *streaking* (Figure 6-5). Here a wire loop or cotton swab is first placed in contact with the environmental

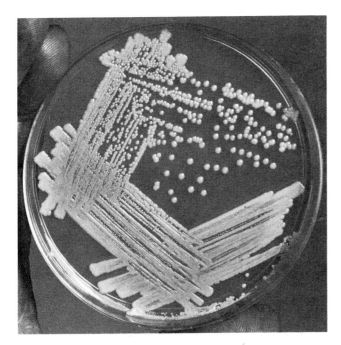

Figure 6-5 Streak plate showing thinning out of the bacteria with each additional streaking until well-isolated colonies develop.

source being examined so that the loop or swab picks up a random sample of the microbes present. The loop or swab is then rubbed over one edge of the agar surface contained in a *petri dish*. A petri dish is a small, flat, usually round container with vertical sides and a cover; it permits the liquid agar to harden in a readily available flat surface (Figure 6-2). The loop or swab deposits thousands of bacteria of many different types on the surface. Next, a sterile wire inoculating loop is slid through the deposited bacteria and then streaked over one-fourth of the untouched agar surface. This step deposits hundreds of bacteria along the line of the streak. The loop is sterilized and slid through the second streaking, followed by streaking over a fresh one-fourth of the plate. This procedure may be repeated one more time. Each streak increasingly dilutes the mixed population of bacteria until single cells are deposited along the streak lines. After incubation for one or several days, individual colonies will develop where the single cells were deposited. Bacteria from each colony can then be transferred to a separate sterile medium to produce a pure culture. To ensure that the culture is pure, a second streak plate may be made from a single colony; if all colonies appear identical, the culture is assumed to be pure.

Types of Culture Media

Bacteria vary widely in their nutritional requirements and hundreds of different formulations of culture media have been developed. Many types of culture media have been formulated to provide the optimum nutrition for cultivated microorganisms. Other media are formulated to favor the growth of one type of microorganism over other types; they are called *selective media*. Selective media may contain ingredients that inhibit the growth of all but a certain group of microorganisms and are used when attempting to isolate these microbes from an environment heavily contaminated with other types of microorganisms. An example of a selective medium is one that contains 7% salt (NaCl); this factor will inhibit or impede the growth of most microorganisms but not the growth of staphylococci, which will characteristically outgrow other bacteria on the medium. Various types of media contain dyes or other chemicals that react with specific cellular components or products produced by a given bacterium. These reactions produce a specific color change in the medium or the microbial colony. Such media are called *differential*, for they help to differentiate one type of bacterium from others that might be growing on the same surface.

Bacterial species vary in the types of carbohydrates they are able to use. Differential media are available with specific carbohydrates or other organic compounds as sources of carbon and energy. These media also contain an indicator dye that will change color when the pH of the medium changes. Thus when a bacterium is able to use the specific carbohydrate, and grows sufficiently in the medium to produce enough acid or alkali to change the color of the indicator dye, the color change can be used to assist in identifying the bacterium. Some microbes also produce gases that can be detected by trapping the gas in small inverted vials (*Durham tube*) that are placed in tubes of broth (Figure 6-6). The production of gas during metabolism is used as an identifying feature for some bacteria.

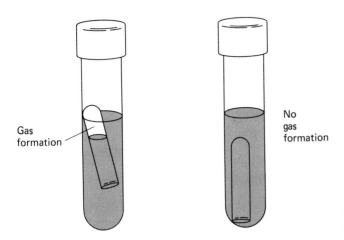

Gas formation

No gas formation

Figure 6-6 A method used to detect gas production by a bacterium.

IDENTIFICATION OF BACTERIA

Once a pure culture is obtained, a series of tests can lead to identification of the isolated bacterium. To begin with, a trained microbiologist is able to select those colonies from the primary isolation media that are most likely to represent disease-producing bacteria. The morphology and staining characteristics can readily be determined by microscopic examination and a pure culture is then inoculated into a selected variety of differential and selective culture media. By comparing the reactions on these media with the known characteristics of different species of bacteria, it is usually possible to determine which disease-producing microbe was isolated from the patient. Sometimes it is necessary to use specific antibodies to make a precise identification of some microorganisms; this concept will be discussed in Chapter 13.

Besides specifically identifying the microbe that is causing the disease, it is important to know which antibiotics will inhibit its growth and could be used for therapy. Antibiotic susceptibility testing (see Chapter 9) is usually performed concurrently with the identification tests. Time is usually important in determining the identification and antibiotic susceptibility of a disease-causing microorganism, for this knowledge may determine the most effective form of treatment for the patient. Using standard procedures, it may require from several hours to several days to complete identification tests on most bacteria. This factor becomes significant in the care of a critically ill patient. Today modern technology is applied in various forms to shorten the time required to obtain the needed information for optimal treatment of the patient.

RECENT LABORATORY INNOVATIONS

Some of the recent clinical laboratory innovations involve miniaturized units that allow rapid inoculation of many different types of differential media or enzyme substrates that give rapid identification information (Figure 6-7). Such units, although

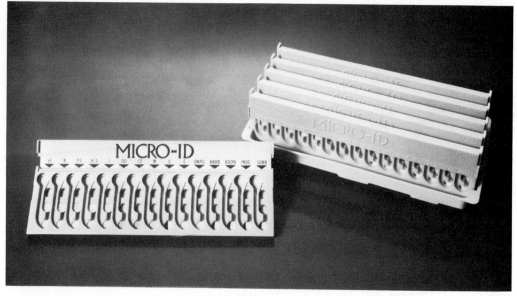

(a)

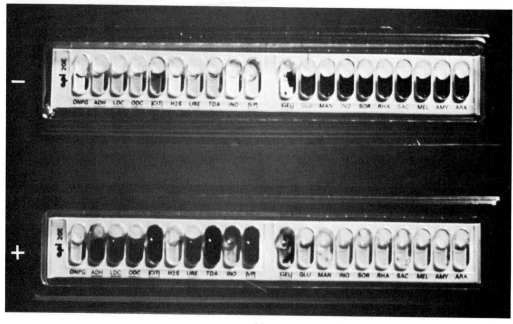

(b)

Figure 6-7 A composite of presently available miniaturized, or kit-type, procedures used to identify bacteria in the laboratory. Each of these systems requires isolated organisms in pure culture. The time required for completion of the test varies from 5 to 6 hours for the MICRO-ID (a) and API (b) systems to 24 hours for systems such as Enterotube (d). (a) The MICRO-ID system showing a series of small plastic cuplets which contain identifying chemicals as indicated (courtesy Warner-Lambert Company). (b) The API system showing both a negative (upper set of reactions) and a

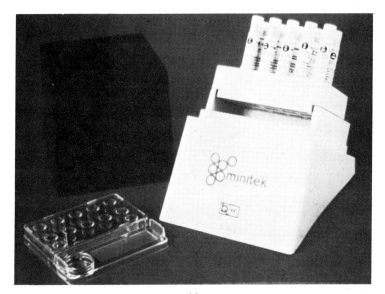

(c)

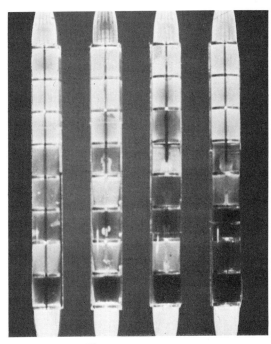

DEXTROSE

LYSINE

ORNITHINE

H$_2$S–INDOLE

LACTOSE

P. A.–DULCITOL

UREA

CITRATE

(d)

positive (lower set of reactions) test for the 20 biochemicals used in the identification scheme (Courtesy Analytab Products). (c) Small paper disks containing any of many desired biochemicals are placed into the plastic holder and then inoculated with bacteria; this Minitek system has great versatility. (d) The Enterotube was one of the earliest kit-type approaches to bacterial identification; in this system the inoculating needle (seen in the center of the tube) is drawn through a series of small media chambers and the unit is then incubated.

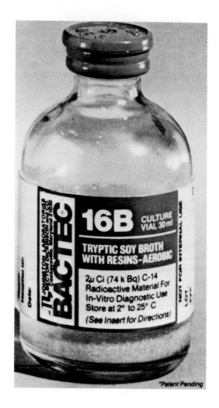

Figure 6-8   Radiolabeled medium used in the BACTEC system for the rapid
detection of the presence of pathogens in human body fluids.

not inexpensive, save technician time and reduce the amount of media and space required to run the tests. Instrumentation is now available that can detect the presence
of bacteria in normally sterile body fluids, such as blood. Samples of body fluid are
introduced into vials of medium containing carbohydrates that have radioactive carbon atoms (Figure 6-8). As the bacteria grow in this medium, radioactive CO_2 is released. This CO_2 can be detected by a sensitive instrument (Figure 6-9), often after as
little as 4 to 8 hours of incubation. Other instruments, such as the Autobac (Figure
6-10), can be used to determine antibiotic susceptibility in periods as short as 4 hours.
Thus by using newer technological advances, it is often possible to provide a physician with vital information within a few hours regarding the nature of the
microorganism that may be causing the infection in the patient.

    Several advances in automation involve the coupling of microgrowth chambers
with sensitive electronic detectors of chemical changes. These systems can be inter-
faced with computers that collect and analyze the data. Such instruments are able to
provide a probable identification of the microbe, plus information on antimicrobial

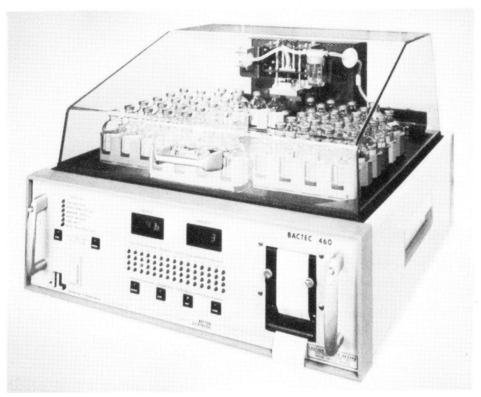

Figure 6-9 The BACTEC instrument used to monitor the development of radiolabeled CO_2 from growing bacteria. This instrument continuously monitors each bottle of medium (see Figure 6-8) and prints a report of all positive cultures.

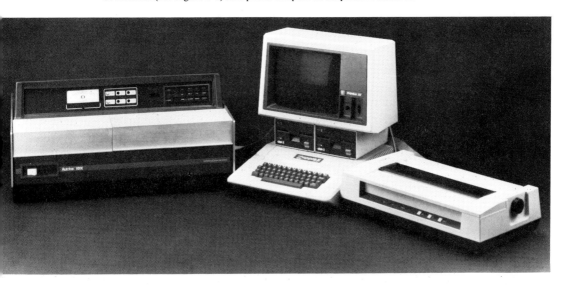

Figure 6-10 The AUTOBAC microbiology system. The unit on the left is a photometer-computer system that can be used to measure the growth of microorganisms. When properly implemented, this system will both identify bacteria isolated from patients and provide the antibiotic susceptibility of such isolates. The units on the right allow instant information retrieval of all cultures processed in the AUTOBAC. (Courtesy Warner-Lambert Company)

susceptibility in hours instead of the days required by older traditional methods. New and innovative instruments are being developed each year to aid in the clinical micro-biology laboratory and medical personnel will need continual updating to keep in-formed of these advances.

MICROBIAL GROWTH

The generation time of a microbial cell is the time required for one complete cell division. Some microbes are able to divide as rapidly as once every 12 to 15 minutes; others require from 15 minutes to several hours; and a few are slow growing and may require up to 1 to 2 days per cell division. When proper nutrients are available and other conditions are favorable, the growth of microorganisms can be a dynamic event with profound effects on the surrounding environment. If a bacterial cell were to continue to divide once every 30 minutes, for instance, there would be 64 cells in 3 hours, 17 million cells in 17 hours, and 280 trillion cells in 24 hours. If this growth rate could continue for 48 hours, the mass of cells produced would weigh several thou-sand times the weight of the earth. Obviously such rapid growth cannot continue for very long periods. Yet under certain conditions such rapid growth may occur for a short time.

Growth Curve

When microbial cells are placed in fresh nutrient broth under favorable growth con-ditions but with a limited supply of available nutrient, multiplication follows the typi-cal growth pattern shown in Figure 6-11. This type of growth is referred to as a *batch* or *limited growth* system. When bacteria are first placed in a fresh medium, a period of adjustment is followed by increased metabolic activity that precedes cell division. It is called the *lag phase* of growth. Afterward the cells begin to divide at a constant rate with the number and mass of cells doubling every generation. During this time growth is exponential and forms the *logarithmic phase* of the growth curve. This ex-ponential phase lasts 6 to 12 hours for most rapidly growing bacteria. Such rapid growth depletes the available nutrients and toxic waste products quickly accumulate. These factors cause a decrease in, and ultimately cessation of, cellular division. The accumulated cells may then remain for a period of time in a static condition—that is, not increasing in the numbers of viable cells. This is called the *stationary phase* of the growth curve. The stationary phase is followed by a period in which the cells gradu-ally die off—the *decline* or *death phase*. Like growth, the rate at which cells die is a function of both the types of cells and the environment.

Although the characteristic growth curve shown in Figure 6-11 probably only

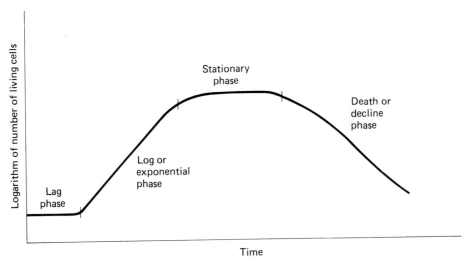

Figure 6-11 Phases in the growth curve of a pure bacterial culture in a closed system.

occurs under selected conditions, modifications do happen in nature and in some clinical circumstances. Products like bottled milk, for instance, if not properly refrigerated, could support the growth of microorganisms in the logarithmic phase, thus causing the rapid souring, while the change in the number of bacteria follows the normal growth curve. In clinical conditions, such as a wound, where an abscess is forming (see Chapter 11), a niche may exist that is filled with dead tissue and body fluids that could support the rapid growth of bacteria for a time. In most abscesses the bacteria have reached the stationary phase of the growth curve; in this condition they do not take in many nutrients or other substances from the surrounding environment. Thus antibiotics given to such a patient to cure the infection do not effectively penetrate into the abscess and may not be taken up by the bacteria if they do. Consequently, such therapy may fail to reduce the infection. In order to resolve this problem, it is nearly always necessary to drain abscesses in order to remove the waste products that are inhibiting the growth of the bacteria and preventing penetration of antimicrobial agents. Fresh nutrients then diffuse into the area and the remaining bacteria begin to multiply. If an antibiotic is given next, it will be taken up by the growing bacteria, inhibit their growth, and help cure the infection.

Growth of bacteria in an open environment, such as soil, water, or even the intestine, generally does not follow the curve shown in Figure 6-11. In these circumstances, bacterial growth is most often continuous or balanced so that the number of viable microorganisms remains fairly constant over long periods of time. Examples of such continuous growth systems in pathogenic microbiology are less common than are batch growth conditions. Humans, however, have "normal" bacteria that inhabit their body surfaces and grow continuously (see Chapter 10) and balanced microbial growth may occur to some extent in chronic disease conditions.

Influence of Environment on Microbial Growth

Moisture

Microorganisms grow only when adequate moisture is present. Because microbes exist as single cells, they depend on the continual diffusion of nutrients in solution across their plasma membrane. Due to the small size of microbial cells, however, the thin film of moisture often present on many substances is enough to support some microbial growth. Keeping materials free of moisture by dehydration is one of the most common methods to control the growth of microorganisms and, in turn, prevent the spoilage or decomposition of food or other materials. Frequently dehydrated foods, such as powdered milk, contain large numbers of viable organisms. A lack of moisture, however, maintains the microorganisms in a static state so that multiplication cannot occur.

Temperature

Each microorganism has adapted to grow within a specific temperature range (Figure 6-12). Some are able to grow at low temperatures and are called *psychrophiles* (cold loving). Even though some can grow at temperatures as low as −7°C, most psychrophilic microbes grow best at about 20°C and grow poorly above 30°C. Because of normal body temperatures, psychrophiles are generally unable to cause in-

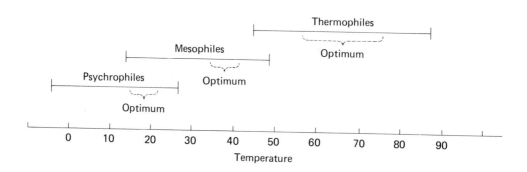

Figure 6-12 Categories of microorganisms based on growth at various temperature ranges. Optimum range indicated.

fections in humans. Still, they may cause spoilage of foods or other products stored at low temperatures.

Many microorganisms grow best at temperatures between 20 and 40°C and are called *mesophiles* (middle loving). Most microorganisms that cause infections in warm-blooded animals are mesophiles and usually have optimum growth temperatures of 35 to 37°C.

Certain microbes are able to grow at temperatures above 45°C and are called *thermophiles* (heat loving). Generally thermophiles are unable to cause infections in humans. These organisms are found in such places as natural hot springs; occasionally they cause problems by growing in hot-water systems or in some industrial processes where high temperatures are used. Some thermophiles are able to grow at temperatures close to 90°C.

Oxygen

Many different microorganisms require free oxygen (O_2) for growth and are called *aerobes*. Aerobes will only grow in environments where atmospheric or free oxygen is available, although some aerobes (*microaerophile*) grow best when only small amounts of oxygen are available.

Certain microorganisms are able to grow in the absence of O_2 and are called *anaerobes*. Several categories of anaerobes exist. Some are able to use O_2 if it is present but can also grow in the absence of O_2; they are termed *facultative anaerobes*. Other bacteria, called *obligate anaerobes*, can grow only in the absence of O_2. For many obligate anaerobes, O_2 is toxic and care must be taken to remove O_2 from the media in which they are cultured. An additional group of microorganisms require CO_2 for growth and are called *capnophilic*. Capnophilic bacteria are found among both anaerobes and aerobes. Microorganisms from each of these oxygen-associated categories are able to grow in various habitats of the human body and may cause diseases.

Other factors

Bacteria are able to survive and often grow in water with low concentrations of ions because of the protective effects of their rigid cell wall against damage due to increased osmotic pressure. This factor is important, for it allows successful water-borne transmission of many diseases. Most bacteria cannot grow in solutions of very high ionic concentrations. Consequently, certain foods are preserved by the addition of high concentrations of salts or sugars.

The pH (relative acidity or alkalinity) of the environment also influences the growth and survival of microorganisms. Most microbes that cause disease in humans grow best at or close to neutrality (pH 7), which is the pH of most normal body fluids.

SUMMARY

1. Bacterial nutritional needs in the laboratory are met by adding appropriate nutrients to a solidifying material called agar. By adding specific substances to the agar, media can be made to enrich, select, or inhibit the growth of desired microorganisms. Use of agar media has simplified the process of obtaining bacteria in pure culture. Such pure cultures are essential for the investigation of organisms and their role in disease processes.
2. Culture conditions, such as temperature, atmosphere, moisture, and pH, all impact the growth of microorganisms. Whatever the conditions, cultures of microorganisms follow a reproducible pattern of growth known as a growth curve.

Methods Used to Study Microorganisms

7

The progress and development of the science of microbiology had to await the availability of tools, techniques, and procedures that could be applied to the study of such small life forms. This chapter describes those methodologies and tools that facilitated the growth of microbiology as a laboratory science. The first section deals with a most valuable tool, the microscope, which has enabled direct visualization of many microbes and indirect observation of others.

MICROSCOPIC METHODS

A microscopy is essential in order to see microbial cells and to determine their morphological characteristics. Two general types of microscopes are available: the light microscope and the electron microscope. Light microscopes use visible light waves as the source of illumination and are able to produce meaningful magnifications to about 1000 times. The electron microscope uses an electron beam as the source of illumination and is able to magnify well in excess of 100,000 times. Most light microscopes are relatively easy to operate and are used in most general and teaching laboratories. Electron microscopes, on the other hand, are large, expensive, complex instruments that are restricted to specialized laboratories with highly trained personnel.

Light Microscopes

The earliest microscopes were essentially little more than fairly sophisticated magnifying glasses. Through these systems a careful observer, such as Leeuwenhoek (see Chapter 1), could view objects at a magnification of about 400 times. A more powerful system of magnification was developed in Denmark by Zacharias Jansens. His system was an imaginative application of optical principles that resulted in the development of the compound microscope. Today virtually all microscopes used in microbiology are compound light microscopes; in other words, they use a series of lenses to magnify the object. The magnifying lenses are called the *objective* lens and the *ocular* or eyepiece lens. The objective lens is the primary magnifying lens and is positioned close to the material or object to be viewed. The ocular lens is positioned close to the eye of the observer and produces a secondary magnification of the image produced by the objective lens. Light is focused on the object by *condenser lenses* that are not part of the magnification system. The magnifications of the objective and ocular lenses provide the total magnification of the compound microscope. The maximum magnification that can be obtained, under most conditions, from a single glass lens is about 100 times ($100\times$); and most compound microscopes have objective lenses that give magnifications of $10\times$, $40\times$, or $100\times$. These lenses are mounted on a rotating base called a nose piece so that each lens can be easily moved into position as needed. Most ocular lenses give magnifications of $10\times$, although lenses of $1.5\times$ to $20\times$ are available. Thus by using the $10\times$ ocular lens with the various objective lenses, total magnifications of $100\times$ (10×10), $400\times$ (40×10), or $1000\times$ (100×10) are obtainable. The lower magnifications are used to observe large areas of the object or relatively large objects and higher magnifications for more detailed observations of selected areas of the object. Magnifications of at least $400\times$ are needed for the observation of most microbial cells and $1000\times$ is customarily used. An outline of an optical microscope is shown in Figure 7-1.

It might be asked: Why not use such lens combinations as a $100\times$ objective and a $50\times$ or $100\times$ ocular lens to obtain magnifications of $5000\times$ or $10,000\times$ and so on? Theoretically it can be done; however, no added value is achieved because this greater magnification shows no added detail. It is called "empty" magnification. The reason is that the *resolving power* (the ability to distinguish between two adjacent objects) is primarily a function of the wavelength of the type of illumination used. This relationship is defined according to the following formula:

$$\text{Resolving power} = \frac{\text{wavelength of light}}{\text{NA}}$$

where NA is the numerical aperture of the lens. The greater the resolving power, the greater is the useful magnification that can be obtained; and obviously the shorter the wavelength of light used and the larger the NA of the lenses, the greater is the resolving power of the microscope. The midwavelength of visible light used in optical microscopes is 0.5 μm. The maximum resolving power obtainable with usual lenses is about one-half the length of the light waves or about 0.25 μm. The relationship between wavelength and resolving power is shown in Figure 7-2.

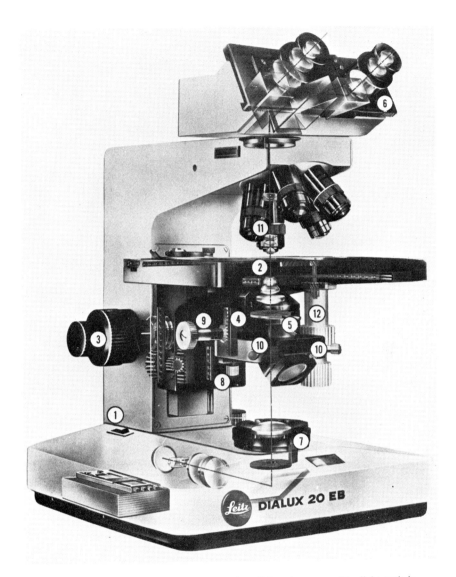

Figure 7-1 A cutaway diagram of a modern light microscope. The light path is shown and the essential parts of the system are indicated: (1) light switch; (2) mechanical stage where the object to be viewed is placed; (3) focus adjustment; (4) substage light condenser; (5) light diaphragm control for condenser; (6) ocular or eye piece; (7) light-focusing lens; (8) condenser adjustment; (9) condenser focus adjustment; (10) condenser light filter; (11) objective lens—this microscope has 5 objectives attached to a rotating turret housing; (12) substage adjustment control. (Courtesy E. Leitz, Inc.)

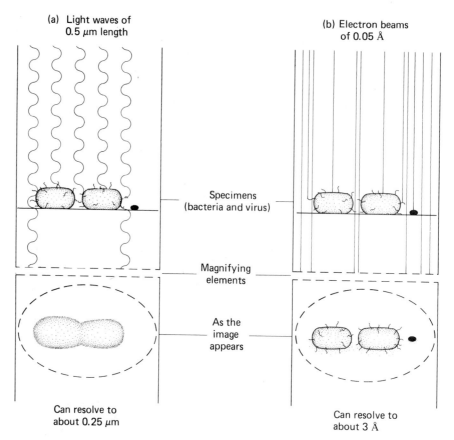

Figure 7-2 The effects of wavelength of radiation source on resolving power of a microscope. (a) Visible light does not detect objects smaller than 0.25 μm, and in this example does not show the fimbriae, the virus, or the space between the two bacteria. (b) The electron beams do detect the fimbriae, the virus, and the space between the bacteria.

Types of Optical Microscopy

Bright-field

In this most common form of microscopy the light is focused directly on the object and the resulting shadow is magnified and observed. Thus the image appears as a shaded object in a bright field (background). Most small objects, such as microorganisms, have only slight optical contrast from their surroundings and cast a very faint shadow. To enhance this contrast, bacteria are stained with various dyes.

Dark-field

Here light is directed onto the object at an angle so that only the light reflected from the object is magnified and observed. The image appears bright in a dark background. This form of microscopy is particularly useful for observing the movement of microorganisms, for no staining is needed.

Phase-contrast

This type of microscopy uses a special optical system that renders the details of unstained cells much more visible. It is particularly useful in observing living cells. Different components of a cell have slight differences in their refractive indices. These differences cause light rays to be bent or refracted as they pass from one portion of the cell to another. The refracted light is intensified by the optical system of a phase-contrast microscope and forms an image in which much of the fine detail of the cellular components can be seen. Staining is not needed and movement of cellular components can be observed.

Fluorescence

This type of microscopy allows us to observe materials that fluoresce—that is, materials that give off light of one color when subjected to light of another color. Most fluorescence microscopes use ultraviolet light as the primary light source; light given off by the fluorescent material is orange, yellow, or green, depending on the type of fluorescing material. To prevent injury, the ultraviolet light must be filtered out before its rays reach the eyes of the observer. Some microorganisms contain naturally fluorescent materials, but in most applications of fluorescence microscopy the microorganisms to be observed must be stained with special fluorescent dyes. The dyes rhodamine, auramine, and fluorescine are most common. They are used directly or are attached to specific antibodies (see Chapter 13), thus allowing attachment to selected microbial cells or only to specific subcomponents of these cells. This procedure has made fluorescence microscopy a useful tool in diagnostic laboratories. Rapid detection and identification of an unknown microbe are possible by adding a known fluorescent-tagged antibody to a clinical specimen and then watching for the presence of fluorescence. This procedure not only allows a specific identification of microbes but also increases the accuracy and speed of their detection.

Electron Microscopes

Electron microscopes can provide much greater magnifications than optical microscopes because they use an electron beam as the source of illumination. The electron beam has a wavelength of only 0.05 Å that produces a great resolving power. Due to technical problems, however, electron microscopes cannot actually resolve to 0.05 Å. Although several special microscopes can resolve to 3 Å, most have a resolving power of about 10 Å. This latter figure allows useful magnifications of well over 100,000×.

Two general types of electron microscopes exist: *transmission* and *scanning*.

Transmission electron microscope (TEM)

This microscope sends a high-voltage electron beam through the center of a vacuum column. The beam strikes the object to be viewed, which then casts a shadow of the object. As the beam continues down the column, electrons are deflected by a magnetic field to produce the desired magnification. The greater the deflection, the greater is the magnification. Ultimately the electron beam strikes a fluorescent screen at the bottom of the column, where an outline of the shadow of the object becomes visible. A photographic film is located under the fluorescent screen and a photograph of the object can be made by moving the screen and allowing the electrons to expose the film. The transmission electron microscope has made it possible to see organisms as small as viruses and much of the internal structure of cells (see Figures 3-6, 5-9, 5-15, 33-1, and 40-4). This information has been a tremendous aid in increasing our understanding of how biological systems function.

Various methods can be used to coat or stain the objects with electron-dense materials. These metals or salts increase the ability of the electron microscope to show contrast and details of minute structures. Certain limitations are inherent in the transmission electron microscope, however. Because the specimen must be observed in a vacuum, it requires dehydration, a factor that, along with the treatment with electron-dense staining materials, frequently causes some distortions. Moreover, the electrons cannot readily penetrate very dense or thick materials; consequently, the specimen must be spread in a thin film or cut into very thin sections in order to allow observation of internal components.

Scanning electron microscope (SEM)

The scanning electron microscope also uses an electron beam. The beam, however, is not magnetically amplified within the column as with the TEM but is focused into a narrow beam that rapidly scans back and forth over the specimen. The electrons reflected from each scan of the beam are picked up by an electron collector in the same orientation as they are reflected. These electrons produce an electrical current that is sent from the collector to amplifiers where each scan is amplified and the image is reconstructed line by line on a television screen. The scanning electron microscope is able to produce magnifications up to $100,000 \times$. Nevertheless, much of the work with these microscopes is done at lower magnifications. Important advantages of the scanning electron microscope include its capability to create images in a three-dimensional reproduction and only slight distortion of the specimen (because the specimen need not be cut into thin sections or intensely treated). As a result, numerous materials or microorganisms can be viewed in their natural orientation (see Figures 5-15, 6-3, 10-1, 11-4, 15-1, 17-3, and 19-1).

Today innovations in electron microscopes are appearing rapidly. Instruments are now available that have the capabilities of both the transmission and the scanning microscopes. Other electron microscopes are equipped with x-ray analysis equipment that permits areas of the specimen to be analyzed for the types of chemical elements it possesses.

Preparation of Microorganisms for Microscopy

When observing with the bright-field microscope, microorganisms, suspended in water or broth, are spread in a thin film over an area of a microscope slide and al-

TABLE 7-1 STEPS IN THE GRAM STAIN

		Results	
Step	Procedure	Gram +	Gram −
Initial stain	Crystal violet for 30 seconds	Stains purple	Stains purple
Mordant	Iodine for 30 seconds	Remains purple	Remains purple
Decolorization	95% ethanol for 10–20 seconds	Remains purple	Becomes colorless
Counterstain	Safranin for 20–30 seconds	Remains purple	Stains pink

lowed to dry. The slide is then passed two or three times through a flame, which fixes the cells to the surface, and the cells are stained. *Simple*, *negative*, and *differential* staining procedures may be used. Simple staining involves adding a stain to the cells for a time, followed by rinsing of the slide to remove excess stain. The most commonly used simple stains are *methylene blue*, *crystal violet*, and a red dye called *safranin*. Negative staining is a procedure that stains the background but not the cells. Either a black dye, called *nigrosin*, or India ink is mixed with the bacteria and spread in a thin film on a microscope slide. The stain will form a dark film over the background but will leave the cells as clear structures. Negative staining is generally used to show the presence of bacterial capsules. Differential staining procedures use more than one stain and are able to define bacteria or bacterial components, based on their staining characteristics. The most widely used differential staining procedure is the gram stain. This process divides bacteria into two major groups, gram positive and gram negative, depending on the structure of their cell walls (see Chapter 3). The steps and reactions of the gram stain are shown in Table 7-1. The *acid-fast* stain is a differential stain that helps identify the bacteria that cause tuberculosis or leprosy. The process is discussed in Chapter 22. Other special staining procedures help to visualize specific cellular structures, such as spores.

COUNTING MICROORGANISMS

Often it is necessary to determine the number of microorganisms present in a culture or material for research or industrial purposes or for an assessment of the quality of food products and the general sanitary state of a given environment. The major direct and indirect methods of counting microorganisms are discussed next.

Direct Microscopic Counts

This is a quick and relatively easy method of determining approximate numbers of microorganisms. Special counting chambers, such as the Petroff-Hausser (Figure 7-

3), that have measured grids marked on the surface and a cover slip held at a precise distance over the slide can be used. The space between the slide and the cover slip is filled with a fluid containing microbial cells; then the number of cells in a specified number of squares of the grid is counted. Because the volume of fluid over each square is known, the number of microorganisms per unit volume can be determined. Suspended microbial cells are best seen with a phase-contrast microscope.

Another method of direct microscopic counting is to spread a small known volume of fluid uniformly over a 1 sq cm area of a slide. The fluid is dried and stained and the number of cells counted with the high-power (40×) lens of a bright-field microscope. This procedure is often used in counting the number of bacteria in milk.

Direct counting methods have certain disadvantages: poor accuracy, counting both living and dead cells, difficulty of seeing small cells, and inability to count cells in low concentrations.

Plate Counts

Among the most frequently used methods of counting bacteria are the plate-counting procedures. Such processes are quite accurate in determining the number of living bacteria in a fluid and can measure low concentrations of cells. One method of ob-

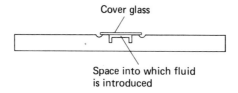

Cover glass

Space into which fluid
is introduced

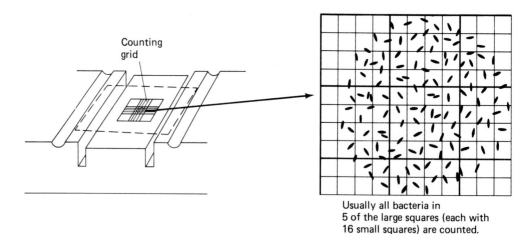

Counting
grid

Usually all bacteria in
5 of the large squares (each with
16 small squares) are counted.

Figure 7-3   A Petroff-Hauser cell counter for making direct microscopic counts of the number of bacteria in a fluid.

taining plate counts is the *spread-plate method*. Here about 0.1 ml of the test fluid is spread evenly over the surface of an agar plate. After incubation for 24 to 48 hours, colonies develop where each viable bacterium was deposited. Another process is the *pour-plate method* in which a measured volume, usually 0.1 or 1.0 ml, of test fluid is mixed with a melted agar medium that has been cooled to 48°C. The agar is then poured into a petri plate, where it solidifies. The bacteria are trapped in the agar and each develops into a colony after incubation for 1 or 2 days.

The number of bacteria is so great in most solutions that need to be tested that, if undiluted samples were used, so many colonies would develop that they would fuse to form a solid mass of bacteria. So it is necessary in most cases to dilute the sample before plating. This step is done by diluting the original sample through a series of tubes. Using separate agar plates, 0.1 to 1 ml is added from each tube. The colonies are counted on those plates that produce between 30 and 300 colonies. These numbers have been shown to give the most reliable indication as to the correct number of cells. The number of cells in the original undiluted sample can be determined from the number of colonies counted in a known volume at the known dilution. This procedure is shown in Figure 7-4.

Indirect Counting Methods

When repeated microbial counts must be made from the same type of liquid, as is often the case in research projects or industrial processes, an indirect method of determining the approximate number of cells can be used. The most frequently used indirect measurement is to determine the degree of turbidity produced in the broth by bacterial growth. The amount of turbidity is directly proportional to the mass of cells present and hence indirectly proportional to the number of cells. The amount of turbidity can be accurately measured by placing a tube of the microbial culture in an instrument called a *spectrophotometer* that electronically measures the amount of light that is able to pass through the fluid. A turbidity reading can be correlated with a reference number obtained by doing spread-plate counts at different intervals during the growth curve at the same time that the turbidity is determined (Figure 7-5). Once this curve is obtained, estimates of the number of cells from similar cultures can be made in just a few minutes with the spectrophotometer.

ENVIRONMENTAL SAMPLING

In many areas, such as a hospital environment, it may be important to know how many bacteria are present in the air, on a surface, or in a fluid. It is necessary to maintain environments with very low numbers of microorganisms in such hospital areas as operating rooms, nurseries, intensive care units and protective isolation rooms. Various procedures are used to control microbial contamination in these areas and several air and surface microbial sampling techniques have been developed in order to monitor the effectiveness of these procedures.

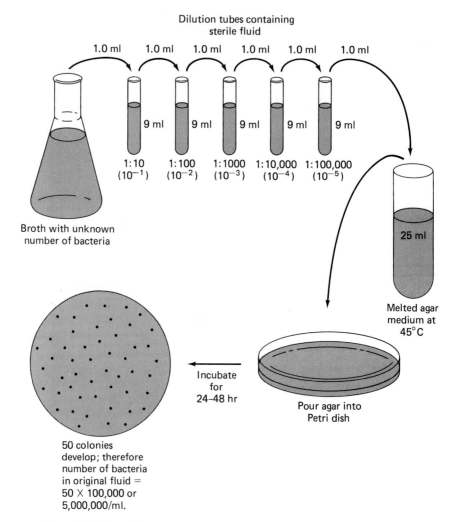

Figure 7-4 Determining the number of bacteria in a broth sample by serial tenfold dilutions and pour plates.

Air Sampling

One of the simplest methods to detect airborne microorganisms is to expose open petri plates containing nutrient agar to the air for an hour or two. This is called the *settling plate method*. A certain percentage of the microbes in the air settles onto the surface and after incubation forms colonies that can be readily counted. Settling plates give only approximations of the actual number of bacteria present. More precise results are obtained with *impaction air samplers*. Impaction samplers draw a given volume of air through a series of limiting openings so that the velocity of air is

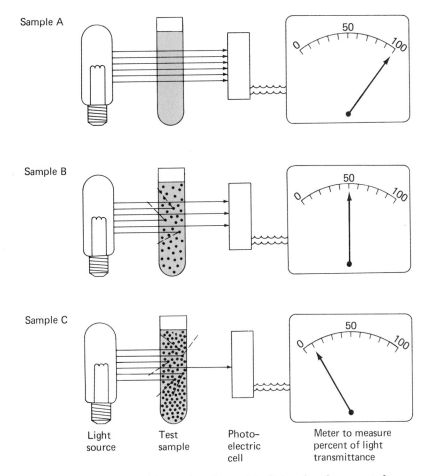

Sample A

Sample B

Sample C

| Light source | Test sample | Photo-electric cell | Meter to measure percent of light transmittance |

Figure 7-5 Estimation of the number of bacterial cells based on the amount of turbidity as measured with a spectrophotometer. Sample A is clear broth and shows 100% light transmittance. Sample B has moderate cell concentration and sample C has a heavy cell concentration; they allow decreased amounts of light transmittance proportional to the number of cells.

increased to a point where airborne particles are impacted onto nutrient agar surfaces (Figure 7-6). The number of colonies developing on the agar surface gives a fairly accurate count of the number of airborne microorganisms in the sampled air.

Surface Sampling

The two most common surface sampling methods are *swabbing* and *contact plates*. Swabbing procedures are used for uneven surfaces, corners, or crevices. The swab is prepared by firmly twisting a material like nonabsorbent cotton over one end of a

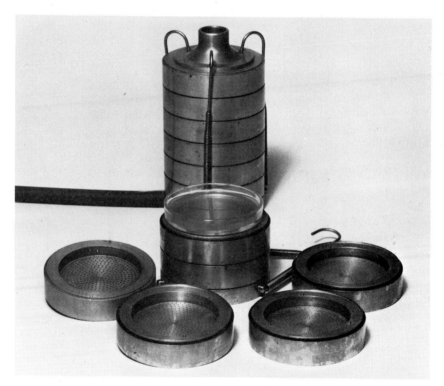

Figure 7-6 The Andersen cascade impaction air sampler. This sampler consists of six metal stages (assembled in background and partially disassembled in foreground) each pierced with 400 holes. The holes in the top stage are larger (far left) and become progressively smaller through to the bottom stage. A petri dish containing nutrient agar is placed under each stage and air is drawn through the unit at the rate of 28 liters per minute. Airborne bacteria are impacted onto the agar surfaces, and as the velocity of air increases as it flows through the progressively smaller holes in the descending stages, the larger particles are impacted onto the upper plate and the progressively smaller particles onto the sequential lower plates. This sampler resembles the respiratory tract, where larger particles are impacted in the upper regions and smaller particles are impacted in the lower region.

wood applicator stick that is then sterilized. In order to take a sample, the tip of the swab is rubbed slowly and thoroughly over a measured surface area three times. The swab is returned to a known volume of solution and vigorously rinsed. Next, a measured sample of the solution is assayed by the spread- or pour-plate method. About 50% of the bacteria on a surface is picked up via the swabbing method.

Another process that is also 50% efficient involves the rodac (an acronym for *r*eplicate *o*rganism *d*etection *a*nd *c*ounting)-type plate and is the most widely used method of contact sampling (Figure 7-7). Such plates, however, are primarily limited to flat surfaces. Rodac-type contact plates are disposable plastic items that are filled with an agar medium to form a 25-cm (2-inch)-square convex surface above its sides.

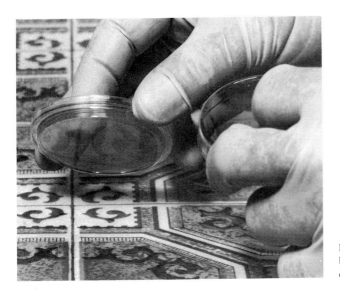

Figure 7-7   A rodac-type contact plate being used to collect a surface sample off of a floor.

A contact sample is taken by pressing the surface of the contact plate on the surface to be sampled, using slight pressure for several seconds. The contact plates are then covered and incubated. The number of bacterial colonies can be counted directly on the surface of the plate. When sampling surfaces treated with chemical disinfectants, neutralizers, such as lecithin or Tween 80, must be added to neutralize any disinfectant that might be transferred to the agar surface, where it would inhibit bacterial growth. Rodac plates are commonly used to monitor the bacterial contamination of burn wounds. Used as described, they are less destructive of the injured tissue than swabbing procedures.

Sampling of Fluids

When fluids may contain moderate-to-large numbers of microorganisms, counts can be made by the spread or pour-plate methods, using appropriate dilutions. If very small concentrations of bacteria are present, as is often the case with drinking water, the bacteria may be concentrated by passing a measured volume through a filter that will retain the bacteria. This filter is then placed on the surface of an agar plate and the bacteria trapped on the filter will grow to form colonies that can be counted.

SUMMARY

A number of laboratory procedures and tools have proven invaluable in the development and understanding of microbiology. Many systems, such as microscopy, staining, enumeration procedures, and air and surface sampling, continue to enhance the growth of microbiology.

Sterilization and Disinfection

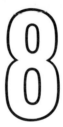

The control of microorganisms in health care services is extremely important and persons working in these areas should have a fundamental understanding of the principles of sterilization and disinfection. This chapter describes the methods used to control microorganisms on body surfaces and nonliving materials. The following chapter discusses chemotherapy, the control of microorganisms that infect living tissues. Physical and chemical methods used to destroy microbes on inanimate objects are generally nonspecific; that is, they destroy a wide variety of different types of living cells. On the other hand, chemotherapeutic agents must be able to destroy selectively only the microorganism and not the host cells.

In certain applications, such as the preparation of bandages or instruments to be used in surgery, successful control requires the complete removal or destruction of all microorganisms. In other applications, such as disinfecting a hospital ward, it is only practical to remove the disease-producing microorganisms or reduce their number to such a low level that the chance of infection is remote.

DEFINITION OF TERMS

Various terms are used to describe the processes involved in the control of microorganisms. Some terms are absolute, others overlap in meaning, and some are relative, having slightly different meanings in different areas of application. The term *sterilization*, which refers to a process that destroys all living organisms, is an absolute term. *Disinfection* refers to a process used to destroy harmful microorganisms but not including the resistant bacterial spores; a *disinfectant* is an agent that produces this result. *Sepsis* means the presence of microorganisms in blood or tissues; thus the term *antiseptic* refers to a substance that opposes or is able to reduce the likelihood of sepsis. Antiseptic refers to substances that, when applied to microorganisms, render them harmless either by killing them or preventing their growth; it generally refers to substances applied to living tissues. The suffix *-cide* is added to imply a killing action—that is, *bactericides* kill bacteria, *fungicides* kill fungi, *germicides* kill a wide range of microorganisms, and so forth. The suffix *-static* refers to agents that stop the growth of microorganisms; for example, a *bacteriostatic* agent prevents the growth of bacteria. Such terms as disinfectant, antiseptic, and bacteriostatic overlap significantly and all might possibly be applied to the same agent. The term *contamination* has different meanings in different settings. In the general clinical environment contamination refers to the presence of disease-producing microorganisms in or on a substance. In more specialized areas, when referring to fluids for intravenous administration or surgical instruments and so on, the presence of any microorganism would be considered contamination. The term *sanitation* is often used in public health regulations and refers to a condition favorable to health; its meaning is relative and must be defined for each application.

PHYSICAL METHODS OF MICROBIAL CONTROL

Moist Heat under Pressure

Over 90% of all medical and laboratory products are sterilized by steam under pressure. This procedure is accomplished in a pressure chamber called an *autoclave* (Figure 8-1). Steam may be generated within the chamber or introduced from an external source under pressure. As steam enters the chamber, air must be expelled through an escape valve. Once air is expelled, the escape valve is closed and the steam pressure is increased to 1.1 kg/cm^2 (15 lb/sq in.). Under these conditions the temperature rises to 121°C. At this temperature, with moisture, bacterial spores are killed in 15 minutes. When using an autoclave, it is necessary to allow time for the temperature to penetrate through all the material and then remain at 121°C for 15 to 20 minutes. A large bundle of such items as surgical drapes or bandages may require exposure times of 30 to 60 minutes or even longer to ensure sterility throughout the package. Items like bandages or surgical instruments that must remain sterile should be wrapped in covers to prevent them from becoming contaminated once removed from the autoclave. Not all materials can be autoclaved. Moisture associated with autoclaving causes such products as dry powders to become soggy, for instance, and the heat involved may damage many plastic products or electronic instruments used in hospitals. Fluids that contain heat-sensitive components cannot be sterilized by autoclaving, but other fluids are routinely sterilized. The pressure, however, must be released slowly to prevent excessive boiling and evaporation. Containers must not be tightly sealed, for such sealing may prevent the movement of steam to and from their contents.

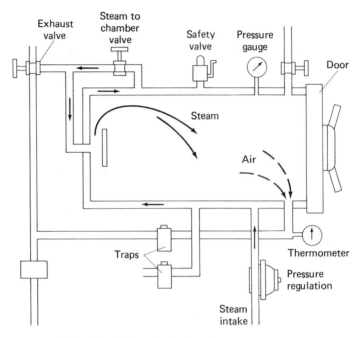

Figure 8-1   Schematic drawing of a steam autoclave.

Various tests are used to determine if sterility has been attained. Papers impregnated with heat-sensitive chemicals that change color when exposed to a critical temperature are useful but not totally reliable indicators of sterility. The most reliable
indicator is a *spore strip test*. Here paper strips impregnated with bacterial spores are
placed in the center of the materials being autoclaved. After the sterilization cycle is
completed, the spore strip is placed in a broth medium. If no growth occurs in the
broth after incubation, the material is assumed to be sterile. The spore strips are
placed between wrapped bundles so that they can be removed without unwrapping
the sterilized materials. Convenient-to-use spore strip test kits are commercially
available (Figure 8-2).

Moist Heat Not Under Pressure

Boiling and live steam, not under pressure, destroy most vegetative forms of bacteria
in several minutes. Bacterial spores and certain viruses may survive boiling temperatures for several hours, however.

The moderate heat of pasteurization is useful in treating some liquids, such as
milk or beverages. Pasteurization occurs via either of two procedures: the holding or
the flash method. In the holding method the liquid is heated to 62.8°C for 30 minutes; the flash method heats the fluid to 71.7°C for 15 seconds. Pasteurization does
not sterilize but does kill disease-producing bacteria that might be transmitted in the

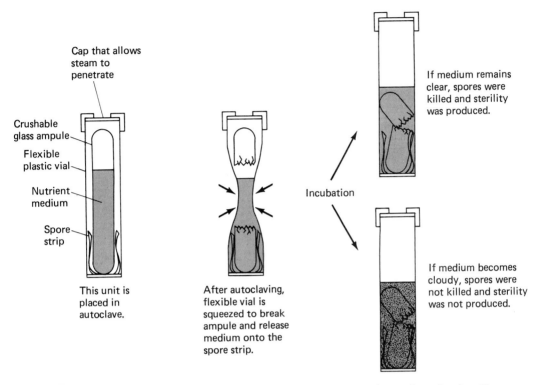

Cap that allows
steam to
penetrate

Crushable
glass ampule

Flexible
plastic vial

Nutrient
medium

Spore
strip

This unit is
placed in
autoclave.

After autoclaving,
flexible vial is
squeezed to break
ampule and release
medium onto the
spore strip.

Incubation

If medium remains
clear, spores were
killed and sterility
was produced.

If medium becomes
cloudy, spores were
not killed and sterility
was not produced.

Figure 8-2 A commercial-type spore strip for testing if the autoclave cycle produced sterility.

liquid. It also greatly reduces the number of other bacteria in the liquid and thus significantly retards the rate of spoilage of products like milk.

Dry Heat

Dry heat requires higher temperatures for longer periods than moist heat in order to cause sterilization. Hot-air ovens are used as dry heat sterilizers and an exposure at 180°C for 2 hours is needed to kill bacterial spores. Dry heat is used for sterilizing such items as glassware, powders, and oils.

Direct exposure of instruments or inoculating loops to open flames for brief periods, a procedure called *flaming*, is an effective means of sterilizing. Incineration of waste products readily destroys any contaminating microorganism that might be present.

Ultraviolet Light

Ultraviolet (UV) light is highly germicidal at wavelengths of 2600 Å. This wavelength of light is absorbed by DNA molecules and the imparted energy causes a rearrangement of some chemical bonds. In particular, new chemical bonds are formed between adjacent thymine bases on the same chain of the DNA molecule, which, in turn, renders the UV-irradiated microorganism nonfunctional. If the UV-inactivated microorganisms are subsequently stored in the dark or are exposed to white light, the chemical bonds might be restored to their original positions and the microorganisms would again become viable.

Sunlight contains UV light; consequently, it has definite germicidal properties. UV light is also produced by mercury vapor lamps. When placed in airducts or over surfaces, these lamps greatly reduce the number of viable microorganisms in the field of irradiation. UV light does not penetrate solids, a factor that has limited its use to disinfecting surfaces, clear liquids, and air. High-intensity UV lamps located in air supply ducts to such critical areas as operating rooms, nurseries, and intensive care areas can greatly reduce the chance of infections being transmitted to these areas by the airborne route. Also, air leaving contaminated areas, such as isolation rooms, morgues, or laboratories, can be exposed to UV light to prevent the spread of disease-producing microorganisms from such sources. UV light is damaging to human tissue and direct exposure must be avoided.

Ionizing Radiation

Forms of ionizing radiation, such as x rays and gamma rays, are able to transmit much more energy than UV light and hence have greater killing effects on microorganisms. Ionizing radiations can penetrate such products as fabrics, plastics, liquids, and foods to produce sterilization. Currently ionizing radiation is used to sterilize products like surgical sutures and disposable plastic items. Meats are effectively sterilized by ionizing radiation, and are much more nutritious and palatable than heat-processed canned meats, and have a comparable shelf life. Such sterilized meats have been used by astronauts during space flights, but as yet this process has not been approved for general use.

Filtration

Filtration is an effective means of removing most microorganisms from liquids and air. Liquids like serum or solutions containing heat-sensitive materials can be freed of microbial cells by passing them through filters with pore sizes small enough to retain bacterial cells. Such filtration, however, usually does not remove any viruses present in the fluid. Filters made of asbestos, fused glass fragments, or diatomaceous earth have been used for many years. Currently biologically inert, precisely produced cellulose ester membrane filters are widely used (Figure 8-3). Such filters are available in pore sizes as small as 0.025 μm. One with a pore size of 0.22 μm effectively removes all bacteria from a fluid. Filters of this type are also used to trap and concentrate bacteria that are dispersed in large volumes of liquids. This procedure is useful in bacterial testing of drinking water.

Airborne microorganisms can be effectively removed from air by filtration. Filters made of various fiber media are widely used in air ducts to remove both inert and

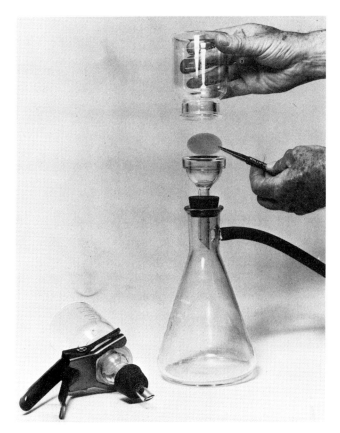

Figure 8-3 Placing of a membrane filter into a filter holder. After being assembled, the unit is covered and sterilized.

microbial particles. Varying densities of filter media can remove the desired size and amounts of airborne particles. Special filters, referred to as absolute or HEPA filters (high-efficacy particulate air filters), consist of a tightly woven fiberglass medium and effectively remove 99.9% of all airborne particles down to the size of 0.3 μm. HEPA filters remove all types of airborne microorganisms. Even though viruses are as small as 0.02 μm, when airborne they are usually attached to larger particles of dust or dried mucus that are readily trapped by HEPA filters. Air filters are used in air supply systems servicing such hospital areas as operating rooms, nurseries, and intensive care units.

CHEMICAL METHODS OF MICROBIAL CONTROL

Hospitals, clinics, and laboratories rely heavily on chemical antiseptics and disinfectants to reduce or eliminate harmful microorganisms on skin or inanimate objects. Thousands of different chemical formulations are commercially available as disinfectants and no single product is suitable for all applications. Several different chemical disinfectants are needed to accommodate the needs of most clinics or hospitals. Persons working in hospitals need to be aware of what disinfectant to use for each type of application. Even though thousands of commercial products are available, most disinfectants belong to one of the categories discussed in the following pages.

Factors Affecting Disinfectants

Disinfectants destroy or prevent the growth of microorganisms via generalized effects produced on the microbial cells. Some disinfectants are surface-active agents that disrupt the normal functioning of cytoplasmic membranes; others cause denaturation of proteins, such as enzymes, that are essential for cell growth and function. The action and uses of some common groups of disinfectants are shown in Table 8-1.

The ability of a chemical disinfectant to act on a microorganism and the extent of that action depend on the following factors.

Concentration of disinfectant

Generally the more concentrated the disinfectant, the shorter is the killing time. At low concentrations the compound may be only bacteriostatic whereas at higher concentrations it may be bactericidal. The concentration needed to kill microorganisms varies from microbe to microbe and from disinfectant to disinfectant.

Time

Not all microbes are killed at the same time after the addition of a disinfectant. Therefore the disinfectant must remain in contact with the contaminated material long enough to allow for the killing of all microbes (Figure 8-4). During most short applications chemical agents do not sterilize; however, if the time is extended to periods of 12 to 24 hours, sterilization is often possible.

Temperature

The killing effects of disinfectants are increased at higher temperatures. Most disinfecting procedures are standardized and carried out at room temperature. Allowances—by extending the time of exposure—are necessary when disinfecting materials at low temperatures.

PH

The acidity or alkalinity of the environment also influences the interaction of disinfectants with microorganisms and may increase or decrease the action, depending on the agents. Thus the effects of pH must be considered separately for each disinfectant.

Types of microorganisms

Some variations in susceptibility between species of microbes occur. Microbes are sometimes grouped as to their susceptibility to disinfectants into the following three groups:

TABLE 8-1 MODE OF ACTION, USES, AND PROPERTIES OF MAJOR CATEGORIES OF CHEMICAL DISINFECTANTS

Agents	Major action	Common uses	Other properties	Use-Dilution (%)
Alcohols	Lipid solvents Denatures proteins	Skin antiseptics Surface disinfectants	Rapid action Flammable Dries skin	70
Mercurials	Inactivates proteins	Skin antiseptics Surface disinfectants	Weak cidal activity Inactivated by organic matter	0.1
Silver nitrate	Denatures proteins	Antiseptic for eyes and burns	Inactivated by organic matter Limited range of microbes affected	1
Phenolic compounds	Disrupts cell membranes Inactivates proteins	In antiseptic skin washes Disinfect inanimate objects	Not inactivated by organic matter Stable Some objectionable odors	0.5–5
Iodine	Inactivates proteins	Skin antiseptic	Soluble in alcohol Rapid action Mixes with soaps	2
Chlorine compounds	Oxidation of enzymes	Water treatment Disinfect inanimate objects	Inactivated by organic matter Flash action Corrosive Irritates skin	5 (as bleach)
Quaternary ammonium compounds	Surface active Disrupts cell membranes Denatures proteins	Skin antiseptic Disinfect inanimate objects	Neutralized by soap Odorless Nonirritating	Less than 1
Glutaraldehyde	Inactivates proteins	Cool sterilizing agent for heat-sensitive instruments	Unstable Toxic High activity in alkaline range	1–2

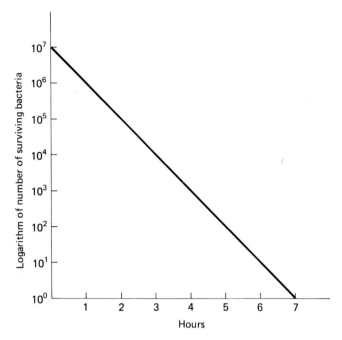

Figure 8-4 An example of the death rate of a bacterium when treated with a constant concentration of disinfection at a constant temperature and pH, and plotted logarithmically.

Group A, the vegetative forms of most bacteria and enveloped viruses that are easily killed by disinfectants

Group B, the more difficult to kill tubercule bacillus and nonenveloped viruses

Group C, the highly resistant bacterial spores and viruses, such as those that cause hepatitis.

Presence of extraneous matter
The presence of materials like soil, blood, and pus may react with some disinfectants and reduce their ability to react with microbes. For this reason, it is strongly recommended that surfaces and materials to be disinfected be thoroughly cleaned before treatment with the disinfectant.

Proper exposure
Care must be taken to ensure proper exposure of all parts of the object to the disinfectant. Tightly packaged material or closed containers, for instance, may not allow complete penetration or contact with the disinfectant.

Groups of Chemical Disinfectants

Organic solvents

Compounds of this group include chloroform, toluene, and alcohols. Their action is to disrupt the structure and function of plasma membranes and to denature proteins. Chloroform and toluene are most often used as additives to solutions that must be kept free from microbial growth. The widely used alcohols are among the most useful disinfectants or antiseptics. They are highly effective against vegetative bacterial cells, including the tubercle bacillus, but are less effective against spores. Alcohol is very useful as a skin disinfectant because it effectively kills bacteria, has a cleansing effect by removing accumulated lipids, and evaporates without leaving a residue. Ethyl and isopropyl alcohol are equally effective and concentrations of 70% should be used. Concentrations below 70% begin to lose some effectiveness. Isopropyl alcohol is most often used, for it does not come under the governmental regulations placed on alcohols used in beverages.

Heavy metals

Various mercury-containing compounds, called *mercurials*, were widely used as disinfectants in the past. The disinfectant mercuric chloride is quite toxic to humans and is now rarely used. Other mercurial preparations known as mercurochrome, merthiolate, metaphen, and mercresin are less toxic. Merthiolate is sometimes used as a preservative for vaccines and metaphen may be used to irrigate the urethra. These preparations, however, are not as effective as many others and are usually corrosive to metallic instruments. In general, other disinfectants are preferred over the mercurials.

Some silver compounds are useful disinfectants, the most common being silver nitrate. A 1% silver nitrate solution is used in the routine irrigation of eyes of newborn babies to prevent gonorrheal infections. This procedure is required by law in all fifty states. Dressings applied to burns are sometimes soaked in a 0.5% solution of silver nitrate to help control bacterial infections. Colloidal silver compounds that slowly release silver ions are used in some antiseptics and in some filters for water purification.

Phenol and phenol derivatives

The natural product phenol, also called carbolic acid, is fairly toxic to tissues, is corrosive, and has a disagreeable odor; yet historically it has served as an important disinfectant. Pasteur recognized the ability of phenol to prevent decomposition of organic matter. This observation prompted Lister to use the product to prevent infections of surgical wounds. Carbolic acid in dilute solution is an effective skin disinfectant and will not cause tissue injury if exposure is limited to less than an hour. Various phenol derivatives, called phenolics, have been developed that are effective disinfectants and yet do not have many of the objectionable traits of phenol. Although phenol is rarely used today, the following phenolic compounds are common.

Cresols. Cresols are obtained from coal tars, are less toxic than phenol, and have strong germicidal actions. Cresols can be mixed with soaps without losing germicidal activity. For many years a mixture of 2% cresol and liquid soap was sold under the trade name of Lysol. This old-type Lysol had a characteristic cresol odor that was familiar to most persons living before the 1940s. In later years mixtures of soaps and improved phenolic compounds with less odor have been marketed under the trade name of Lysol. They are effective products for disinfecting inanimate objects or organic wastes.

Hexachlorophene. This phenolic compound is especially effective against staphylococci and streptococci and can be used against many other microbes as well. Hexachlorophene retains its antimicrobial effectiveness when mixed with soaps or detergents, is nonirritating to skin, and leaves a protective film after application. It is bactericidal at high concentrations and bacteriostatic at lower concentrations. During the 1960s hexachlorophene had many medical and nonmedical applications. Newborn infants were routinely bathed in mild solutions of hexachlorophene, a procedure that greatly reduced bacterial colonization and subsequent infection by staphylococci. In the early 1970s evidence from animal studies suggested that hexachlorophene may be absorbed into the blood and cause brain damage. And even though no evidence exists for its toxic effects on newborn humans, restrictions have been placed on its use. Many hospitals stopped using hexachlorophene in newborn care only to see an increase in the number of staphylococcal infections. Today most hospitals use hexachlorophene in smaller amounts when treating newborns and are still able to control staphylococcal infections effectively. Hexachlorophene, however, is no longer allowed in over-the-counter products, such as deodorants and cleansing agents. At 3% concentrations it is mixed with soaps, detergents, and lotions to form effective antiseptic skin-cleaning products for medical applications. Such products as Phisoderm, Phisohex, and Hexagerm are examples of hexachlorophene-containing products. These products are widely used in hospitals and clinics for routine washing and disinfection of hands, surgical scrubs, and preoperative cleansing of skin. In addition to the immediate effect when applied, hexachlorophene leaves a protective film on the skin for several days. Used with discrimination, hexachlorophene is a valuable product in controlling microorganisms in the medical environment.

Chlorhexidine. A 4% concentration of chlorhexidine gluconate mixed with detergent and 4% alcohol is now being widely used as a surgical handscrub, cleanser for superficial skin wounds, and handwashing agent. It is highly effective against both gram-positive and gram-negative bacteria and fungi. It leaves a protective film on skin and no irritation to skin has resulted from extensive use. Hibiclens is an example of a chlorhexidine containing product.

Halogens

The halogens *iodine* and *chlorine* are among the most useful chemical disinfectants. Chlorine is widely used in treating water. If free chlorine is added directly to water, a reaction occurs to form hypochlorous acid (HOCl), an active disinfectant. Chlorine compounds, such as hypochlorites, that slowly release free chlorine are also effective disinfectants of water. Hypochlorites are the common household bleach agents, such as Clorox and Purex. Chlorine compounds are routinely used to sanitize food and dairy-processing equipment and to treat swimming pools. Chlorine bleaches are useful household disinfectants and can be used on dishes, utensils, toilets, or other noncorrodible materials. Chlorine compounds should not be used on skin or open lesions; moreover, they are corrosive to metals. Chlorine is readily inactivated by organic matter and dilute solutions easily lose their effectiveness when excessive organic matter is present in solutions or on surfaces.

Iodine is among the most effective skin antiseptics. A preparation known as *tincture of iodine*, a 2% concentration of iodine dissolved in alcohol, is widely used as a skin antiseptic and to treat minor wounds. A 2% solution of iodine in water is also an effective antiseptic. Iodine forms complexes with soaps and detergents without losing its antiseptic qualities; such products are called *iodophors*. Iodophors are soluble in water and gradually release the iodine. They are not as active as tincture of iodine but have the advantage of being less irritating and nonstaining. They also have the cleansing effect of soap or detergent. Iodophors are used as antiseptic soaps, preoperative skin disinfectants, and general disinfectants in medical and industrial environments.

Surface-active agents

Various surface-active compounds have detergentlike characteristics and cause the destruction of microbial membranes. The *quaternary ammonium compounds*, often referred to as *quats*, are the most common surface-active agents. These agents are effective against a wide range of vegetative bacteria. They are not effective against spores, some vegetative bacteria, and the more stable viruses. These compounds are used for disinfecting floors, walls, furniture, and other inanimate objects. They have the advantages of being odorless, colorless, tasteless, inexpensive, nontoxic, soluble in water, and active in low concentrations.

Common detergents and soaps are surface-active agents that can effectively clean large numbers of microorganisms from skin or other surfaces but are generally nontoxic to microorganisms. As a rule, thorough washing with such agents removes in excess of 90% of the microbes present.

Formaldehyde

Formaldehyde is a gas that acts as a fumigant and a gaseous disinfectant. It dissolves in water to 37%, which is then called formalin. Solutions containing 5 to 10% formalin are widely used for preserving and fixing tissue specimens. Animals dissected in biology classes are fixed in formalin; and as most students in these classes can attest, formalin has a disagreeable odor and is irritating to tissues. Because of these objectionable properties, it has limited use as a disinfectant in clinics and patient-related activities.

Glutaraldehyde

This compound is related to formaldehyde and is germicidal against a wide range of microorganisms. It is used as a cold sterilizing agent for many items that would be damaged by heat. It is widely used for sterilizing dental equipment, pieces of equipment used in inhalation therapy, and equipment with optical lenses. Glutaraldehyde is most germicidal in the alkaline pH range and so a 0.3% sodium bicarbonate solution is added to a 2% glutaraldehyde solution just before it is to be used. An alkaline pH results and the solution is then said to be activated. Activated glutaraldehyde retains its potency as a disinfectant for about 4 weeks. Materials to be sterilized must be clean and completely immersed in 2% activated glutaraldehyde for 12 hours. Glutaraldehyde is irritating to tissues and has a mildly disagreeable odor; thus its use is limited to inanimate objects.

Hydrogen peroxide

A 3% solution of hydrogen peroxide (H_2O_2) is sometimes used to clean wounds. It is nonirritating to the tissues and has only a brief, mild disinfecting action due to the rapid breakdown to water and oxygen.

Ethylene oxide

Ethylene oxide vaporizes readily at room temperatures and is a highly effective sterilizing agent in the gaseous form. It is active against all microorganisms, including bacterial spores. The major advantage of ethylene oxide gas is its ability to sterilize at room temperature and without high levels of moisture. It is slow acting, however, and 12 hours are required to destroy spores at 70°C. Also, ethylene oxide is explosive when mixed with air; for this reason, it is always diluted with an inert gas, such as carbon dioxide. A 10 to 15% concentration of ethylene oxide is used for sterilization. Special chambers or especially adapted autoclaves are used for this form of gas sterilization. Such items as plastic ware, catheters, sutures, electronic instruments, and heart-lung machines that may be damaged by heat are sterilized with ethylene oxide. In the past few years this form of sterilization has become an essential procedure in most hospitals. Items sterilized with ethylene oxide must be well aerated to remove any residual gas.

Other disinfectants

Acids and alkalies have antimicrobial activities due primarily to the free hydrogen or hydroxyl ions. Such acids as benzoic or propionic, or their salts, are added to foods to help retard spoilage. Some aniline and acridine dyes have bacteriostatic activities and are used in treating lesions on the skin and mucous membranes.

Evaluation of Disinfectants

The official method of evaluating a disinfectant is the *Phenol Coefficient Method.* This method compares the effectiveness of the test disinfectants to that of phenol against bacterial strains of *Salmonella typhi, Staphylococcus aureus*, and *Pseudo-*

monas aeruginosa. The time required to kill these bacteria by using dilutions of the test disinfectants compared to dilutions of phenol gives the comparative strength of the two compounds. By comparing all disinfectants to phenol, it is possible to gain a comparison of their relative potency. The phenol coefficient method does not give information on the dilution of a given disinfectant that might be suitable for a given object or surface. A second test, called the *Use-Dilution Method*, is now officially used to determine the concentration of a disinfectant that is needed to kill bacteria effectively. In this test 10 small stainless cylinders contaminated with the test bacteria are placed in the test dilutions of the disinfectants and left for 10 minutes. If all bacteria are killed on all 10 cylinders, the dilution of disinfectant is considered suitable for use.

SUMMARY

The removal of all living microorganisms from an environment (sterilization) or the removal of most pathogens (disinfection) is usually accomplished by physical or chemical means. Heat, radiation, and filtration are most commonly used to obtain sterile conditions whereas the bactericidal actions of alcohols, phenols, halogens, and aldehydes is frequently applied for disinfection. Both industrial and household uses of these procedures are intended to reduce the number of microorganisms in our environment so that health and safety are maintained.

Chemotherapeutic Agents

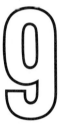

Antimicrobial chemotherapeutic agents are chemicals that can selectively interfere with the growth of microorganisms and yet not interfere significantly with the functions of the cells of the infected animal host. This type of activity is known as *selective toxicity*. Generally diseases caused by bacteria are more effectively controlled by chemotherapeutic agents than diseases caused by fungi, protozoa, or viruses. A primary reason is that bacteria are procaryotic cells and possess some structures and metabolic processes that often differ greatly from those of the eucaryotic cells of the animal host. Based on these cellular differences, it was possible to develop chemicals that specifically interfere with procaryotic cell functions but not with the activity of eucaryotic cells. The differences between the eucaryotic fungal or protozoal cells and the eucaryotic host cells are not as great. It has therefore been difficult to find chemicals that selectively inhibit one type of eucaryotic cell without interfering with others. Viruses use host cell functions to carry out their replication activities and as yet few chemical agents can interfere selectively with viral activity but not with the functions of the host cells.

Early historical developments of chemotherapeutic agents were covered in Chapter 1. The continued development of new chemotherapeutic agents over the past 40 years is one of the most important achievements of medical science and has resulted in saving millions of lives and alleviating untold suffering.

The ideal chemotherapeutic agent would possess the following characteristics:

1. Be highly toxic to a large number of pathogens
2. Have no toxicity to the host

3. Not induce the development of resistant mutant microbes
4. Not induce hypersensitivities in the host
5. Not interfere with the normal host defense mechanisms

Unfortunately, the ideal chemotherapeutic agent has not yet been found. Most have some toxicity to the host and induce varying degrees of hypersensitivity or allow the development of resistant mutant microbes. Thus some tradeoff is given for all applications of chemotherapeutic agents and benefits to the patient must be weighed against possible adverse side effects.

Some chemotherapeutic agents are manmade and are referred to as *synthetic* agents. Others are natural products of microorganisms and are called *antibiotics*.

SYNTHETIC AGENTS

Chemotherapeutic agents may act by mimicking essential components needed in normal cellular reactions. When present, the chemotherapeutic agent is taken into a cellular reaction in place of the normal component. Once integrated, the chemotherapeutic agent prevents the cell from functioning or developing in a normal manner. Extensive efforts have been carried out to develop synthetic chemicals that would interfere with specific microbial functions; yet relatively few useful compounds have been developed. Most useful synthetic agents are related to the *sulfonamides*.

Sulfonamides

Since their discovery in the mid-1930s, the sulfonamides have been important agents in treating a variety of bacterial infections. Sulfonamides, sometimes simply called sulfa drugs, are various derivatives of a molecule called *para-aminobenzene-sulfonamide* or just *sulfanilamide* (Figure 9-1).

Mechanism of action

The sulfonamides are structurally similar to *p-aminobenzoic acid* (PABA) and function as competitive inhibitors of this compound. PABA is an essential component in the synthesis of folic acid, which is an essential metabolite for both mammalian and procaryotic cells. Mammalian cells, however, depend on preformed folic acid whereas procaryotic cells must synthesize their own using PABA. This difference in the source of folic acid allows sulfonamides to function as effective chemotherapeutic agents. In bacteria the sulfonamide molecule is able to substitute for PABA during the synthesis of folic acid and this results in nonfunctional folic acid.

The enzymes that convert PABA to folic acid are unable to distinguish between PABA and sulfonamide. So if only a small amount of a sulfa drug is present, most of the enzyme continues to interact with PABA and the cell continues to grow but at a reduced rate. As the concentration of sulfa increases, there is a greater and greater

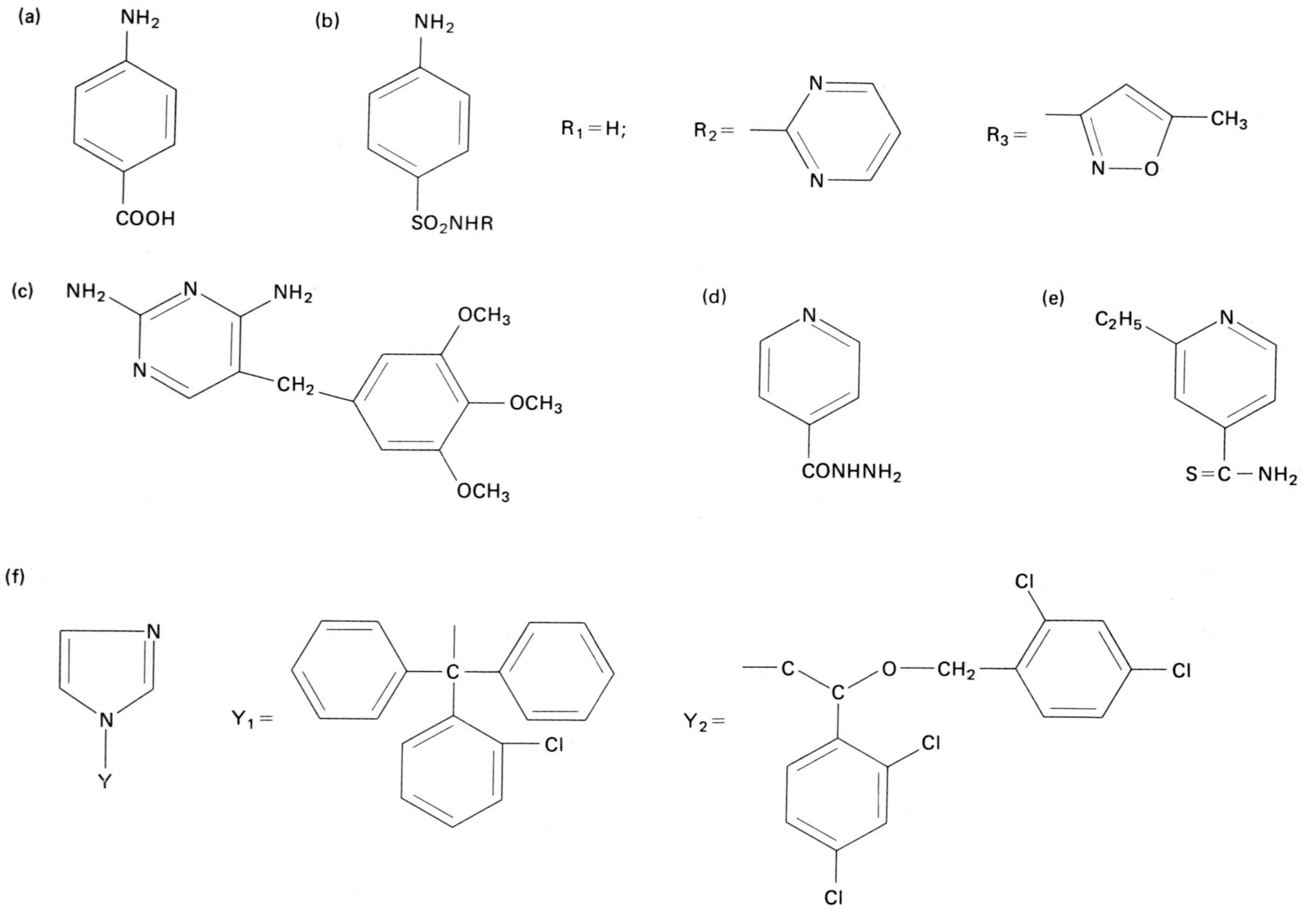

Figure 9-1 Structure of some synthetic antimicrobial agents: (a) p-aminobenzoic acid, a bacterial metabolite. (b) Sulfonamide, an analog of p-aminobenzoic acid. Chemically modified at position "R," the sulfonamide becomes a "sulfa drug," e.g., R_1 = sulfonamide, R_2 = sulfadiazine, R_3 = sulfamethoxazole. (c) Trimethoprim, most commonly used in fixed combination with sulfamethoxazole. (d) Isoniazid and (e) Ethionamide which are used almost exclusively as therapy against tuberculosis. (f) The imidazole nucleus, modifications of which produce antifungal agents, e.g., Y_1 = clotrimazole, Y_2 = miconazole.

possibility that the enzyme will find only the sulfa drug to interact with and the cell will stop growing. Such chemical interactions, which depend on the relative concentration of the inhibitor and the normal substrate, are known as *competitive inhibition reactions* (Figure 9-2). That is, there is competition between the two substrates for the active site on the enzyme molecule.

In bacteria, just as in humans, the short-term absence of a necessary metabolite does not result in death. However, for a single cell, such a condition results in the cessation of growth. Yet if the needed metabolite is again made available to the cell within a reasonable time, it will once more begin to grow. Such a condition is analogous to placing a culture of bacteria in the refrigerator; although the cells do not immediately die, the cold reduces their rate of metabolism to a point where growth is essentially stopped. When the culture is again placed in the incubator, growth soon returns to normal. This condition of suspended growth is known as *bacteriostasis* and

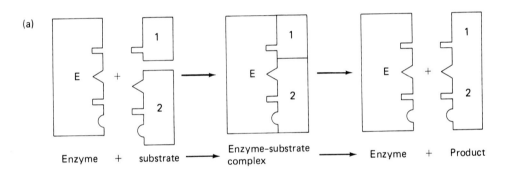

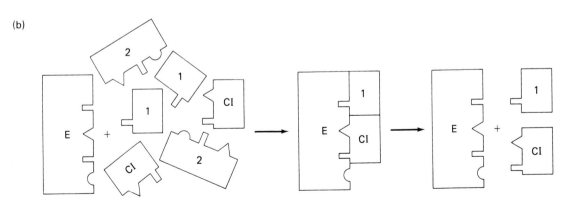

Figure 9-2 Representation of competitive inhibition of enzyme function by a substrate analog. (a) Normal enzyme substrate interaction leading to product formation. (b) The addition of a competitive inhibitor to the reaction results in competition for active site on the enzyme. (In this example the competition is between CI and 2.) The successful formation of product depends on the relative concentrations of CI and 2.

antimicrobial drugs that lead to such a reversible growth state are called *bacteriostatic* agents. Therefore sulfonamides are an example of a bacteriostatic drug.

Clinical applications

Because of the extensive use of sulfonamides during the late 1930s and throughout the intervening years, numerous bacteria are now resistant to these antimicrobial drugs at concentrations normally achieved in patients. For this reason, antibiotics are preferred over sulfa drugs in most clinical treatments today in spite of the relatively low level of toxicity due to these agents. The major exception is in the treatment of urinary tract infections; here sulfonamides can reach high levels of concentration and are generally effective. Combinations of antibiotics and sulfonamides have been used to suppress the number of bacteria in the intestinal tract prior to surgery. The major toxicity problems associated with sulfonamide use are due to some hypersensitivity reactions and the tendency of sulfonamides to crystallize in the kidney with resulting damage to the renal tubules.

One of the newer sulfonamide drugs is actually a combination of a sulfonamide (sulfamethoxazole) and a similar compound (trimethoprim) that also competitively inhibits an enzymatic reaction in the biosynthesis of folic acid. This compound, trimethoprim-sulfamethoxazole, is sold by several names, such as Bactrim or Septra, and has increased application in a number of serious disease conditions due to organisms of the genera *Shigella*, *Haemophilus*, and *Pseudomonas*.

Other Synthetic Agents

Several synthetic agents are widely used in treating tuberculosis and leprosy. The *sulfones* are a group of compounds, related to the sulfonamides, that are effective against infections caused by the acid-fast bacilli. Their use today is limited almost entirely to the treatment of leprosy. *Para-aminosalicylic acid* (PAS), an analog of PABA, is an effective bacteriostatic agent for the treatment of tuberculosis but has limited effectiveness against other diseases. *Isoniazid* (INH) is effective and the most widely used agent in the treatment of tuberculosis. It is often used in combination with other antituberculosis agents. The exact mode of action of INH is not known. *Ethambutol* (Embutal or EMB) is another effective antituberculosis agent that is always used in combination with PAS or INH. In fact, therapy for active tuberculous disease should always include multiple antituberculous agents. The structures of several sulfonamides and related synthetic chemotherapeutic agents as well as p-aminobenzoic acid are shown in Figure 9-1.

ANTIBIOTICS

Penicillins

Penicillin is a term applied to a group of closely related compounds produced by various fungi of the genus *Penicillium*. Some penicillins are the natural product; others have been chemically altered in the laboratory. Penicillin, the first antibiotic discovered, has been the most useful. During the late 1930s and early 1940s, when penicillin was first used, it became known as the miracle drug because it could often cure otherwise fatal diseases rapidly. The most dramatic effects of penicillin use were seen on some major killer diseases, such as pneumonia, scarlet fever, staphylococcal diseases, and the veneral diseases gonorrhea and syphilis. The natural penicillins are primarily effective against gram-positive bacteria, gram-negative cocci, and the syphilis spirochete. Because of its great success, there was a strong tendency during the late 1940s and 1950s to use penicillin in treating a wide variety of infections. This widespread and often indiscriminate use, particularly in the hospital environment, led to the emergence of many penicillin-resistant staphylococci. By the late 1950s the effectiveness of penicillin in treating staphylococcal infections had greatly diminished. At this time it was discovered that the basic central structure of the penicillin molecule could be produced by *Penicillium* molds under special controlled conditions. Various chemical side chains could then be added to this basic structure to modify its action (Figure 9-3). Through extensive, empirical investigations and testing, a series of altered or semisynthetic penicillins were found that have enhanced antimicrobial activities. Several are able to kill bacteria that are resistant to the natural penicillin; others are effective against a wider range of bacteria. A list of some semisynthetic penicillins and their uses is given in Table 9-1. Figure 9-4 is a diagrammatic representation of the development of many available penicillin compounds.

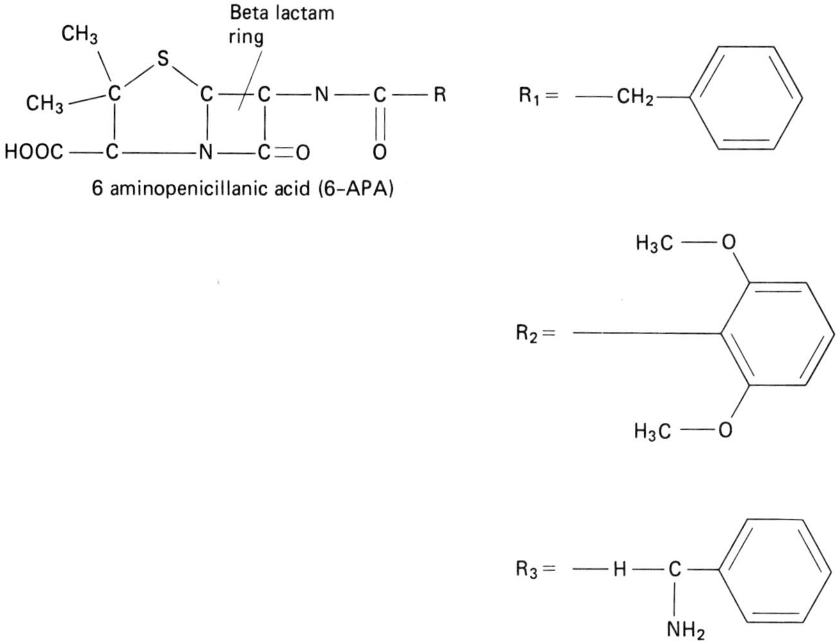

Figure 9-3 The structure of penicillin. The common portion of all penicillins is 6-APA. This molecule may be modified at "R" to produce a wide variety of "synthetic" penicillins, as exemplified by R_1 = penicillin G, R_2 = methicillin, R_3 = ampicillin.

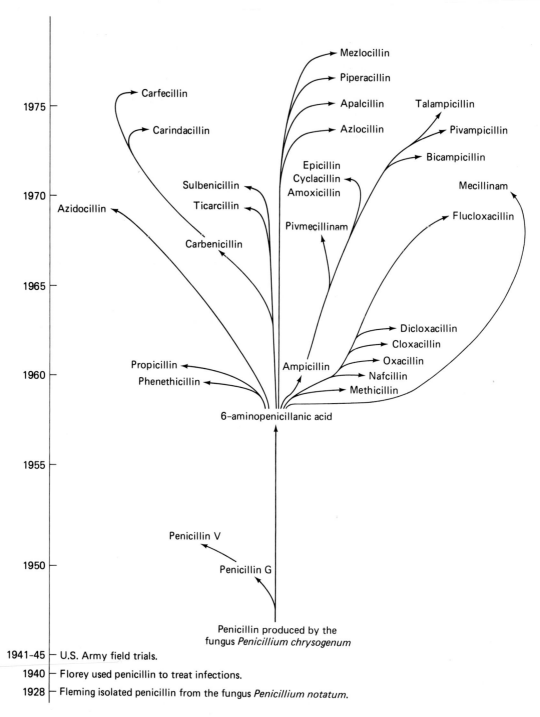

Figure 9-4 A schematic representation showing the approximate historical date and genesis of many of today's penicillins. This diagram shows relatedness among penicillins.

TABLE 9-1 PENICILLINS COMMONLY USED IN TREATMENT
OF BACTERIAL INFECTION

Name	Source	Common uses
1. Penicillin G (Benzylpenicillin)	Natural	
2. Penicillin V	Natural	Oral penicillin (acid stable)
3. Methicillin	Semisynthetic	3 through 6 used in treatment of infections caused by penicillinase-producing staphylococci. Cloxacillin can be given orally
4. Oxacillin	Semisynthetic	
5. Nafcillin	Semisynthetic	
6. Cloxacillin	Semisynthetic	
7. Ampicillin	Semisynthetic	A broad-spectrum penicillin used against gram-negative bacteria and for patients with endocarditis
8. Carbenicillin	Semisynthetic	8 and 9 specific use penicillins, used to treat *Pseudomonas* infections
9. Ticarcillin	Semisynthetic	
10. Piperacillin	Semisynthetic	A new penicillin used in treatment of gram-negative bacterial infections

The action of penicillin is to interfere specifically with the formation of new bacterial cell wall synthesis during cell division. The cross-linkages of the peptidoglycan strands are prevented from forming. And without a complete cell wall the high internal osmotic pressure of the bacterial cell results in rapid cell lysis. Because mammalian cells have no cell walls, penicillin is generally nontoxic to these cells and can be used in relatively large concentrations. Complications do occasionally result in persons who are allergic to penicillin, however.

Bacterial resistance to the penicillins results mostly from bacterial production of enzymes called penicillinases. Penicillinase splits the beta-lactam ring of the penicillin, producing an inactivate molecule (Figure 9-3). Some penicillins, such as penicillin G, are unstable in stomach acid and cannot be taken orally whereas others, such as penicillin V, are acid stable and can be absorbed intact from the gut. Penicillin is the treatment of choice when susceptible bacteria are causing infection because it is both less toxic to the host than other antibiotics and, in general, less expensive. It should not, of course, be used in persons who are hypersensitive to penicillin. The appropriate semisynthetic penicillins, such as methicillin, nafcillin, or oxacillin, are the agents of choice in treating penicillin-resistant staphylococcal infections. When a broader spectrum of activity is needed, ampicillin, carbenicillin, or ticarcillin might be used.

Aminoglycosides

The aminoglycosides include streptomycin and antibiotics with a similar chemical structure. Streptomycin (Figure 9-5) is bactericidal against various gram-positive and gram-negative bacteria as well as the tubercle bacillus. It was the first major antibi-

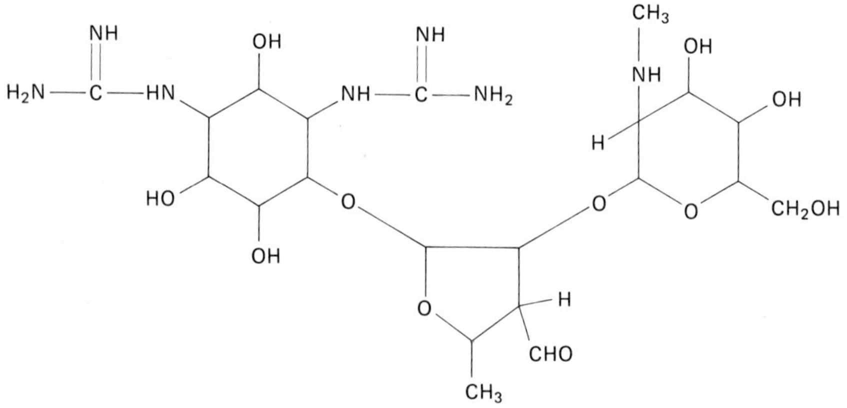

Figure 9-5 Chemical structure of streptomycin, first of the aminoglycoside antibiotics to have wide clinical application.

otic developed after penicillin. When it became available in the mid-1940s, it was effective against many gram-negative bacteria that were not susceptible to penicillin as well as against tuberculosis. It was the first effective antituberculosis agent to be developed.

These antibiotics function by attaching to the small 30 S component of the 70 S procaryotic ribosomes. Such attachment interferes with the proper initiation of protein synthesis. The 80 S ribosomes of eucaryotic cells are not readily affected. Aminoglycosides cannot be given orally and must be injected, which usually requires that the patient be hospitalized. Resistant mutant bacteria develop when the site of attachment on the 30 S ribosomal component is altered. Other organisms are resistant because the cells are impermeable to the aminoglycosides and some cells become resistant when they are infected with plasmids carrying genes that direct the synthesis of enzymes that modify and inactivate the antibiotics.

Aminoglycosides are among the most toxic of the commonly used antibiotics. Toxicity may lead to kidney damage, hearing loss, or other physical impairments. In order to prevent the excessive accumulation of antibiotics in patients receiving aminoglycosides, it is necessary to monitor the concentration of the compound present in the body fluids. Such determinations, called *antibiotic assay*, are usually performed on the blood of patients receiving these or other toxic antibiotics. Using this technique, it is possible to monitor the amount of antibiotic given the patient and to maintain levels below the toxic concentrations.

Several widely used aminoglycoside antibiotics are amikacin, neomycin, kanamycin, netilmicin, gentamicin, and tobramycin. These antibiotics have a broad antibacterial spectrum and are used to treat infections that do not respond well to other chemotherapeutic agents. Spectinomycin, which is similar to the aminoglycosides, has a very specific use in the United States. It is used in the therapy of penicillinase-producing *Neisseria gonorrhoeae*, which causes gonorrhea.

Tetracyclines

The tetracyclines are a group of closely related antibiotics that are bacteriostatic against a wide range of both gram-positive and gram-negative bacteria as well as rickettsiae, chlamydiae, and mycoplasma. Because of this wide range of activity, they are called *broad-spectrum* antibiotics. Tetracyclines inhibit protein synthesis of growing bacteria by combining with the 70 S ribosomes and interfering with the binding of *t*RNA to *m*RNA.

Some natural and semisynthetic tetracyclines are chlortetracycline (Aureomycin), oxytetracycline (Terramycin), doxycycline (Vibramycin), and minocycline (Minocin). Although differing in structure and name, these compounds are effective against the same microorganisms. These antibiotics are very useful in treating infections that are not responsive to penicillins and can be taken orally; however, they may produce such side reactions as irritation of the intestinal tract, liver damage, and discoloration of teeth when taken before permanent dentition is formed.

The use of tetracycline during the early years of the antibiotic era led scientists to the discovery of a phenomenon generally applicable to broad-spectrum antibiotics. When these compounds are used indiscriminately or for long periods of time, normal bacterial flora, as well as pathogens, are frequently destroyed. The loss of normal flora often allows bacteria that are resistant to the antibiotic and that are normally maintained at reduced numbers by the competitive effect of other normal flora to increase rapidly in numbers. The large increase in the number of these organisms frequently results in disease, one that will not respond to the antibiotic being used but that may regress in patients where the antibiotic is discontinued.

Chloramphenicol

Chloramphenicol is a broad-spectrum antibiotic that is effective against a wide range of bacteria as well as rickettsiae and chlamydiae. It is, however, quite toxic to humans and is generally used only when other antibiotics are not effective. It is the drug of choice under some circumstances, such as in typhoid fever. Chloramphenicol binds specifically to the 70 S ribosomes of procaryotic cells and blocks protein synthesis by preventing the formation of peptide bonds.

Erythromycin

Erythromycin is the most active of a group of related antibiotics called *macrolides* (Figure 9-6). The spectrum of activity of the macrolides is similar to penicillin. Erythromycin may be either bacteriostatic or bacteriocidal, depending on the concentration. The mechanism of action is similar to chloramphenicol. This antibiotic is most often used as a substitute for penicillin in patients who are allergic to the latter drug. It is also the agent of choice in treating whooping cough and the relatively recently recognized Legionnaires' disease. Toxicity is usually not severe, but microbial resistance is common.

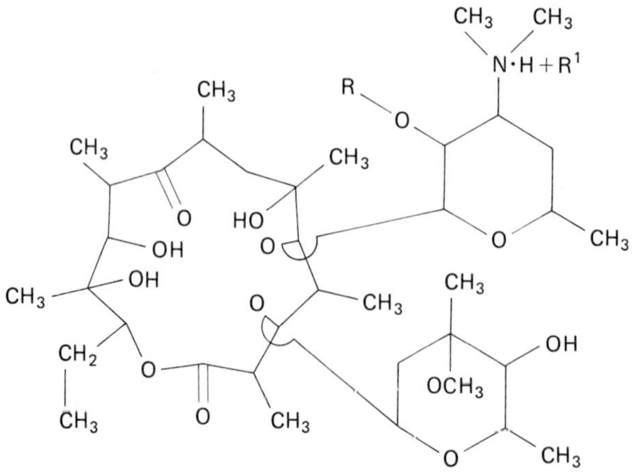

Figure 9-6 Structure of erythromycin, most commonly used of the macrolide antibiotics.

Lincomycin and Clindamycin

These antibiotics have a spectrum of activity similar to penicillin but a basic chemical structure different from other antibiotics. They have relatively low toxicity and are useful in treating patients who are allergic to penicillin. The mechanism of action is similar to chloramphenicol and erythromycin. Clindamycin has been particularly useful in treating disease caused by gram-negative anaerobic bacteria.

An increasing use of clindamycin has led to an important observation regarding undesirable reactions during or following antibiotic therapy. Certain patients who had been receiving clindamycin developed a severe, often fatal intestinal disease known as *pseudomembranous enterocolitis*. It was discovered that this antibiotic caused a severe loss of normal bowel flora except for several resistant bacteria, one of them an anaerobe known as *Clostridium difficile* (see Chapter 20). Overgrowth by this organism resulted in the disease. It is now known that this condition can result following the use of almost any antimicrobial agent.

Rifampicin (Rifampin)

Rifampicin is a semisynthetic compound produced from the natural antibiotic rifamycin. It inhibits the growth of gram-positive, gram-negative, and acid-fast bacteria, can be taken orally, and is effective in low concentrations. It specifically blocks the transcription of *m*RNA. It has been particularly effective in treating tuberculosis and leprosy. Use of this drug usually results in the rapid selection of resistant bacteria, a feature that suggests using a therapeutic approach that will reduce the number of such resistant organisms. In order to do so, it is customary, when using some antibiotics, to use them in combination and give them simultaneously to the patient. The rationale for such an approach lies in an understanding of the genetics of mutation as discussed in Chapter 5. If, for any given phenotypic characteristic, the chance of developing a mutant organism that would be resistant to any given antimicrobial were 10^{-6}, and the chance of developing resistance to a second antibiotic were 10^{-7}, then, on the basis of probability, the likelihood that the organism would develop resistance to both antimicrobial agents at the same time would be 10^{-13}, a number so small that such resistance would probably not occur.

Cephalosporins

The structure and activity of cephalosporins resemble penicillin's. They are effective against both gram-positive and gram-negative bacteria. Their advantage lies in their broad spectrum of activity as well as their relative resistance to some penicillinases.

Research and development in the area of antibiotics are proceeding more rapidly with the cephalosporins than with any other group of antibacterial compounds, perhaps because it is relatively easy to alter the molecule chemically at several points (Figure 9-7), thus producing "new" antimicrobial agents. These modifications have produced a relatively large number of antibiotics with exceptionally broad spectra, including *Pseudomonas aeruginosa* (Chapter 26). A number of these agents, such as moxalactan, cefoperazone, cefotaxime, cefoxitin, and cefamandole, are presently in limited clinical use.

Bacitracin

Bacitracin is a polypeptide that interferes with the development of the cell wall. It is effective against many gram-positive bacteria. The high toxicity of this agent has primarily limited its use to topical ointments.

Polymyxins

These antibiotics are simple polypeptides that are quite toxic to humans. Their mode of action is to disrupt the functions of plasma membranes of gram-negative bacteria. They are used to treat some of the more resistant gram-negative bacilli, although toxicity severely restricts their use.

Polyenes

Polyenes specifically change the permeability of membranes of fungi and are useful as antifungal agents. Nystatin and amphotericin B are the major antifungal agents in this category. Nystatin is limited to topical applications because of its toxicity.

Griseofulvin

This antibiotic specifically inhibits the growth of certain fungi by interfering with DNA replication. It is effective in treating fungal infections of the skin.

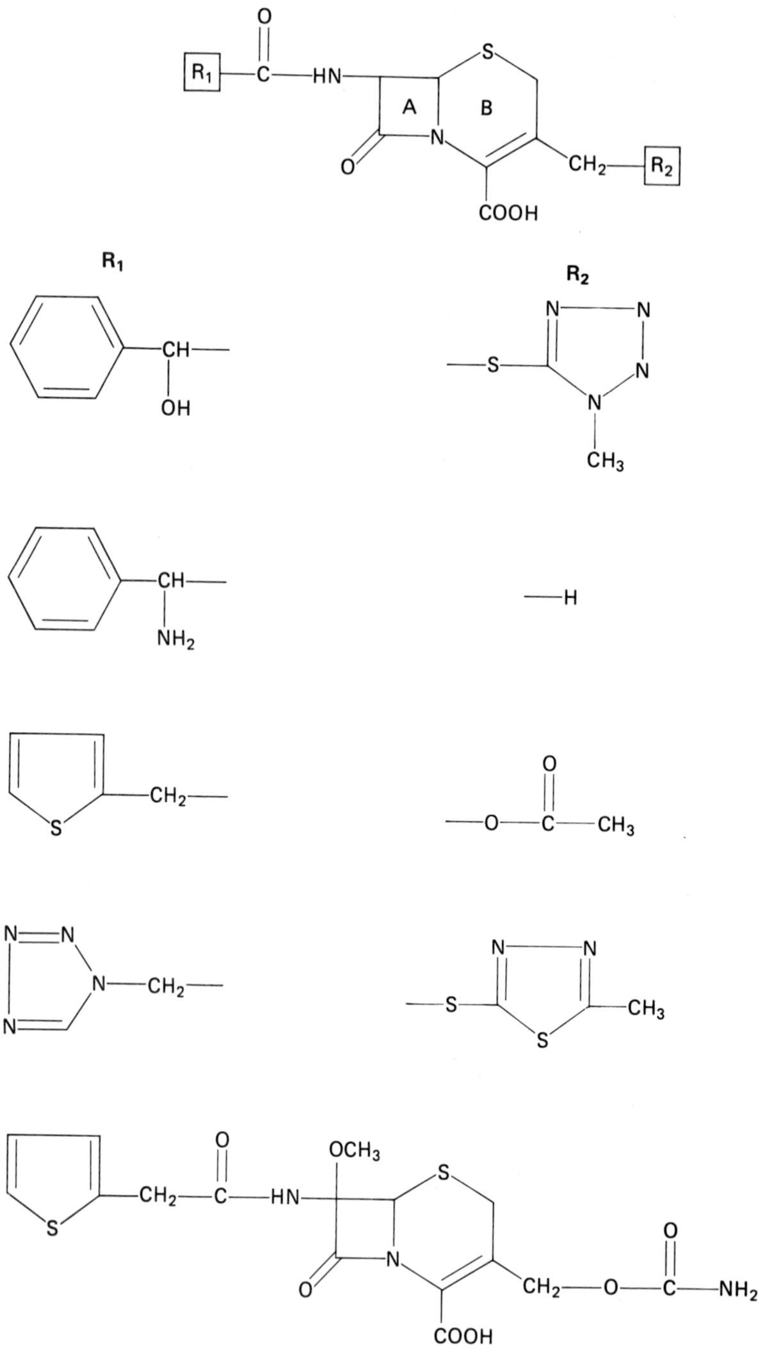

7-aminocephalosporanic acid

Cefamandole

Cephalexin

Cephalothin

Cefazolin

Cefoxitin

Figure 9-7 Chemical structure of some commonly used cephalosporin antibiotics. The 7-aminocephalosporanic acid molecule can be modified at R_1 and R_2 (as shown) to produce the indicated antibiotics. Cefoxitin, one of the newer cephalosporins, has a modification of the basic 7-aminocephalosporanic acid molecule in addition to R_1 and R_2.

Imidazoles

Imidazoles constitute a relatively new approach to fungal therapy. There are several such agents, miconazole and ketoconazole being perhaps the best known. These agents are a welcome addition to the rather limited antifungal therapeutic options. Their structure (Figure 9-1) is simple and similar compounds have been used to treat diseases due to protozoa and helminths for several years. Their advantages are a limited toxicity and the fact that some can be taken orally. Fungal diseases of the skin, as well as the deep, systemic mycotic diseases, respond to these agents.

MICROBIAL RESISTANCE

A major problem associated with chemotherapy is the selection of resistant microorganisms. Microorganisms may spontaneously mutate against a given trait in their environment once in every 10^5 to 10^{10} cell divisions. Because of their rapid multiplication rates, the chance of microbial mutations against a given antimicrobial agent is quite probable. In this situation, the mutant may rapidly multiply in the presence of the antibiotic and produce many resistant progeny. In addition to spontaneous mutations, genetic resistance may be passed from one bacterium to another by small, circular extrachromosomal DNA fragments called *resistance plasmids* or R factors (see Chapter 5). A resistance plasmid may contain the genetic information that codes for resistance to one or several antibacterial agents; when the plasmid is passed to a new cell, the trait of antibiotic resistance is also passed.

Certain resistant mutants function by producing enzymes that destroy or alter the chemotherapeutic agent. Others become resistant from changes occurring on the receptor sites to which the chemotherapeutic agent binds. Still others may develop resistance by changes occurring in the permeability of the cell to the chemical agent.

TREATMENT

The procedure used in treating a disease should be designed so that the chance of a cure is maximum and the chance to develop a resistant microbial mutant is minimum. To do so, it is first necessary to determine which chemotherapeutic agents are effective against the disease-causing microbe. This process requires isolating and testing for the susceptibility of the pathogen to different chemotherapeutic agents. The most commonly used method of determining antibiotic sensitivity is to place antibiotic-impregnated disks on a Mueller-Hinton agar surface that contains a film of the test bacterium (Figure 9-8). A zone of inhibition of bacterial growth is produced around the disk that contains effective antibiotics. This type of testing requires 24 hours; with critically ill patients, it may be desirable to initiate treatment as soon as possible. Such empirical therapy is commonly used in clinical situations where time may be critical to the patient and where it is possible to make a logical choice of antibiotics based on

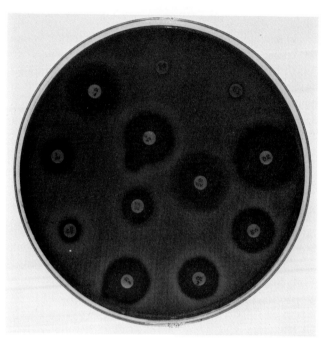

Figure 9-8 Antibiotic susceptibility test. The surface of the growth medium is inoculated such that the bacteria will grow as a confluent lawn. Paper disks containing the antibiotic are then placed on the inoculated surface. The susceptibility of the antibiotics is determined by measuring the diameter of the zone of bacterial growth inhibition.

previous experience. Table 9-2 lists those antibiotics that are presently tested against bacteria isolated from human infections. More than one set of antibiotics is necessary for testing because not only is there considerable variation in the in vitro susceptibility of bacteria, but the concentration of antibiotic obtainable in the many body spaces also varies. Some antibiotics, for instance, can be used to treat a urinary tract

TABLE 9-2 ANTIBIOTICS SUGGESTED FOR SUSCEPTIBILITY TESTING AGAINST DIFFERENT GROUPS OF BACTERIA

Gram-positive cocci	Enterococcus	Pseudomonas	Enterobacteriaceae
Amikacin	Ampicillin	Amikacin	Amikacin
Cephalothin	Chloramphenicol	Carbenicillin	Ampicillin
Chloramphenicol	Erythromycin	Chloramphenicol	Cefamandole
Clindamycin	Penicillin G	Gentamicin	Cefoxitin
Erythromycin	Tetracycline	Polymyxin B	Cephalothin
Gentamicin		Sulfisoxazole	Chloramphenicol
Kanamycin		Tetracycline	Gentamicin
Penicillin G		Tobramycin	Polymyxin B
Methicillin			Tetracycline
Tetracycline			Tobramycin
Vancamycin			Trimethoprim-sulfamethoxazole

infection in which the concentration of antibiotic can reach high levels whereas those same antibiotics may not reach a high enough concentration in the lung to be useful in treating pneumonia. The several test sets of antibiotic agents also reflect the fact that a finite number of compounds can be conveniently tested at any one time. Rapid susceptibility tests, often requiring less than one day, are now available through automated systems using sensitive electronic instrumentation for reading results. Some of these rapid tests were described in Chapter 6.

When an effective antibiotic has been determined, treatment should be initiated as soon as possible or modified to appropriate antibiotics when empirical therapy was initiated. Antibiotics must be given in sufficiently high concentrations to result in a cure and treatment should continue for some time after the symptoms of the infection have subsided. This procedure gives the best chance of a complete cure and minimizes the chance of selecting resistant mutant microorganisms. If low rather than adequate concentrations of antibiotics are given, it is much more probable that resistant mutants will develop. If treatment ends too soon, the infection may reoccur and further increase the probability of resistant mutants developing. Delay in initial treatment may allow the infection to penetrate to deeper body tissues where abscesses may develop and block the diffusion of the antibiotic to the site of the infecting microbe. If bacteria in an abscess are in the stationary-growth phase, antibiotics that are effective only against growing microbes will not work. In these situations, the abscess must be drained before effective treatment can be given.

COMPLICATIONS

Many antibiotics have direct toxic effects on humans and such effects must be considered and weighed against any possible benefits. Allergies or hypersensitivities may develop against an antibiotic like penicillin and patients should be questioned about such allergies before treatment is started. Unfortunately, there are few reliable tests to detect allergies to antibiotics.

Besides eliminating disease-causing microorganisms, antibiotics often destroy many bacteria of the normal flora of the body. A superinfection by an antibiotic-resistant, indigenous microorganism that is usually held in check by the normal flora may result. Such conditions frequently occur in the intestinal tract of persons on antibiotic therapy and mild intestinal disturbances are sometimes considered a necessary tradeoff for the successful treatment of a more serious infection.

SUMMARY

1. The concept of selective inhibition is the principle underlying the application of chemotherapy to microbial infections. Careful study of microbial structure, physiology, and metabolism has led to the development of a wide variety of

antimicrobial agents useful in combating the infectious diseases of both humans and animals.

2. Both bacteriostatic and bactericidal antimicrobial agents are available. Their action is primarily aimed at the inhibition of essential metabolic activity, interruption of cell wall synthesis, disruption of cell membrane integrity, or suppression of nucleic acid function. Use of these agents has provided a surprising advantage to humans in their quest for good health.

Interactions Between Host and Microorganisms

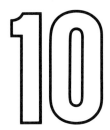

HOST-PARASITE RELATIONSHIPS

Interactions between human hosts and microorganisms are complex and are influenced by many factors. This textbook deals with human diseases and human interactions with microbes, but the principles apply to a large degree to all animals. In fact, much of what we know about human disease and interactions with microorganisms has evolved through research on lower animal species.

The concern here is not with the many indirect beneficial or detrimental effects of microorganisms on humans in the general biological cycles in nature, such as nitrogen fixation or spoilage of food, but with those situations in which the microbes are either present in or on the tissues of humans or are involved in human diseases.

Over the years various terms have been used to describe and categorize microbes into different groups relative to their interaction with human or other hosts. Some of these terms need to be introduced at this time. The beginning student should bear in mind that it is difficult to categorize biological phenomena neatly without some overlapping, particularly when attempting to categorize the complex interactions between microbes and human hosts.

The term *pathogen* refers to a microorganism that is able to produce disease; *pathogenic* is used as an adjective when referring to such microorganisms. *Nonpathogens* are microbes that are not able to cause disease. It will become apparent that the dividing line between pathogens and nonpathogens is not distinct and a large gray area exists in which microbes may be either pathogenic or nonpathogenic, depending on the interactions of many traits of both the microbe and the host. For a further understanding of the concept of a pathogen, it is necessary to introduce the term *virulence*, which means disease-producing powers or potency of a pathogen. When referring to the disease-producing capabilities of a microorganism, it is sometimes more convenient to refer to them as having high, moderate, low, or no virulence. The word *pathogenicity* is frequently used interchangeably with the term virulence. The term *pathogenesis* means the development of a disease and is used when referring to the mechanisms, sequence of changes, and processes that occur in the development of a disease.

The terms *infection* and *disease* are often used interchangeably; however, the technical definition of infection is when a microbe is able to overcome the defense barriers and live inside the host; tissue damage may or may not result. Disease refers to those conditions where the host's tissues are damaged or their function is altered by the microorganisms. When referring to infections, it is often convenient to use the term *clinical* or *apparent infection* when signs and symptoms of the disease are apparent and *subclinical* or *inapparent infection* when no apparent signs or symptoms are produced. The term *colonization* is used when referring to the ability of a microorganism to establish itself on a body surface (Figure 10-1).

Another term that helps describe interactions between a host and microorganisms is *parasitism*. A *parasite* is an organism that lives in or on the host and derives its sustenance from the host. If this parasitic relationship is beneficial to both the host and the parasite, the relationship is called *mutualism*. If the parasite causes no damage to the host, it is referred to as a *commensal*. Of course, a parasite that causes disease is a pathogen. It is possible for a parasitic microbe to change from the commensal to the pathogenic relationship and vice versa. When the host's defense mechanisms are weakened, a commensal organism of moderate or low virulence that is normally unable to cause disease in a healthy person may then be able to multiply at a faster rate or gain access to deeper tissues and cause a clinical disease; under such conditions the microbe is referred to as an *opportunist*. Under other conditions the balance between the host and a potentially virulent microbe may be such that the microbe is able to multiply and persist in the host as a commensal; yet when this microbe is transmitted to a new host, a clinical disease may result. In such cases, the first host is called a *carrier*. Most microorganisms found in nature are not parasites and are able to use nonliving materials as nutrients; these microbes are called *saprophytes*. Most saprophytes are nonvirulent; some, however, are able to cause diseases in humans.

The outcome of an infection is a result of the integrity of the host's defense mechanisms (discussed in subsequent chapters), the number of microorganisms, and the virulence of the invading microorganisms. The defense mechanisms may be stimulated to greatly increased effectiveness by previous immunization to a given pathogen. Perhaps of greater concern in clinical medicine today is the host (patient) whose natural defense mechanisms have been impaired or suppressed by other illnesses, genetic defects, stresses, or treatments; such a person is referred to as a *compromised*

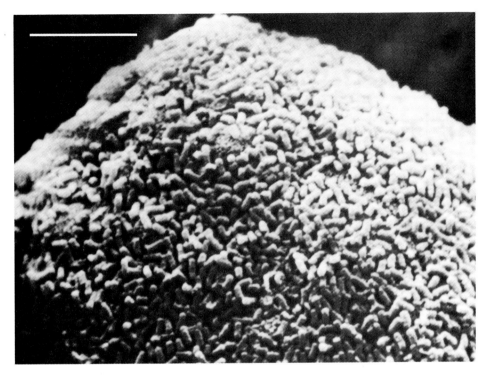

Figure 10-1   A strain of the bacterium *E. coli* specifically adhering to and colonizing the intestinal epithelium, at the tip of a villous in the ileum, of a pig. Scanning electron micrograph; bar equals 10 μm. (B. Nagy, H. W. Moon, and R. E. Isaacson, *Inf. Imm. 13*:1214–1220, Figure 3, with permission from ASM)

host. In most cases, for a microorganism to be a successful pathogen, it must possess those qualities that will allow it to enter the tissues and be able to resist the host's defense mechanisms, to multiply, and to cause damage to or malfunction of tissues of the host.

The relationships between microorganisms and the host are presented in Figure 10-2. The varying levels of the host's defense mechanisms are shown at the left with the immunized host, resistant to highly virulent microorganisms, shown at one extreme and the compromised host, highly susceptible to low virulent microorganisms, shown at the opposite extreme. The varying levels of microbial virulence are shown at the bottom of Figure 10-2. The high degree of resistance of the immunized host is specific only against the type of microorganism against which it has specific antibodies. A normal nonimmunized host may have varied responses to microorganisms of high and moderate virulence and a high degree of resistance toward infections by microbes of low virulence.

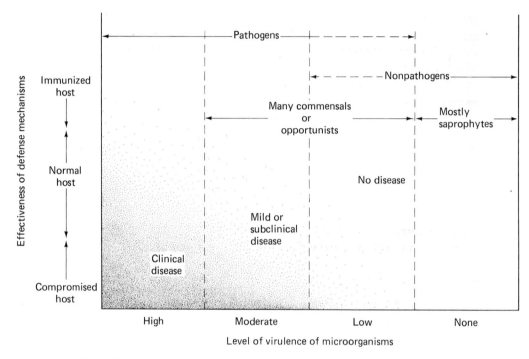

Figure 10-2 The interaction of microorganisms of varying levels of virulence with hosts of varying levels of resistance, and the resultant clinical outcome (the density of the dots represents the approximate severity of the disease).

An additional dimension, along with the virulence of the microbe and levels of resistance of the host, is the number of microbes. This added dimension is shown in the following conceptual formula:

$$ID = \frac{N \times V}{HF}$$

where ID means infectious disease, V is the virulence of the microorganism, N is the number of microorganisms, and HF stands for host factors or the level of effectiveness of the host's defense mechanisms. Based on the interrelationships presented in this formula, the following examples could be postulated. Moderate to small numbers of low-virulent microorganisms would not produce disease in a normal host, but they may be able to produce disease in a host with impaired defense mechanisms; however, a large number of such organisms may be able to produce disease in a normal host. In the case of compromised patients, the "host factors" component of the formula is reduced, causing these individuals to become more susceptible to infections. The problem of the compromised patient is of increasing concern today, for many newer medical treatments and procedures, while providing significant improvements in many medical conditions, do interfere with the normal defenses of the patient against microbial infections. An example is the treatment of a cancer patient with drugs that both slow down or stop the growth of the cancer cells and interfere with the ability of white blood cells to fight infections. Although the compromised patient may be given many meaningful years of added life by these new products, the patient's balance with microbes in his or her environment has been altered and this factor must be considered in the overall management of the case. Many infections encountered in medical practices today result from low-virulence microorganisms that are normally found on the tissues of the host (normal flora) but are able to cause infections due to the compromised conditions of a person's defense mechanisms.

NORMAL MICROBIAL FLORA OF HUMANS

The term *normal microbial flora* refers to those microorganisms that are the normal inhabitants of healthy individuals. Most would be considered harmless commensal microorganisms; yet some are potential pathogens—that is, opportunists—and do cause diseases when the balance between them and the host is altered. Under normal conditions, however, humans are able to live in healthy balance with the microorganisms that constitute their normal flora. In fact, some microbes that make up the normal flora may be beneficial to the host by interfering with the growth or attachment of pathogenic microbes.

The common types of microorganisms normally found on different parts of the body are mentioned in this section. The names of many microorganisms referred to here will be unfamiliar to most beginning students but are being introduced at this time so that this section may serve as a reference source. Many microbes that may be part of the normal flora but that are also able to cause specific disease syndromes will be discussed in greater detail in subsequent chapters.

Bacterial Sites

Skin
The type and number of bacteria vary from one area of skin to another. The superficial layers of the skin (squamous epithelium) contain many dead cells that are colonized predominantly with a bacterium of low virulence called *Staphylococcus epidermidis.* This part of the skin may also contain small numbers of the more virulent *Staphylococcus aureus*. Low concentrations of *Streptococcus pyogenes* and some gram-negative bacilli may also be present. Gram-positive bacilli, referred to as diphtheroids, are of very low virulence and are widespread as a normal inhabitant of the skin. An anaerobic bacterium called *Propionibacterium acnes* inhabits the sebaceous glands and is not destroyed by most methods used to disinfect the skin. This bacterium is a common contaminant in blood or other tissue samples collected by

passing a needle through the skin. Fortunately, this bacterium is a very low grade pathogen, but it may work synergistically with other bacteria in the development of pimples.

Nasal cavity

The nares may contain large numbers of such bacteria as *Staphylococcus epidermidis*, *Staphylococcus aureus*, and diphtheroids. A nonpathogenic gram-negative coccus called *Branhamella catarrhalis* and an opportunistic pathogen called *Haemophilis influenzae* are periodically present. Large numbers of diphtheroids and *Branhamella catarrhalis* also inhabit the pharynx. The pathogenic bacteria *Streptococcus pyogenes*, viridans streptococci, *Streptococcus pneumoniae*, *Neisseria meningitidis*, and *Haemophilis influenzae* may periodically be carried in the pharynx. The trachea, bronchi, bronchioles, and alveoli are usually free of microorganisms in healthy persons as a result of effective defense mechanisms that rapidly remove contaminating microorganisms (see Chapter 11).

Mouth

The mouth contains large numbers of diverse types of bacteria and marked variations are associated with the presence or absence of teeth or tooth decay. Some bacteria are of low virulence and may cause troublesome infections if introduced into deeper tissues—for example, from a bite. Other bacteria are able to cause tooth decay and many are nonvirulent. Several types of microorganisms commonly found in the mouth are listed in Table 10-1. When collecting clinical specimens from the throat or lower respiratory tract, care should be taken to minimize contamination of the swab or aspirate with oral secretions, for the large number of bacteria in the mouth will often obscure the pathogen being sought.

Stomach

The high acid content of the human stomach keeps the number of viable microorganisms in this organ low. Certain microbes, however, are able to survive passage through the stomach.

TABLE 10-1 GENERA OF BACTERIA MOST COMMONLY FOUND IN THE HUMAN ORAL CAVITY

Anaerobic	Facultative anaerobic
Actinomyces	*Haemophilus*
Bacteroides	*Lactobacillus*
Peptostreptococcus	*Neisseria*
Veillonella	*Staphylococcus*
	Streptococcus

Intestines

The microbial content of the small intestines changes drastically from relatively few bacteria in the upper portion to massive numbers in the lower section. The contents of the colon provide an ideal environment for the growth of many species of microorganisms. It has been estimated that over 100 different species of bacteria may be common inhabitants of the lower colon. Their concentration may reach 10^{11} cells per gram of fecal material, which represents about a third of its total weight. Intestinal flora become established early in life and generally humans live in healthy balance with these microorganisms. Such microorganisms may offer several benefits to humans by producing certain vitamins and by aiding in food digestion. These masses of common bacteria may also help suppress the growth or block the attachment of pathogens that might enter the intestinal tract.

The common bacteria of the colon can be categorized as facultative anaerobes and obligate anaerobes. The facultative anaerobes include the gram-negative bacilli commonly called the enteric bacilli, which include such genera as *Escherichia*, *Klebsiella*, *Enterobacter*, and *Proteus*. Also present are staphylococci and streptococci. The yeast *Candida albicans* is frequently present. For many years it was assumed that the facultative anaerobes were the major inhabitants of the colon, for they were readily cultivated by the standard aerobic-culturing procedures. The use of improved anaerobic culture methods, however, has shown that over 99% of the colon bacteria are obligate anaerobes. They include various species of the genera *Bacteroides*, *Fusobacterium*, *Clostridium*, *Peptostreptococcus*, and *Peptococcus* (see Table 26-1).

Genitourinary tract

Some bacteria are found in the lower portion of both male and female urethra. Normal bladders, ureters, and kidneys are free of microorganisms. The female genital tract has a complex and varying microbial flora. With menarche the vaginal and cervical tissues become populated with lactobacilli that produce lactic acid and maintain the pH of these tissues at 4.4 to 4.6. This acid environment inhibits the growth of the gram-negative enteric bacteria but allows growth of such microorganisms as bacteroides, diphtheroids, staphylococci, enterococci, and *Candida albicans*. The microflora of the vaginal canal undergo some cyclic fluctuations with hormonal variation.

TRANSMISSION OF MICROORGANISMS

Contagious disease results from the ability of a pathogenic microorganism to multiply in a host, to exit from that host, be transmitted to one or more secondary hosts, and enter and cause disease in the secondary hosts. The term *communicable* is also used in describing such diseases.

Exit of Microorganisms from the Host

Microorganisms found in the mouth and respiratory tract are expelled to some extent during normal speech and breathing. Singing and shouting expel larger numbers and coughing and sneezing expel massive numbers. Many microorganisms are dispersed on small bits of mucus and saliva. The moisture evaporates within a very brief period and the remaining particle is called a *droplet nucleus*. These microbe-laden particles may remain suspended in air currents to be carried to new hosts. In addition to being aerosolized, saliva may serve as a vehicle for microbial transmissions by kissing or expectoration. Bacteria attached to the skin scales are continually being shed from the body. Massive numbers of microorganisms are present in feces and are readily spread to new hosts living under conditions of poor sanitation. Urine and other secretions of the urinogenital tract may contain some microorganisms, but host-to-host transmission from these tissues usually results only from direct contact. Blood from a healthy person is free of microorganisms; however, blood from persons with certain diseases contains pathogenic microorganisms that may be taken up and transmitted by blood-sucking arthropods or by blood transfusions. Milk may act as a vehicle for the microorganisms shed from a lactating female with an infection of the mammary glands. The possible routes of exit of microorganisms from the body are shown in Figure 10-3.

Routes of Transmission and Entry of Microorganisms into the Host

Most microorganisms shed from a healthy person will be the same as those found on persons about them; thus the exchange of these microorganisms is of little consequence. If a person is a carrier of a pathogen or has an active infection, however, the spread of that person's microorganisms may cause infection in a new host. Some pathogens are transmitted to humans from animals or birds and, in the case of some fungal infections, the infectious spores are carried from the soil to humans by airborne route. Various modes of transmission are shown in Figure 10-4 and the possible routes of microorganism entry into the body are shown in Figure 10-5.

Airborne transmission

A majority of the infectious diseases of humans are of the respiratory tract and most of them are transmitted through the air. Microorganisms are vigorously aerosolized due to the increased coughing, sneezing, and secretion of mucus associated with a respiratory infection. Many aerosolized microbes become associated with droplet nuclei whereas others are deposited on such surfaces as floors, clothing, and bedding. The microorganisms present on various objects may become aerosolized on dust particles due to physical movement or air currents and may be inhaled by persons in the area. This form of transmission is most efficient in enclosed, crowded buildings and is an important source of infections in hospitals. Airborne bacteria may also cause infections by settling onto open wounds during surgery or when changing bandages.

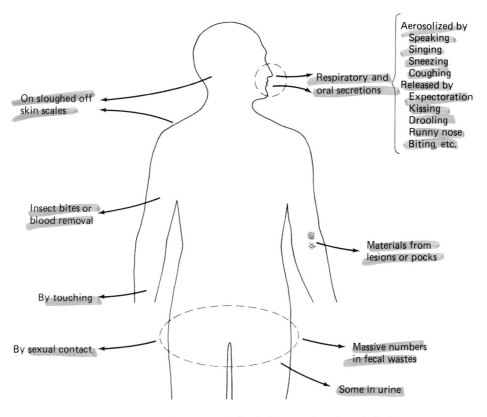

Aerosolized by
  Speaking
  Singing
  Sneezing
  Coughing
Released by
  Expectoration
  Kissing
  Drooling
  Runny nose
  Biting, etc.

Respiratory and oral secretions

On sloughed off skin scales

Insect bites or blood removal

Materials from lesions or pocks

By touching

By sexual contact

Massive numbers in fecal wastes

Some in urine

Figure 10-3 Possible routes of exit of microorganisms from the body.

Mouth

Many microorganisms enter the body by the ingestion of contaminated foods or water, by kissing, or by placing contaminated objects in the mouth.

Bites

A significant number of infectious agents are transmitted from host to host by biting insects. After the insect has ingested contaminated fluids from an infected host, the pathogen may proliferate in the insect. When such an insect bites a new host, large numbers of the pathogen may be inoculated into the body tissues. Some insects transmit the pathogen mechanically by first feeding on an infected host and then feeding on a new host with its contaminated mouth parts.

Some infections, such as rabies, are transmitted by the bites of mammals. Because of the large and varied numbers of microorganisms in mouths, troublesome infection may result from bites, particularly human bites.

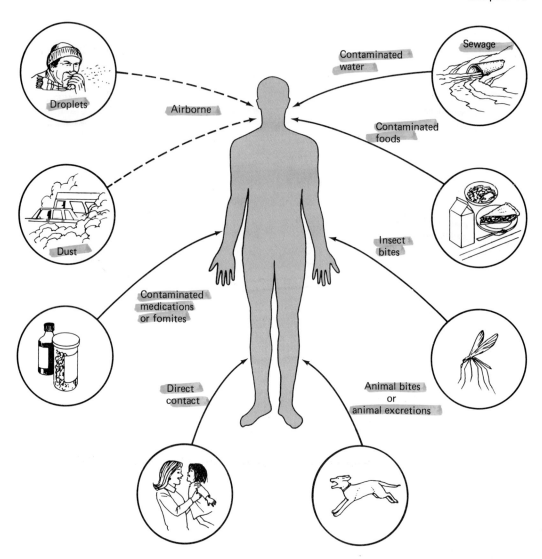

Figure 10-4 Possible routes of transmission of microorganisms to humans.

Contact

Although some preceding modes of transmission are by contact, it is desirable to expand this concept further because of its significance in routine medical care. *Direct contact* entails the touching of infected tissues with uninfected tissues. Some pathogens require intimate contact for their successful transmission and are most effectively passed from person to person by sexual intercourse or kissing. A person with a skin lesion may readily transmit the infection by direct contact. This mode of transmission is of special concern to medical personnel, for they may inadvertently transmit their infection to patients; conversely, a patient may transmit an infection to at-

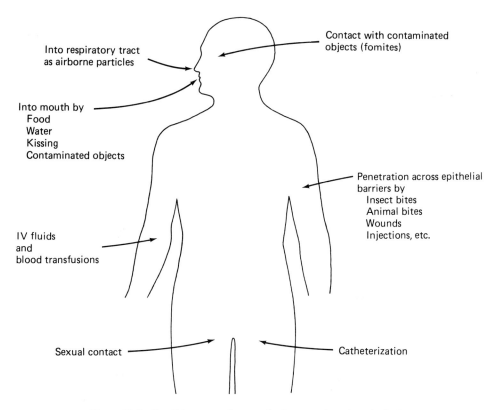

Figure 10-5 Possible routes of entry of microorganisms into the body.

tending personnel. *Indirect contact* requires intermediate objects, called *fomites*, to transmit the pathogen. The fomites become contaminated by coming in contact with pathogens from an infected patient. Then at some later time the fomites transfer some of these pathogens when coming in contact with a second individual. In medical practice such items as hands, clothing, instruments, toys, and books may serve as fomites in transferring infections between patients. Disposable items, proper handwashing and gloving, gowning, and similar procedures to prevent transmission of infections in hospitals or clinics should receive continual emphasis. Water and food are the most commonly involved fomites in our everyday environment.

Endogenous spread
The preceding examples describe the *exogenous* spread of microbes—that is, microbes coming from a source outside the host. It is also possible for microbes to spread from one part of a host to another, a process called *endogenous spread*. Many opportunistic pathogens found in the upper respiratory tract, mouth, or intestinal tract may be spread to open lesions or other tissues and cause serious infections. Some common examples are the spreading of intestinal bacteria into the urethra to

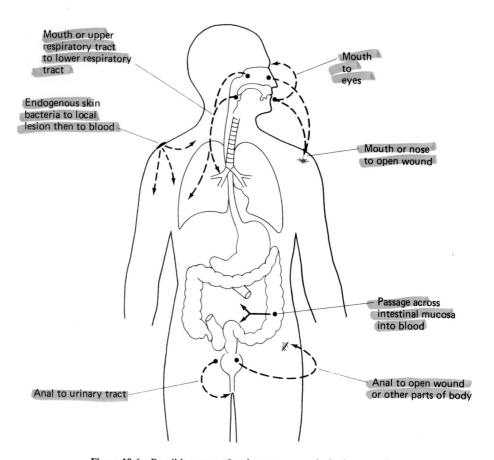

Mouth or upper
respiratory tract
to lower respiratory
tract

Endogenous skin
bacteria to local
lesion then to blood

Mouth
to
eyes

Mouth or nose
to open wound

Passage across
intestinal mucosa
into blood

Anal to urinary tract

Anal to open wound
or other parts of body

Figure 10-6   Possible routes of endogenous spread of microorganisms.

cause a urinary tract infection, the "leakage" of intestinal bacteria across the intestinal mucosa into the blood and lymphatic systems, and the spread of oral microbes to eyes by moistening contact lenses with saliva or to wounds by licking. Possible routes of endogenous spread of microorganisms are shown in Figure 10-6.

SUMMARY

1. The interaction between a host like humans and the microbial world can best be viewed much as a seesaw where the fulcrum is moved in favor of one or the other as the balance of normality is altered. Thus classic nonpathogens can become pathogens to a host suffering from environmental pressures whereas a virulent microorganism may at best coexist with a host that is well adapted to its environment.

2. All life forms, humans included, are endowed with a contingent of micro-organisms collectively referred to as normal flora. These organisms, although capable of producing disease, frequently provide a beneficial component to life and participate in maintaining a normal environment for their hosts.

3. Microorganisms are transferred from one host to another through a variety of mechanisms, including food and water, human or animal bites, contact, and aerosols.

Nonspecific Host Defense Mechanisms

11

Humans are endowed with a wide variety of mechanisms that help protect them from the many microorganisms encountered during their lives. These mechanisms include the external tissues that act as a first line of defense to help prevent microorganisms from penetrating into the deeper body tissues. If microbes do penetrate the external barriers, however, they encounter a second line of defense that includes internal mechanisms like phagocytosis, antimicrobial fluids, and inflammation. These defense mechanisms, referred to as *nonspecific* defense mechanisms, are an innate part of the body and will function immediately against any microorganism or particulate material that might land on or enter the body tissues. Nonspecific defense mechanisms are the subject of this chapter.

Antibodies are important additional defense mechanisms, sometimes called the third line of defense, that are acquired only after the first exposure of the host to an invading microorganism or its virulence factors. Antibodies are specific because they will only react against the type of microorganisms that originally stimulated their formation. The protection afforded by antibodies is called *acquired immunity* and will be discussed in the following two chapters.

The term *immunity* generally refers to resistance to a disease as a result of acquiring antibodies. In the broader usage, however, the term may encompass all forms of resistance to diseases. *Nonspecific immunity*, for example, is often used to refer to the resistance resulting from mechanisms other than antibodies and *racial*, *innate*, *natural*, or *inherent immunity* refers to resistance to a given disease as a result of genetic traits of the host.

NONSPECIFIC EXTERNAL DEFENSE MECHANISMS

The external defense mechanism consists of those components of the body that prevent microorganisms from attaching to body tissues or penetrating into the deeper, more susceptible tissues.

Bacterial Interference

Often the attachment site for a given pathogen is very specific and if the attachment site on a tissue is already occupied by one bacterium, it cannot be readily occupied by a second bacterium. In this regard, we are becoming increasingly aware that many bacteria that make up the normal flora of the host occupy many of these tissue receptor sites. They thus interfere with the attachment of many potentially harmful pathogens and perform a valuable service in helping to protect the host. Also, the normal microbial flora may compete with the invading pathogen for available nutrients and hence suppress their growth.

Physical Barriers and Chemical Agents

The resident and transient microbial flora of the tissues and organs described are generally incapable of producing disease if the physical integrity of the tissue barriers remains intact. The intact epithelial membranes, both epidermis and mucous membranes, are the most important defense mechanisms that humans possess against microbial invasion. The parts of the body exposed to the external environment are endowed with a variety of mechanisms to prevent microorganisms from penetrating to the more susceptible internal tissues. The more important mechanisms are described next.

Skin

Intact skin provides a barrier that cannot be penetrated by most microorganisms. Most pathogenic bacteria are unable to survive on clean healthy skin for any length of time, partly because of the acid pH of the skin, which is inhibitory to most pathogenic bacteria, and partly because of bactericidal acids secreted in the sebaceous glands. An exception is the bacterium *Staphylococcus aureus*, which is able to persist on the skin and is a frequent source of infection when the integrity of the skin is altered.

Mucous membranes

Body cavities are lined with mucosal membranes that consist of one or more layers of living cells. The cells are bathed by a mucous film that helps remove microbes. These surfaces, however, while offering a valuable protective barrier against most microorganisms, are more easily penetrated by some microorganisms than is the intact outer epidermis.

Eyes

Along with the barrier effect of the intact tissues, the secretion of tears and the movement of eyelids provide a continuous flushing action that disposes of contaminant microorganisms. Tears also contain an enzyme called *lysozyme* that destroys certain gram-positive bacteria.

Outer ear canal

This surface is lubricated with a waxy deposit that contains effective antibacterial components.

Alimentary canal

The physical integrity of the mucosal epithelium is extremely important in preventing the spread into the blood or deeper tissues of the massive numbers of bacteria found in the mouth and lower intestinal tract. Along with this barrier effect, the flow of saliva and swallowing continually dilute bacteria in the mouth. Stomach acid destroys large numbers of microorganisms that are swallowed. Secretion of mucus along the intestinal tract aids in trapping and removing microorganisms. The mucous secretion contains some antibacterial substance and antibodies to help further reduce the numbers of microorganisms.

Genitourinary tract

The intact mucosal epithelium presents a physical barrier and the flushing action of urine keeps most microorganisms restricted to the lower portion of the urethra. The protective role of the acid pH of the female genital tissues was discussed earlier.

Respiratory tract

The respiratory tract is endowed with a unique series of defense mechanisms against the continuous onslaught it experiences from a wide variety of airborne microorganisms. The positions of various defense mechanisms are shown in Figure 11-1. Nasal hairs are of some value by inducing turbulence of the inhaled air and by acting as very crude filters. The nasal turbinates provide a large exposure surface and cause increased air turbulence. The turbulence results in increased impaction of the larger airborne particles against the surface of the turbinates.

Much of the surface of the nasal cavity is lined with ciliated epithelium. Ciliated epithelium contains large numbers of ciliated cells. Each ciliated cell contains several hundred cilia (hairlike structures) that are rapidly and continuously beating. Interspersed between every four to five ciliated cells is a mucus-secreting cell. A film of mucus forms on top of the ciliated epithelium and serves as a sticky surface to trap the airborne particles impacted onto it. Mucus also contains antimicrobial substances. The rhythmic movement of the cilia moves this mucous film, with the entrapped particles, into the pharyngeal area where the mucus can be disposed of, usually by swallowing. A significant portion of the larger airborne particles is removed by these mechanisms of the upper respiratory tract.

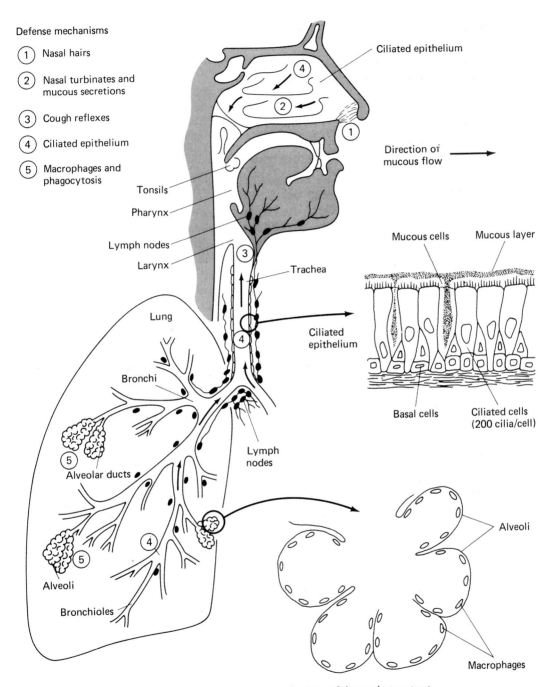

Defense mechanisms

1. Nasal hairs
2. Nasal turbinates and mucous secretions
3. Cough reflexes
4. Ciliated epithelium
5. Macrophages and phagocytosis

Ciliated epithelium

Direction of mucous flow

Tonsils

Pharynx

Lymph nodes

Larynx

Trachea

Mucous cells

Mucous layer

Ciliated epithelium

Basal cells

Ciliated cells (200 cilia/cell)

Lung

Bronchi

Lymph nodes

Alveolar ducts

Alveoli

Bronchioles

Alveoli

Macrophages

Figure 11-1 Defense mechanisms of the respiratory tract.

The smaller airborne particles are carried into the trachea, bronchi, and bronchioles where many are impacted onto the ciliated epithelium that completely lines these passages. The direction of mucous flow is from the lungs to the opening of the trachea. As mucus accumulates at the top of the trachea, it is removed by "clearing the throat" and disposed of by swallowing. When mucus begins to accumulate or particles become trapped along this ciliated epithelium, the cough reflex is triggered and coughing aids in dislodging and removing these materials from air passageways. Only the smallest microbe-containing airborne particles (those between 5 to 10 μm) are able to penetrate into the air sacs (alveoli) of the lungs. Large numbers of phagocytic white blood cells, called alveolar macrophages, are located in the air sacs and are able to ingest and destroy most microorganisms deposited in healthy lungs. Overall the mechanisms of the respiratory tract, when functioning properly, effectively protect the host against many potential airborne pathogens.

NONSPECIFIC INTERNAL DEFENSE MECHANISMS

After a pathogenic microbe has become attached to the tissues of the host, it may be able to pass into the cell because of its own invasive mechanisms or it may be introduced into the deeper, more susceptible tissues through sections of epithelium that have been injured. Once beyond the protective outer barrier of the body, the invading microorganisms encounter a series of internal host defense mechanisms. Because these mechanisms are closely associated with the activities of the *white blood cells* (WBC), also referred to as leukocytes, the structure and function of these cells, as well as other components of the blood, are discussed next.

White Blood Cells

White blood cells can be divided into three categories: *granulocytes*, *monocytes*, and *lymphocytes*. Specialized types of cells are found within each category. The WBC are involved in such host defense activities as phagocytosis (the ingesting of foreign particles), inflammation, and antibody formation. Often different types of WBC will function in a cooperative effort to produce the final result. These interactions are discussed in the following sections. The development of the different types of WBC is outlined in Figure 11-2.

Granulocytes

These white blood cells get their name from the large number of granules present in their cytoplasm. These granules may contain chemicals that act as stimulators of certain body responses or they may contain enzymes that aid in the digestion of microorganisms and other materials. The granulocytes have lobular nuclei and are 9 to 12 μm in diameter. Because of the extreme lobular nature of their nuclei, they are also called *polymorphonuclear leukocytes* or simply *PMNs*. These cells are formed and mature in the bone marrow and are continually being released into the blood. They

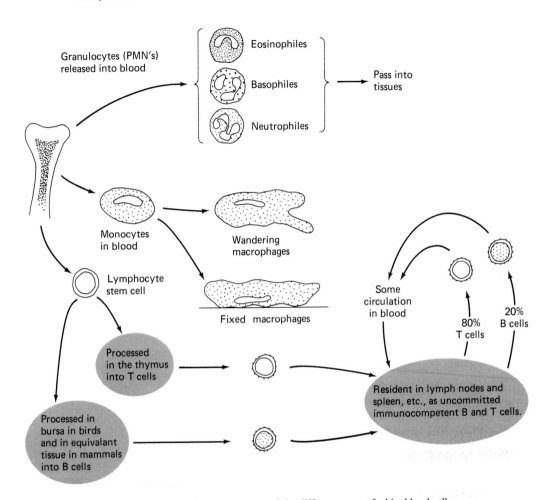

Figure 11-2 Development of the different types of white blood cells.

circulate for several hours and then pass into the tissue spaces, where they remain for a few days and then die. These cells do not divide after leaving the bone marrow and the body is required to produce about 10^{11} new cells per day. Many granulocytes are held in reserve in the spleen and bone marrow; when an inflammation occurs, large numbers are released into the blood and the rate of production of new cells is accelerated. Normal blood contains from 5000 to 9000 WBC mm³ and 70 to 75% of them are granulocytes. When inflammation occurs in the body, the increased output of granulocytes may increase the total number of WBC well above the normal level. This increased WBC count is one of the valuable signs used to diagnose the presence of inflammation in a patient. The different types of granulocytes are *eosinophils*, *basophils*, and *neutrophils*, names derived from their staining characteristics. The full range of functions of the eosinophils is not understood. They seem to be involved with some allergic responses and parasitic infections. They constitute only 2 to 4% of the total WBC found in the blood. The basophils make up less than 1% of the WBC. They contain granules of histamine and may be involved in controlling the movement of body fluids involved in the inflammatory response. Neutrophils are the most numerous WBC, constituting 65 to 70% of the total, and are active phagocytes. Large numbers are involved in the early phases of the inflammatory response.

Monocytes

The monocytes are those cells that possess a large smooth nucleus and a large area of cytoplasm. These cells are formed in the bone marrow. As they are released into the blood, they are called monocytes and are from 14 to 20 μm in diameter. Circulating monocytes make up 1 to 6% of the total WBC. Monocytes collect in or pass into many different body tissues and become known as macrophages. Whether all different types of macrophages come from the same type of monocyte is not known. In the transformation from monocyte to macrophage the cell increases in size to 25 to 50 μm. Some macrophages are motile and are called *wandering macrophages*. These wandering cells move by amoeboid action and are found throughout all tissues and cavities of the body. Other macrophages become attached to the walls of blood capillaries and sinusoids and are known as *fixed macrophages*. All macrophages are active phagocytic cells. They live for months after leaving the bone marrow. Under an appropriate stimulus macrophages may divide or become "activated" in that their phagocytic and antimicrobial capabilities are considerably increased.

Lymphocytes

Lymphocytes make up 20 to 25% of the WBC. Some are small, about 6 μm in diameter; others are about 12 μm in diameter. They are round with a large, smooth nucleus and a small amount of cytoplasm. Lymphocytes develop from *stem cells* that are originally produced in the bone marrow. These cells are released from the bone marrow and develop into two different types of lymphocytes, *B cells* and *T cells*. The stem cells that become T cells first pass to the thymus, where they are influenced by thymic hormones to become T cells. Many T cells circulate throughout the body and constitute about 60 to 80% of the lymphocytes found in the blood. Moreover, many are found in the lymph nodes and spleen. The organ or hormone that influences the stem cells to change into B cells has not yet been identified in humans but is currently thought to reside in the bone marrow. The influencing organ in birds is the *bursa of Fabricius*. A majority of the B cells are found in lymph nodes and the spleen. The T cells and B cells are involved in the production of cell-mediated immunity and the production of antibodies.

Other blood components

Red blood cells, which constitute 45% of the blood volume, will not be discussed, for they have no apparent direct role in fighting invading microorganisms.

A brief introduction into the fluid components of blood will be useful in understanding concepts presented later. When blood is collected and substances are added to prevent clotting, the blood cells can be separated from the fluid by settling out. The remaining fluid is called the *blood plasma*. If blood is allowed to clot, a clear yellowish fluid called *serum* remains. The major difference between plasma and serum is that plasma still contains fibrinogen and other essential components for blood clotting. Both fluids are rich in other proteins. The serum proteins can be separated into two major types called albumin and globulin. The globulin proteins can be further separated into three types called alpha, beta, and gamma. Most antibodies that form against microorganisms are found in the gamma globulin fraction of the blood serum and are called *immunoglobulins*. Figure 11-3 shows the formation of blood plasma

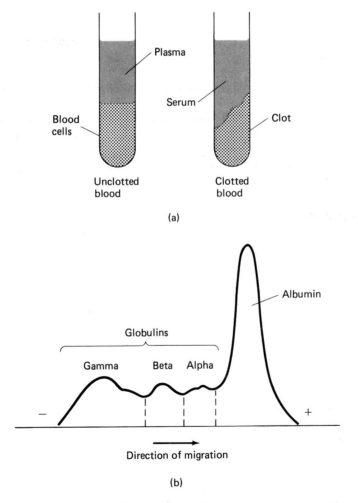

(a)

(b)

Figure 11-3   (a) The source of blood plasma and blood serum. (b) The separation of blood serum into major types of proteins based on the rate of migration through an electrical field.

and serum as well as the separation of serum into its different classes of proteins based on their rate of migration through an electrical field (electrophoresis).

Phagocytosis

Neutrophils and macrophages are the major cells involved in the phagocytosis and destruction of microorganisms (Figure 11-4). Phagocytosis is perhaps the most important defense mechanism of the host once the pathogen has penetrated beyond the epithelial and mucosal barriers. The first step in phagocytosis requires the attachment of the foreign particle to the cell membrane. Some bacteria readily attach to phagocytes and so are readily phagocytized whereas others will not attach and are thus difficult to phagocytize. Phagocytosis is facilitated if the phagocyte is able to trap the bacterium against a rough surface; in this case, phagocytosis can occur without attachment. Attachment and phagocytosis are much more effective if the microorganisms are coated with specific antibodies.

Once attachment of the microbe has occurred, the cell membrane extends around the particle and fuses to form an intracellular membrane-bound vacule containing the microbe. This vacule is called a *phagosome*. The phagosome next fuses with the lysosomes, thereby causing the release of digestive enzymes into the phagosome. This combined structure is called a *phagolysosome*. These enzymes, along with

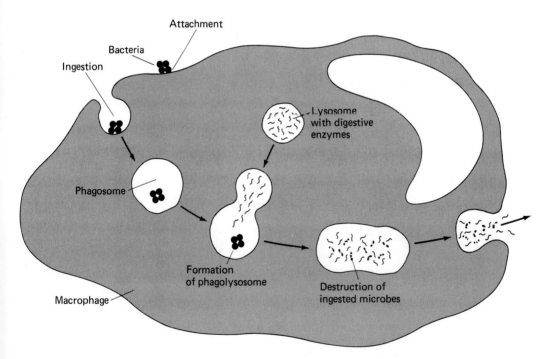

Figure 11-4 Mechanisms of phagocytosis and destruction of bacteria by a macrophage.

the hydrogen peroxide that is also produced by the phagocytic cell, readily destroy most microorganisms or break down other particles of organic material. The phagocytosis and intracellular digestion of a bacterium are shown in Figure 11-5.

Lymphatic System

The lymphatic system consists of a complex network of thin-walled ducts (lymphatic vessels), strategically located filtering bodies called *lymph nodes*, and concentrations of large numbers of lymphocytic cells in various organs or tissues. The lymphatic vessels are widespread and generally parallel to the blood vessels. They are particularly plentiful in the skin and along the respiratory and intestinal tracts. A major function of the lymphatic vessels is to serve as return ducts for the fluid that is continually diffusing out of the blood capillaries into the body tissues. Before the lymph fluid is returned to the blood, it must first pass through several lymph nodes. The major concentrations of lymph nodes that filter fluid coming from the lymphatic vessels of the skin are located in the neck, inguinal, and axillary regions (Figure 11-6). Deeper lymph nodes are located along the respiratory and intestinal tracts—that is, in areas where microorganisms are most likely to invade the deeper body tissues. The lymph fluid flowing out of the lymph nodes flows into larger collecting ducts that eventually drain into the thoracic duct, which, in turn, empties into the bloodstream. The lymph nodes contain a series of narrow passageways (sinusoids) lined with macrophages. The phagocytic activity of these macrophages removes extraneous particulate matter, including most microbes, that may be carried in the lymphatic fluid. Under normal conditions the lymph nodes successfully prevent invading microorgan-

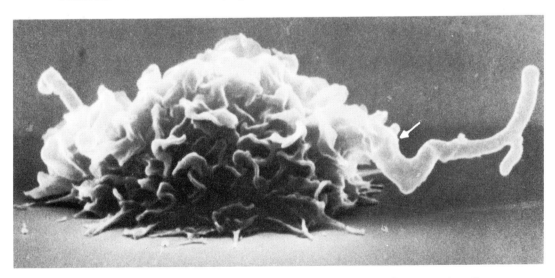

Figure 11-5 Scanning electron micrograph showing a branch-shaped bacterium (*Nocardia asteroides*) being phagocytized by a macrophage. Arrow points to the area where the bacterium is being enfulged. (B. L. Beaman, *Inf. Imm. 15*:925–937, Figure 2, with permission from ASM)

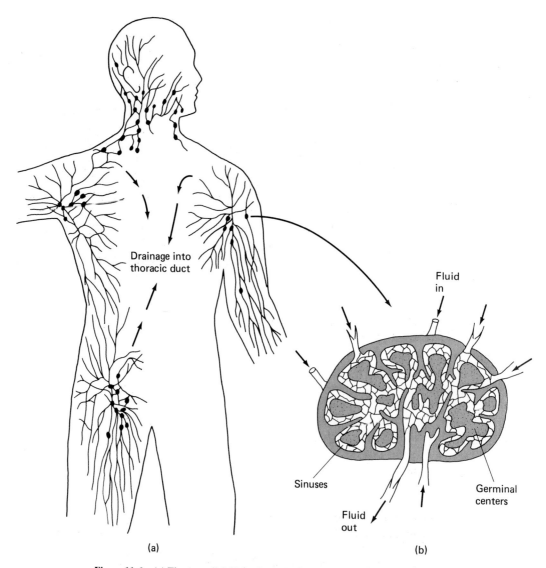

Drainage into
thoracic duct

Fluid
in

Sinuses

Fluid
out

Germinal
centers

(a)   (b)

Figure 11-6   (a) The superficial lymphatic ducts and nodes. (b) Cross section of a lymph node. The fluid filters through the sinuses of the node where large numbers of macrophages are located. The germinal centers contain the antibody-producing cells.

isms from reaching the bloodstream. When large numbers of bacteria become trapped or multiply in the lymph nodes, inflammation may occur with accompanying swelling and tenderness. The presence of swollen lymph nodes is a useful clinical sign for the diagnosis of an infection in the tissues being drained into that node. Lymph nodes also serve as a storage organ for the lymphocytes and are initiating sites for antibody responses.

Reticuloendothelial System (RES)

The RES is a composite name given to those tissues and organs that contain the mononuclear phagocytic cells and has also been referred to as the mononuclear phagocyte system. Many macrophages are found in the loose connective tissue fibers called reticulum and fixed to the endothelial cells that line the sinusoids of such organs as the lymph nodes, liver, spleen, and bone marrow. Both fixed and wandering macrophages, as well as circulating monocytes, are part of the RES. Most microorganisms that find their way into the lymphatic system or into the blood or other tissues of the RES are generally disposed of within a few minutes by phagocytosis.

Inflammation

When tissue injury occurs, whether by physical trauma or the multiplication of microorganisms, a series of reactions is set in motion to remove or contain the offending agents and repair the damage. This series of events is referred to as the *inflammatory response* and is outlined in Figure 11-7. The inflammatory response is initiated by the release of such chemicals as histamine, serotonin, kinins, and prostaglandins. These chemicals are contained in certain tissues and WBC and are released in response to trauma to the tissues. Histamine is one of the most important chemical mediators and is found in high concentrations in circulating basophils and *mast cells*. Mast cells resemble basophils but are scattered throughout various body tissues, with the largest concentration being in the mucosal tissues. These chemical mediators, often called *vasoactive agents*, can rapidly affect the flow of blood and the permeability of blood vessels in the immediate area. Upon release of the vasoactive agents the blood vessels in the surrounding area dilate, which brings an increased flow of blood to the injured tissues. This process occurs within several minutes and is accompanied by an increased permeability of the walls of the blood vessels, which allows an increased amount of plasma and PMNs to move from the vessels into the area of injury. The chemical mediators of inflammation appear to have an attractive influence for PMNs that draws these WBC to the inflammatory site; this process is called *chemotaxis*. After several hours of the inflammatory response the tissue will be reddened, warm, swollen, and painful due to the increased blood and plasma flow into the area. If the stimulus of the response is the growth of microorganisms in the tissues, the PMNs begin collecting in large numbers and will phagocytize and destroy many microbes. Plasma flowing into the area carries clotting factors, including fibrinogen, which begins to form a network of fibrin strands around the injured area. The fibrin and PMNs continue to build up over several days and are joined by other cells to form a barrier around the injured area. It is called the *inflammatory barrier.* The center of the area becomes the battleground in which large numbers of dead bacteria and dead PMNs begin to accumulate in pools of fluids; it is called the *inflammatory exudate* or, more commonly, *pus*. This accumulation of pus circumscribed by the inflammatory barrier is called an *abscess*. As the inflammatory process continues, other types of white blood cells enter the area. Increased numbers of lymphocytes appear and are

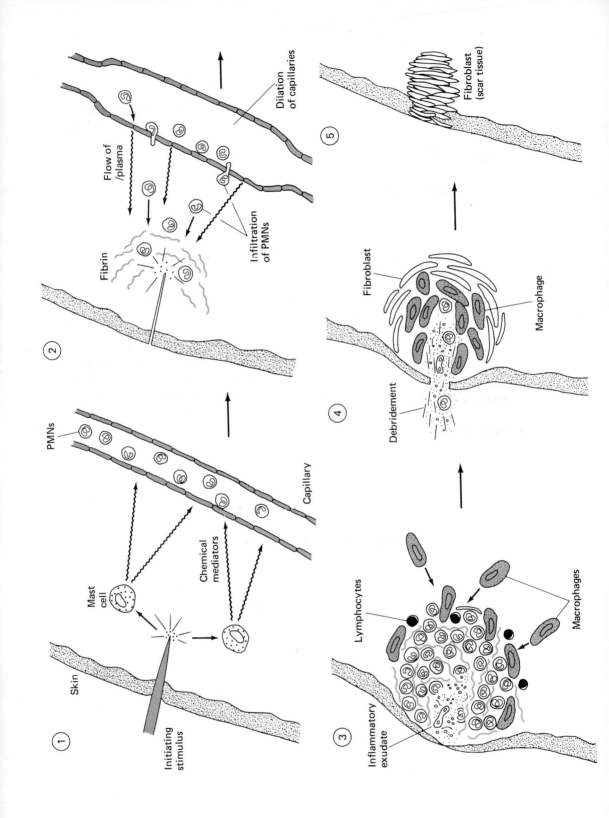

thought to attract and stimulate macrophages. Macrophages next begin to appear in large numbers to aid further in walling off the injured area, to clear up debris through phagocytosis, and to help in repair. If the abscess has formed on the surface, such as skin, the inflammatory barrier and skin may break and allow the pus to be expelled. This drainage is called *debridement*; if not accompanied by damage to the inflammatory barrier between the abscess and deeper tissues, it may help accelerate healing of the lesion. A pimple or boil is an example of such a skin abscess. If the abscess is in deeper tissues and the inflammatory exudate cannot be expelled, healing is much slower. A standoff may be reached in an abscess in that the bacteria are in an environmental niche of dead tissue that affords them protection from host defense mechanisms and, at the same time, they may be in a metabolically inactive state so that antibiotics may not affect them. Often surgical drainage is needed at this time to clean out the debris or pus. The last phase of the inflammatory response is the growth of repair cells called *fibroblasts*. The fibroblasts are long, slender cells that form a wall of scar tissue around the injured area. They continue to form scar tissue until the void where the normal cells were destroyed has been filled. It may be several weeks from the beginning of the response until complete healing has occurred. Scar tissue formation is basically a beneficial response; however, excessive scar tissue formation in vital organs may result in impaired function and excessive scarring is undesirable on exposed areas of the body for cosmetic reasons. The inflammatory response occurs with most injuries; and if microbial infection is not present, healing occurs without pus formation.

SUMMARY

1. Each individual is endowed with a number of barriers to infection that function without respect to the kind of possible disease-producing agent. These barriers are called nonspecific host defense mechanisms.
2. Nonspecific host defense mechanisms often function in sequence such that a breach in one barrier leads to the action of the next. These barriers are anatomical, such as the skin, mechanical, such as ciliary movement, chemical as with lysozyme in tears and cellular, including both granulocytes and macrophages.
3. The reticuloendothelial system has a major responsibility in maintaining body defense against invading microorganisms. Cells and body fluids from this system are primarily responsible for the beneficial inflammatory response associated with many types of infections.

Figure 11-7   The progression of an inflammatory response from the initial stimulation to abscess formation, to healing with the formation of scar tissue.

Acquired Immune Responses

12

Acquired immunity refers to the resistance of a host resulting from the formation of antibodies or antibodylike responses. The immune response is a dual system. One part of this dual system is called the *humoral antibody response* and includes those responses that lead to the formation of antibody molecules that circulate with the body fluids. The other part is called the *cell-mediated immune response* and involves the production of special types of lymphocytes that possess specific reactive sites on their outer surface.

Much new information about mechanisms of the immune responses and characteristics of antibodies has become available in the past 10 to 15 years, but a detailed description is beyond the scope of this textbook. Coverage here is limited to an overall view of the formation and functions of antibodies and the cell-mediated immune response, how these phenomena can be manipulated by the use of vaccines to prevent diseases, and how acquiring these responses can be used to help in the diagnosis of diseases. Some detrimental effects of immune responses on the host are also discussed.

ANTIGENS

The basic concept of the immune responses centers around the ability of the body to react against certain types of foreign substances. Any foreign substance that stimulates the formation of antibodies is called an *antigen*. Antigens are usually proteins or

166

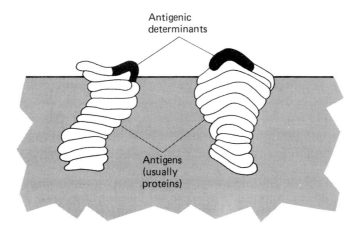

Figure 12-1 Antigens associated with bacterial cells. A single cell may contain a number of different antigens. Antigenic determinants are the smaller segments (dark areas) of the antigens.

carbohydrates of over 10,000 daltons molecular weight; some lipid complexes, however, may also function as antigens. Once an antibody is formed, it will specifically combine only with the type of antigen that stimulated its production. Moreover, the antibody is not formed against the entire antigen but only against certain chemical groups of the antigen called *antigenic determinants*. An antigenic determinant that is separated from the remainder of the antigen is not able to stimulate antibody formation because of its small size, but it can react with antibodies that are already formed. Under these conditions the antigenic determinant is called a *hapten*. Protein antigens and their antigenic determinants that may make up part of a bacteria are shown in Figure 12-1.

TYPES OF ACQUIRED IMMUNE RESPONSES

The circulating or humoral antibody response involves the lymphocytic B cells whereas the cell-mediated immune response involves T cells. When the body is exposed to the complex antigens associated with invading microorganisms, both humoral and cell-mediated immune responses are stimulated. The acquired immune responses are usually beneficial to the host in that they offer added protection against invading microorganisms; these responses, however, may sometimes react against the host or produce certain types of antibodies that cause undesirable side reactions. These undesirable reactions are called *allergies* or *hypersensitivities*. The immune responses are discussed under three general categories: (a) formation of circulating or humoral antibodies, (b) formation of cell-mediated immunity, and (c) allergies and hypersensitivity.

HUMORAL ANTIBODY RESPONSE

Humoral antibodies are released into the blood and are found in most tissue fluids. The antigens associated with microorganisms and foreign proteins, in general, are excellent stimulators of this antibody response. These antibodies are effective in helping destroy invading microorganisms or in neutralizing toxins.

The following sequence of events, outlined in Figure 12-2, occurs when the antigens enter body tissues. Macrophages may phagocytize the antigen at the site of entry into body tissues. The antigen is then carried to a lymph node by the macrophage or the unphagocytized antigen may be carried by lymph fluid or blood to a lymphatic organ where phagocytosis by macrophages first occurs. It is not yet clear how the antigen is processed by the macrophage. Nevertheless, the processed antigens or the antigenic determinants are presented by the macrophage into the surrounding lymphoid tissue where large numbers of B and T cells are located. In order to produce humoral antibodies, the antigenic determinants must combine with a specific receptor site on a B cell. These receptor sites have the same specificity and structure as antibodies. Based on current theories, a large number of receptor sites of different configurations are present in the population of B cells. A given B cell will contain large numbers of repetitive copies of only a single type of receptor site. So within the population of B cells in the body are cells with receptors that will more or less fit any antigenic determinant that might enter the body. When the B cell encounters and combines with its specific antigenic determinant, it becomes activated and begins to multiply, a process that rapidly leads to an increase in the number of identical B cells. This selective increase in the number of a specific type of cell is called *clonal expansion*. It is theorized that during this clonal expansion a pool of genes, which contains the genetic information for the configuration of the receptor site (and the variable region of the antibody molecule—see below), is rearranged to form genes that will code for receptor sites with an exact fit to the antigenic determinant. This allows highly specific antibodies to be formed against virtually any antigen that might enter the body. The activated B cells continue to divide and differentiate into either *memory lymphocytes* or *plasma cells*. A type of T cell called a *helper T cell* appears to be involved in this process in some yet undetermined manner. The plasma cells contain increased amounts of cytoplasm, endoplasmic reticulum, and ribosomes that equip them to produce large amounts of proteins. The main proteins produced by the plasma cells are the circulating antibodies, which are called *immunoglobulins* (Ig). The plasma cells are concentrated mainly in the lymphatic tissues but continue to replicate until large numbers of these antibody-producing cells are scattered throughout the body. In the meantime, the memory cells replicate to a limited extent and also scatter throughout the body; these cells become involved in secondary antibody responses, which will be discussed later.

Classes and Structure of Antibodies

Five different classes of circulating antibodies, or immunoglobulins, have been identified and are designated IgG, IgM, IgA, IgD, and IgE. The properties of these im-

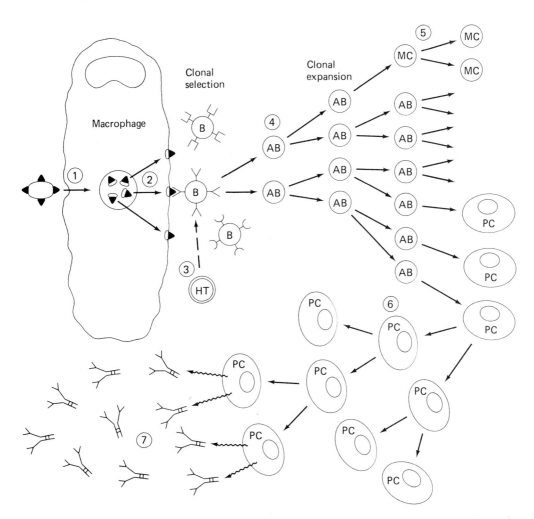

Figure 12-2 The production of humoral antibodies. (1) A bacterium showing repeated copies of one type of antigenic determinant; bacterium is phagocytized by a macrophage. (2) Antigen is processed and presented to a B cell which possesses a receptor that specifically combines with the antigenic determinant (clonal selection). (3) Cooperative influence by helper T cell. (4) Selected B cell becomes activated (AB) and begins to multiply (clonal expansion). (5) Some activated B cells change into memory cells (MC). (6) Most activated B cells change into plasma cells (PC) and plasma cells continue to multiply. (7) Plasma cells secrete large amounts of specific antibodies.

munoglobulins are shown in Table 12-1. The basic unit of an antibody, as typified by IgG, consists of two heavy and two light polypeptide chains connected in a Y-type arrangement (Figure 12-3). The arrangements of amino acids at the top of the four chains of the Y are variable and form the specific reactive sites of the antibody. These specific reactive sites, called the *variable region*, will combine only with an antigenic

TABLE 12-1   PROPERTIES OF FOUR CLASSES OF HUMAN IMMUNOGLOBULINS

Property	IgG	IgM	IgA	IgE
1. No. of Y-shaped units	1	5	2	1
2. Molecular weight	145,000	850,000	385,000	200,000
3. How transferred to offspring	Via placenta	Not transferred	Via milk	Not transferred
4. Half-life (days)	25	5	6	2
5. Where found in body	40% in blood, 60% in extra cellular fluid	90% in blood, 10% in extra cellular fluid	Mostly in secretions	Attached to PMNs or mast cells

determinant that is the same as that of the original antigen that initiated the antibody response. The remainder of the antibody molecule does not vary and is called the *constant region*.

The IgG antibodies are the major type present in the circulation; most are in the blood, but lesser amounts are found in other fluids, such as lymph, synovial, and spinal. IgG is an important long-term antibody that helps protect the host against infections. This antibody is able to cross the placenta in humans in the transfer of passive immunity to the newborn.

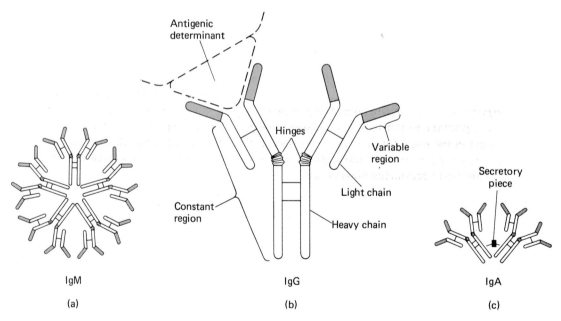

Figure 12-3   The structures of immunoglobulins. (a) Structure of IgM showing pentamer arrangement of the basic immunoglobulin Y-shaped units. (b) Details of the IgG structure (scale enlarged). (c) Dimer arrangement of IgA.

The IgM antibodies consist of clusters (polymers) of five Y-shaped immuno-globulin basic structures. These antibodies appear earlier in the infection than the other classes and offer valuable assistance to the host during the critical early stages of an infection. IgM is found mostly in blood fluids but disappears from the body soon after the onset of the infection and does not cross the placenta.

IgA antibodies are made up of two (dimer) Y-shaped basic structures. These immunoglobulins are readily secreted and, besides being found in the blood, are also found in tears, saliva, mucosal secretions, and similar fluids. IgA offers valuable protection against infections of the superficial tissues, such as the mucosal surfaces of the respiratory, intestinal, and genitourinary tracts.

IgD is found only in low concentrations and seems identical to the specific receptor sites on B cells. IgE is associated with allergies and is discussed later.

Primary and Secondary Humoral Antibody Responses

After exposure to an antigen, small amounts of antibody first appear in a few days, but readily measured amounts usually cannot be detected until a week after stimulation. A steady rise in antibody concentrations occurs over the next 2 weeks until the maximum level is attained at about 3 weeks. The level of antibodies then slowly decreases over ensuing years. The rapid increase of antibodies is a result of the rapid proliferation of the specifically programmed plasma cells. A given IgG antibody will remain in the body for only a few months after it is formed; therefore the prolonged persistence of antibodies must result from the continual dividing and activity of specific plasma cells.

If a person has experienced a primary antibody response to a given antigen and is reexposed at some later date to the same antigen, a rapid antibody response is stimulated and high levels of antibodies, primarily IgG and IgA, are produced within a few days instead of a few weeks. This is called the *anamnestic, booster,* or *secondary response* and is associated with the memory lymphocytes that were produced as part of the primary response. These memory lymphocytes are long lived and some will remain in the body for years. These cells are preprogrammed; when they encounter the same type of antigen that stimulated the primary response, they rapidly change into antibody-producing plasma cells. This mechanism allows the body to replenish its antibody supply before the invading microorganism has had a chance to cause a clinical disease, and in many cases confers life-long immunity to the host. The primary and secondary responses of IgG and IgM are shown in Figure 12-4.

Effect of Humoral Antibodies on Microorganisms

When a microorganism like a bacterium enters the body tissues, antibodies may be formed against such cellular components as different antigenic determinants on the surface, internal proteins, toxins, capsular antigens, or flagella. Thus the antigen–antibody reactions may involve various components of the microorganism with varied effects. Also, antibodies often work in conjunction with other compo-

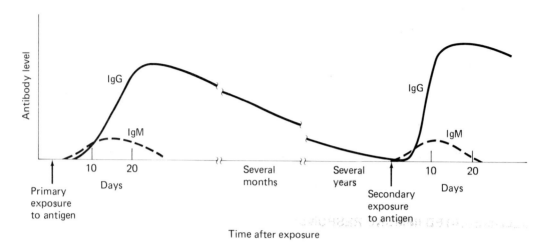

Figure 12-4 Primary and secondary responses of IgG and IgM antibodies.

nents of the host's defense mechanisms, such as phagocytic cells, or complement, to bring about the end results. The following categories cover the most common ways that antibodies function against microorganisms.

Promotion of phagocytosis
Antibodies combining with surface antigens may bind the microbes into clumps by forming antibody bridges between cells. This is called an *agglutination* reaction. These clumps of microbes are much more readily phagocytized than single cells. In addition, some antibodies may first attach to the antigen with their reactive sites and the opposite end of the antibody molecule—that is, the constant region—may specifically attach to the phagocytic cell. This step binds the microbe to the phagocytic cell, which greatly facilitates the process of phagocytosis. Antibodies that render microorganisms more susceptible to phagocytosis are called *opsonins*.

Interference with attachment
Antibodies may combine over the surface of the microbes and prevent their attachment to host cells. They are called *neutralizing* antibodies because they neutralize the ability of the microbe to cause infection.

Neutralization of toxins
Antibodies may neutralize the toxins produced by microorganisms. Such antibodies are called *antitoxins*.

Activation of the complement system
The complement system is a group of nine or more protein components found in normal serum and designated C1, C2, C3, C4, C5, C6, C7, C8, and C9, and so on. When activated, different components of the complement system stimulate and am-

plify such host defense mechanisms as inflammation, chemotaxis, and phagocytosis and cause lysis (breaking up) of certain microorganisms or other cells. The complement system becomes activated when an antigen–antibody reaction occurs and forms a complex with and activates the first component of complement. A few molecules of the activated first component, in turn, activate many more molecules of one of the other components of complement (C4), which, in turn, activates yet a larger number of molecules of the next component (C2), and so on through the other components. This expanding effect, as the reactions cascade through the complement system, allows a small number of antigen–antibody reactions to trigger a greatly amplified effect on the antigen as a result of the host defense mechanisms that are stimulated by the activated components of complement.

CELL-MEDIATED IMMUNE RESPONSE

The cell-mediated immune response involves T cell-type lymphocytes (Figure 12-5). This response is stimulated by many antigens that stimulate the formation of humoral antibodies and the two responses may occur simultaneously against the same type of antigen. But antigens associated with cells, tissue organs (such as organ transplants), or antigens containing high contents of lipids stimulate a vigorous cell-mediated immune response. Like the B cells, there are many different T cells, each with a specific receptor site that is able to combine with a specific antigen. The pool of T cells has some cells with specific receptors to almost any antigen that might be encountered. The antigen is first phagocytized by macrophages where processed and then presented to a T cell. Only a T cell that possesses matching receptors can combine with a particular antigen. Before combining with an antigen, the T cell is inactive; after combining, it becomes active and is called a *sensitized T cell*. The sensitized T cell increases in size and begins to multiply to produce many identical cells (clonal expansion). Sensitized T cells do not secrete immunoglobulins; however, many of these cells circulate in the body fluids and are called *killer T cells*. When killer T cells encounter and combine with an antigen, they begin to secrete a series of polypeptides called *lymphokines*. Lymphokines stimulate a variety of responses that may lead to destruction of the antigen or the cells that contain the antigen. The actions stimulated by the various lymphokines are listed in Table 12-2. The lymphokine called the cytotoxic factor may directly destroy invading microorganisms whereas most other lymphokines attract and stimulate macrophages to contain and destroy invading microorganisms or tissues that possess foreign antigens. An inflammatory response is often part of this reaction and may lead to the formation of scar tissue around the antigen. These nodules of scar tissue and other cells are called *granulomas*. The cell-mediated immune response is sometimes referred to as *delayed hypersensitivity*, for it requires several days for the first phases of this reaction to be seen when an antigen is injected into the tissues of a sensitized host; this phenomenon is the basis of skin tests that are used in the diagnosis of such diseases as tuberculosis (see Chapter 22). A substance called *interferon* is also released by killer T cells and has inhibitory effects

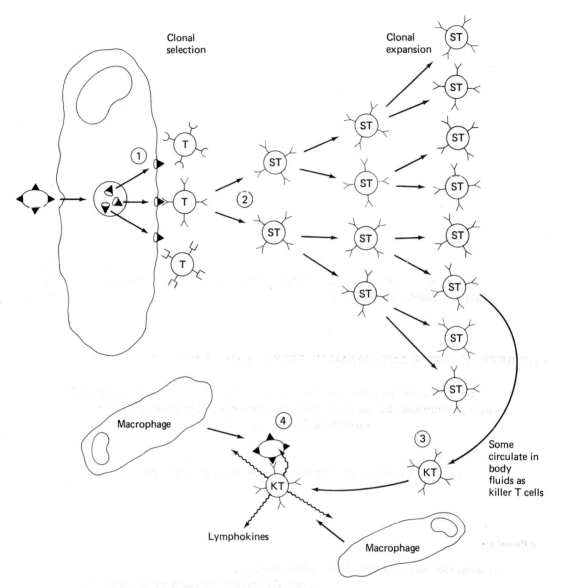

Figure 12-5 Induction of the cell-mediated immune resonse. (1) Phagocytosis, processing, and presentation of the antigen to the specific T cell. (2) The selected T cell becomes sensitized (ST) and multiplies (clonal expansion). (3) Killer T cells (KT) circulate in the body fluids. (4) When killer T cells encounter and specifically react with an antigen, lymphokines are released and aid in the destruction of the antigen.

TABLE 12-2   MAJOR LYMPHOKINES RELEASED BY KILLER T CELLS
AND THE RESPONSES THEY MEDIATE

Lymphokine	Response or action
Cytotoxic factor	Kills foreign cells and adjacent host cells
Transfer factor	Stimulates nonsensitized lymphocytes at the site of the antigen to change into sensitized T cells and aid in intensifying the response
Macrophage chemotactic factor	Attracts macrophages to the site of the antigen
Migration-inhibitory factor	Immobilizes macrophages to keep them from leaving the area of the antigen
Macrophage-activating factor	Greatly increases phagocytic activity and the ability of macrophages to kill foreign cells and break down ingested materials

on the growth of some cancer cells and on the multiplication of viruses. Interferon is also produced by cells that are infected with viruses and is an important defense mechanism against viral infections. Interferon will be discussed in more detail in the section on viruses.

HYPERSENSITIVITIES AND HARMFUL EFFECTS OF ANTIBODIES

Sometimes immune responses are harmful to the host because they react against host tissues or stimulate the release of excessive amounts of chemical mediators. Such reactions are referred to as *hypersensitivities* and *allergies.*

These harmful reactions depend on various interacting factors, such as nature and dose of antigen, route of injection, and the physiological conditions of the host. They may involve either the humoral or the cell-mediated immune systems. Still, the more typical allergic reaction involves a different type of an immune response that produces antibodies of the immunoglobulin E class (Figure 12-6).

Allergies

Antigens that induce allergies are called *allergens.* Many different substances are capable of functioning as allergens. Some of the more common allergens are plant pollens, animal hairs, and food. The mechanism of stimulation and formation of IgE is not well understood but appears to be similar to the mechanisms used to produce the other immunoglobulins. Once formed, IgE molecules do not remain free in the circulation but rapidly attach to either mast cells or basophils. This attachment involves the constant region of IgE and is such that the antibody reactive sites of IgE molecules are pointing out from the cells and are still free to react with the antigen. Once this sequence of events occurs, the host is sensitized to the specific allergen. When the

(a) First exposure to allergen

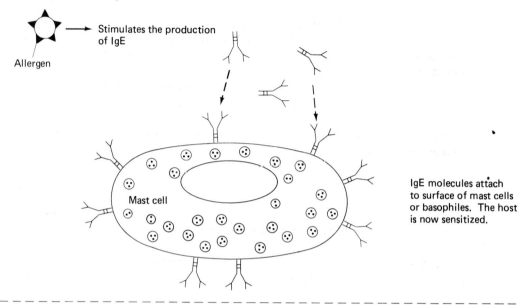

(b) Subsequent exposures
    to the same allergen

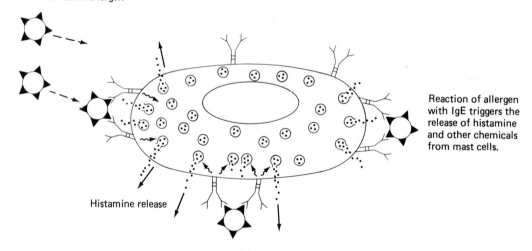

Figure 12-6 An immediate type allergic response. (a) No reaction is seen when IgE is produced and attaches to mast cells by their constant region. (b) Reaction is seen after subsequent exposures to allergen as a result of the release of histamine, etc.

host is subsequently exposed to the allergen, the allergen specifically attaches to the reactive sites of the IgE antibodies that are already attached to the mast cells. This antigen–antibody reaction triggers the release of histamine and other related substances from the mast cells. Histamine has immediate effects on the surrounding tissues, such as dilation and increased permeability of blood vessels, contraction of smooth muscles, and increased mucous secretions. If this reaction occurs along the mucosal lining of the upper respiratory tract, the symptoms are the familiar runny nose, watery eyes, itching, and sneezing of hay fever. If the reaction occurs through contact of allergens with mast cells located in the skin, hives (urticaria) may result. Reactions along the intestinal tract may result in such symptoms as vomiting, abdominal pain, and diarrhea. If the reaction between the allergen and sensitized mast cells or sensitized basophils is of sufficient magnitude, as would occur with the injection of the allergen into the body, systemic anaphylactic shock may occur. This situation involves a massive shift of blood flow from some vital organs and may result in the death of the patient within a few minutes after the injection. An injection of epinephrine may counter the effects of systemic anaphylactic shock.

Allergy testing

Skin testing can be used to determine the type of substance to which a person is allergic. Extracts of suspected allergens are injected intradermally (between the layers of skin) or a drop of the extract is placed on an area of skin that has been lightly scratched. If the person is hypersensitive, an immediate (within minutes) reaction of reddening and swelling will occur at the site of contact with the allergen. Often a person will be tested simultaneously for sensitivity to different allergens by injecting extracts of each into different areas of skin.

Control of allergies

Once the specific allergen is identified, a person can take the necessary precautions to avoid that substance. Food allergies are most easily avoided, but people can also move from a geographic area where an allergen of plant origin is present or can avoid a certain species of animal and so on.

A person may become *desensitized* by receiving injections of extracts of an allergen. When introduced into the deeper tissues by injection, the allergen stimulates the formation of IgG antibodies. These antibodies are then able to react with the allergen on subsequent natural exposures and neutralize its ability to react with the IgE antibodies attached to the mast cells. Thus no allergic reaction occurs.

Perhaps the most popular but least effective method of relieving allergy symptoms is the use of various medications. Antihistamines are widely used and have the direct effect of neutralizing the action of histamine. Other substances that act as decongestants, expectorants, or suppressants of pain and so on may be used in conjunction with antihistamines to bring added symptomatic relief. Corticosteroids may also be effective in treating some allergies but should be used with proper medical discretion, for they have a suppressive effect on the entire immune system and may render the recipient more susceptible to infectious diseases in general.

Delayed Hypersensitivity

Allergies involving cell-mediated immunity occur after exposure to certain types of antigens. Exposure to poison ivy is a familiar example. No visible reaction is seen on first exposure; however, a typical T cell-mediated immune response is stimulated. On subsequent skin contact with poison ivy, the sensitized T cells react with the poison and induce a gradual localized reaction of reddening and swelling that reaches a peak response about two days after exposure.

SUMMARY

1. The acquired immune response results from antigenic stimulation of lymphocytic cells in the body. These lymphocytes are of two general types: B cells and T cells.

2. The humoral immune response is characterized by the production of specific immunoglobulins, called antibodies, produced by B lymphocytes in response to an antigenic stimulus. These antibodies are found in one or more of five classes of immunoglobulins. Each type of immunoglobulin acts uniquely in disease limitation by serving as agglutinins, neutralizing toxins, opsonins, and inhibitors of pathogen attachment.

3. Acquired cell-mediated immunity is largely a function of the T cells. These cells are activated by the presence of antigen so that they fulfill numerous functions in the process of disease control.

4. Some individuals overreact or react in an altered way to the presence of antigen in their environment. Such overactivity is known as hypersensitivity. Hypersensitivity reactions are often damaging to the host and may require considerable effort and expense to control.

Applications of the Immune Responses

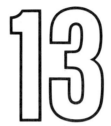

The acquired immunity resulting from the production of circulating antibodies or cell-mediated immunity may offer protection for prolonged periods or even for the lifetime of the host. It is called *active immunity*, for the host actively produces its own antibodies, and it may be stimulated either by natural infections or by artificial exposure to antigens in the form of vaccines.

It is also possible to confer a short-lived immunity by the passive transfer of antibodies from one host to another. This type is called *passive immunity* and occurs naturally when antibodies are passed from mother to offspring or artificially by the injection of antisera.

TYPES OF IMMUNITY

Traditionally the types of antibody-induced acquired immunity are divided into four categories:

1. Natural active immunity
2. Artificial active immunity
3. Natural passive immunity
4. Artificial passive immunity

Natural Active Immunity

This type of antibody immunity develops after recovery from a naturally acquired infectious disease. During the process of the infection large amounts of microbial antigens that stimulate the production of a maximum amount of antibodies are produced. Usually both humoral antibodies and cell-associated immunity are stimulated. These antibodies remain in the body for years. During this time any reexposure to the same pathogen would result in the rapid destruction of the invading microbe. Even if the time between the first exposure and reexposure has been so long that most of the original antibodies have disappeared, the recall or anamnestic response rapidly stimulates the production of new antibodies before the invading microbe is able to cause a serious or even a clinically evident disease. Immunity of this type is more effective against diseases in which the microorganisms must pass through the blood or into deeper tissues compared to infections of such superficial tissues as the respiratory or intestinal mucosa. But even when complete immunity is not maintained, the reinfections are generally much less severe than the original infection. This basic immune response is shown in Figure 12-4.

Artificial Active Immunity

The immune mechanism of the body can be stimulated to produce antibodies when antigens are introduced by artificial means—that is, in the form of a vaccine. The following three general categories of vaccines are used.

Killed vaccines

These vaccines are made by culturing large numbers of a pathogenic microorganism and then subjecting them to treatment by heat or chemicals. When just the right amount of treatment has been given, the components of the microbe that are necessary for multiplication are destroyed, but the antigens are not altered. These killed microbes must be injected into the tissues of the host; there they can be phagocytized by macrophages and passed to the lymphatic tissues, where specific antibodies will be produced. Usually it is not possible to get enough antigen into the tissues with one injection to produce a maximum stimulation of antibodies. Therefore the immunization must be repeated about every other week for a total of three or four injections in order to obtain the maximum antibody stimulation. The effectiveness of this type of vaccine may be enhanced by mixing the killed microbes with such materials as mineral oils or alum. These materials are called *adjuvants* and slow down the clearance of the vaccine from the tissues, thereby providing a longer exposure to the antigen. Generally adjuvants are not used in vaccines for humans, for they may cause some discomfort. Some vaccines use purified fractions of the microbe rather than the entire microbial cells. Several newer vaccines, for example, use only the capsule of the bacteria as the immunizing agent. Such fractionated vaccines help reduce undesirable side reactions caused by endotoxins and other materials found in the intact microbial cells. A new generation of purified antigen vaccines produced by genetic engineering is being developed. Such vaccines will contain only the antigens that stimulate protective antibodies and this factor will help reduce adverse side reactions. This technology is particularly useful in providing purified viral antigens that cannot be produced economically by conventional methods.

The immunity induced by a killed vaccine does not persist as long as the immunity induced by a natural infection. Often the immunity has disappeared or is greatly reduced after several years. Then if a single dose of the vaccine, called a *booster* dose, is given, the anamnestic reaction is stimulated and high levels of antibodies are produced in just a few days. If booster doses are given every few years, an immune state can be maintained continuously.

Toxoid vaccines

Diseases like diphtheria and tetanus are caused by exotoxins and the antibodies formed against the exotoxins, called *antitoxins*, are able to prevent them. Therefore vaccines against such toxin-caused diseases contain inactivated toxins, called *toxoids*, rather than the killed microbial cells. Toxins are converted into toxoids by the addition of chemicals or by exposure to heat. The antibody response to *toxoids* is similar to that produced by killed vaccines in that a series of primary doses and periodic booster doses are needed for maximum and continued protection.

Living attenuated vaccines

Attenuated means weakened or reduced in force. These vaccines contain microorganisms with a low virulence. Under most conditions they produce only a mild or subclinical disease. These attenuated microbes proliferate in the tissue to yield a mass of antigens similar to the amount produced by the natural disease; thus a single dose stimulates a high antibody level that lasts for a prolonged period. In some cases, the living vaccine can be given by a natural route of infection that is easier to administer than by hypodermic injection—for example, the oral administration of the living polio vaccine.

A disadvantage of living vaccines is an occasional mild or even an active infection that may result from the vaccine itself. This factor is of particular concern in persons with defective or suppressed immune mechanisms and such persons should not receive living vaccines. Similarly, pregnant females should avoid receiving living vaccines because the attenuated microbes may cause infection of the developing fetus. The most commonly used vaccines and their recommended administration schedules are listed in Table 13-1.

Natural Passive Immunity

The newborn of many species receive antibodies from their mothers that give them valuable protection during the critical early phase of life. Some mammals, such as calves and pigs, obtain the passed antibodies in a substance called colostrum, which is present in their mother's milk during the first week after delivery. With humans and many other mammals, much of the passive transfer of antibodies occurs across the

TABLE 13-1   CURRENTLY AVAILABLE VACCINES

Vaccine	Type of immunogen		Recommended schedules
Commonly recommended immunizations			
DPT	Diphtheria and Tetanus toxoid with killed *B. pertussis*	P.[a]	3 doses 2, 4, 6 mo
		B.[b]	18 mo, 6 years
Polio	Live attenuated oral, trivalent (types 1, 2, and 3)	P.	2 doses, 2, 4 mo
		B.	14 mo, 6 years
MMR	Live attenuated measles, mumps and rubella	P.	1 dose, 15–18 mo
Influenza	Formalin inactivated virus	P.	All during epidemic years; persons at high risk
		B.	Annual
Immunizations recommended for specified circumstances			
Pneumococcus	Capsular polysaccharide of most common types	P.	Persons over 2 years at high risk
		B.	Unknown
Cholera	Phenol inactivated *Vibrio cholerae*	P.	Travel to cholera area
		B.	6 mo
BCG	Attenuated *Mycobacterium bovis*	P.	Persons at increased risk
		B.	Not recommended
Typhoid	Killed *Salmonella typhi*	P.	Persons at high risk
		B.	3 years
Rabies	Killed attenuated virus	P.	Preexposure, persons at high risk Postexposure, all persons
		B.	Under some conditions
Smallpox	Live attenuated vaccinia virus	P.	Not recommended
Yellow fever	Live attenuated virus	P.	Travel to endemic areas
		B.	10 years
Hepatitis B	Inactivated Dane particles	P.	3 doses, high-risk persons
		B.	Unknown

[a] P = Primary immunization schedule.
[b] B = Booster immunizations.

placental barrier; these are IgG antibodies and at birth the infant has a full complement of the same antibodies found in its mother. The role of colostrum and the passage of antibodies to the infant in human milk are not clearly understood. Some IgA antibodies appear to be passed by this means and may offer protection to the mucosal surfaces of the intestinal tract. Natural passive immunity lasts from 3 to 6 months in humans.

Artificial Passive Immunity

Under certain circumstances a person must receive a supply of antibodies immediately. Here preformed antibodies can be taken from another host and injected into the person needing antibodies. This artificially passed immunity only lasts for several weeks. Before the development of antibiotics, it was a common practice to produce high levels of antibodies in horses or cows, for instance, and then collect their serum and use it as "antiserum" to treat various infectious diseases of humans. Although this procedure had some value, serious side reactions often occurred due to hypersensitivities that developed against the animal serum. Antiserum therapy is still used against some infectious diseases, but it is more effective in treating diseases caused by toxins. Whenever possible, human antiserum, particularly the gamma globulin fraction, is used because it concentrates the antibodies and reduces the chance of hypersensitivity. Antisera effectively treat such diseases as diphtheria, tetanus, and botulism poisoning caused by toxins. In addition, antisera can be produced against various venoms and then used in treating victims of bites by venomous animals. Passive immunity may also be used as a prophylactic (preventative) measure for high-risk persons who may be or have recently been exposed to an infection.

MEASUREMENT OF ANTIBODIES

Role of Antibodies in Diagnosing Diseases

The presence of humoral antibodies in someone's serum indicates that the person has either had a specific disease or has been immunized against that disease. Furthermore, the level of antibodies may give some indication as to how recently this person was exposed to the disease.

An analysis of the levels of specific antibodies present in the serum of a patient is an important diagnostic tool. In diagnosing an infectious disease, it is important to obtain a serum sample from the patient as early as possible, preferably during the first few days of illness. Called the *acute phase* serum, this sample should contain no or only low levels of antibodies against the microorganism causing the disease. Several weeks later a second serum sample should be taken. It is called the *convalescent phase* serum and should contain higher levels of antibodies against the disease-producing microorganisms (Figure 13-1). If the increase in antibody levels between the

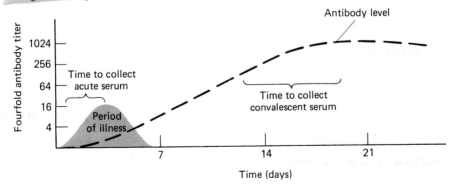

Figure 13-1   The relationship between the period of illness and the time to collect acute and convalescent phase serum samples.

acute and the convalescent phase is significant, usually fourfold or greater, it is assumed that the disease was caused by the microorganism against which the antibodies were formed. Before this diagnostic test can be run, a pathogenic microorganism is needed to serve as the test antigen. Ideally this microorganism is isolated from the patient during the illness. If the signs and symptoms of the disease are compatible with the type of disease caused by the isolated pathogen, the diagnosis of the disease based on this evidence alone is fairly certain. If a specific rise in antibodies occurred against this pathogen, the diagnosis is confirmed. If no specific pathogen was isolated from the patient, however, the signs and symptoms of the disease might be consistent with a disease caused by any one of several different pathogens. Because diagnostic laboratories generally have commercially prepared antigens obtained from the more commonly encountered pathogens, a laboratory could be asked to determine the levels of antibodies in the acute and convalescent phase sera against the suspected pathogens. The pathogen against which a significant rise in antibody level is seen is assumed to cause the disease.

In other situations, it may be desirable to know if a person had previously had a specific disease. A woman in the early stages of pregnancy, for example, may have been exposed to rubella—a disease known to pose a serious threat to the developing fetus should the expectant mother become infected. It would be useful to know if the expectant mother had antibody immunity to rubella. In this case, the serum of the expectant mother could be tested for antibodies against rubella and then the course of action determined. Another application involves the routine blood tests for persons applying for a marriage license in which the serum is checked for antibodies against syphilis. If present, such antibodies indicate that the person may be harboring the syphilis spirochetes. In such cases, proper treatment with penicillin is given to clear up the possible infection.

The analysis of amounts and types of antibodies has many applications in diagnostic medicine, epidemiology, and research work. The study of antigen and antibody reactions in vitro (in test tubes) is called *serology.* Some more commonly used methods of detecting and measuring antibodies and antigens are discussed in the following pages.

SEROLOGIC TESTS

Either a known antigen or a known antibody is needed for most serologic tests. Many routinely used antigens or antibodies (antisera) are available from commercial sources. If a known antigen is used, the serum samples can be tested to determine if they contain specific antibodies against this antigen. On other occasions it may be necessary to identify an unknown antigen. Generally the antigen to be identified is a microorganism that cannot be completely identified by its physiologic or morphologic characteristics. This unknown microorganism is tested against known selected antisera; when specific reactions occur, a specific identification can be made.

The relative amount of antibodies in a serum sample is measured by determining the extent to which the serum can be diluted and still produce an observable antigen–antibody reaction. The term *titer* refers to this relative amount of antibodies. It is common to use either 2, 4, 8, or 10-fold dilutions of serum in determining the antibody titer. If the last tube in which a detectable antigen–antibody reaction occurred was a dilution of 1:256, for instance, then the antibody titer would be reported as 256.

Agglutination Tests

Agglutination tests use whole cells or particles about the size of cells as antigens. When antibodies attach to the antigenic determinants on these cells or particles, they form bridges that result in aggregates of interconnected particles. Such aggregates or agglutinations are visible to the naked eye (Figure 13-2). Agglutination tests are used to detect antibodies against bacterial cells and to determine the types of red blood cells and are also used in various artificially constructed tests. In the artificial tests known antibodies or antigens are attached to small particles of latex or to tanned red blood cells. Such treated particles may then be used in agglutination tests to detect the corresponding antigen or antibody in test specimens.

Precipitation Tests

Precipitation tests use soluble antigens. The interaction of proper ratios of these antigens with specific antibodies results in a fine precipitation reaction. This reaction can best be visualized at the interface of a solution of antibodies and antigens. These tests are carried out in small-diameter tubes in which the antigen is layered over the antiserum. A ring of precipitation will be seen at the interface of the two solutions if specific antibodies and antigens are present. These tests are called *ring tests* and *capillary tube tests* [Figure 13-3(a)].

A convenient and widely used method of demonstrating precipitation reactions is by *immunodiffusion*, a procedure that is also called the *Ouchterlony* method (named after its discoverer). Solutions of specific antigens and antibodies are placed in adjacent wells that are formed in an agar gel. A line of precipitation occurs where the diffusing antigen and antibodies come together. This precipitated antigen–antibody complex becomes fixed in the agar and is readily visualized [Figures 13-3(b) and (c)].

Neutralization Tests

Neutralization tests use living microorganisms that are exposed to antibodies in test tubes. After the antibodies have had a chance to react with the antigens on the microbe—usually for a period of an hour or two—the mixture is inoculated into a suitable experimental host. If the microorganism has reacted with specific antibodies, it

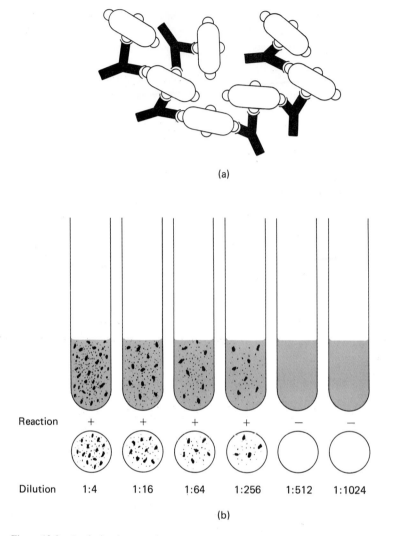

Figure 13-2   Agglutination reactions. (a) Agglutination of bacterial cells by IgG type antibodies. (b) Tube (top) and slide (bottom) agglutination reactions in four-fold dilutions of serum. The reaction is positive through a dilution of 1:256, therefore the titer is 256.

will be unable to multiply in the host; that is, it is neutralized. This test is often used to identify viruses.

Complement Fixation Tests

Earlier it was noted that complement enters into a complex with certain antigen–antibody reactions (p. 172). Once complement has entered into this complex, it is not

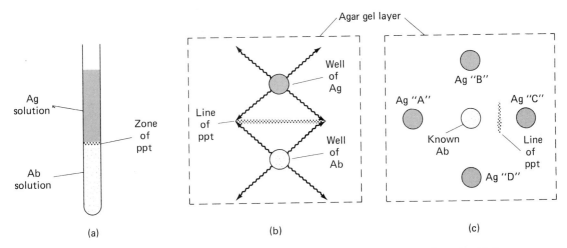

Figure 13-3 Precipitation (ppt.) reactions between antigens (Ag) and antibodies (Ab). (a) A precipitation reaction in a small diameter test tube. (b) Precipitation reaction in an agar gel. (c) Use of the agar gel method to identify unknown antigens that will react with a known antibody; in this case, antigen "C" is identified as the specific antigen.

free to enter into a second reaction; that is, it is fixed. By finding out if the complement has become fixed, it is possible to determine if an antigen–antibody reaction has taken place. The steps of a complement fixation test are outlined in Figure 13-4.

If a serum sample is being analyzed by the complement fixation test for antibodies against a known antigen, it is first heated to 56°C for 30 minutes to destroy any residual complement that might be present. Next, the known antigen and a standard amount of complement are added to the serum. If the serum contained specific antibodies to the antigen, a complex of complement–antigen–antibody would form and the complement would be fixed. This reaction would not be visible. Therefore the next step would be to add an indicator system that would tell if the reaction had occurred. The indicator system uses both a known antigen and a known antiserum. The antigen is sheep red blood cells and the antiserum contains antibodies against the sheep red blood cells. The sheep red blood cells and antiserum are added to the original test system; if a specific reaction had not occurred in the original test, the complement would be available to complex with the indicator system, which would result in the lysis (dissolving) of the red blood cells. This reaction is readily visible. If the sheep red blood cells do not lyse, it is assumed that the original reaction had fixed the complement and so specific antibodies must have been present in the original serum. This is an indirect test for antibodies and adequate controls are needed to show that all components are working properly before any assumption can be made.

Fluorescent Antibody Tests

It is possible to conjugate (attach) certain fluorescent dyes to known antibodies. The antibodies can then be mixed with test microorganisms; if a specific reaction occurs,

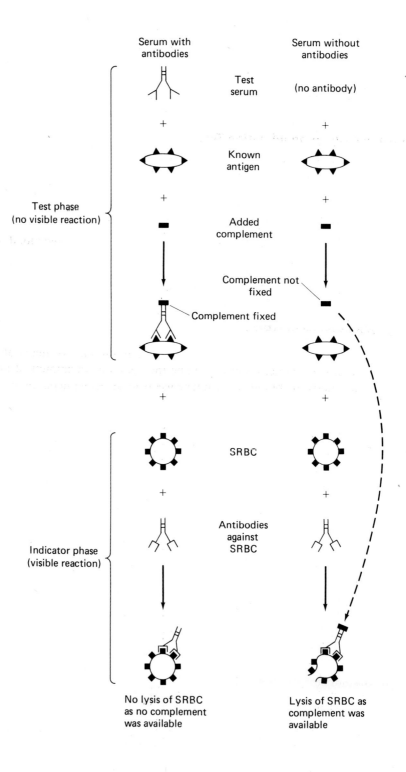

Serum with antibodies   Serum without antibodies

Test serum   (no antibody)

+

Known antigen

+

Added complement

Complement not fixed

Complement fixed

+

SRBC

+

Antibodies against SRBC

Test phase (no visible reaction)

Indicator phase (visible reaction)

No lysis of SRBC as no complement was available   Lysis of SRBC as complement was available the antibodies, along with the fluorescent dye, will attach to the microbial antigens. This reaction is carried out on a microscope slide. When it is placed under a fluorescence microscope (p. 99), the areas where specific antigen–antibody reactions have occurred will fluoresce. Using this method (Figure 13-5), it is possible to identify a specific type of microbe in a mixed microbial population.

Hemagglutination Inhibition Test

These tests, which are relatively simple to conduct, are useful in detecting antibodies against certain types of viral infections. Some viruses specifically attach to red blood cells and cause the cells to agglutinate. This process is called *hemagglutination* and is a useful method for detecting the presence of such viruses. If coated with antibodies, the virus cannot cause hemagglutination. Thus in the hemagglutination inhibition test the serum is reacted with a known virus and then the red blood cells are added. If specific antibodies are present in the serum, they will coat the virus and inhibit the occurrence of hemagglutination. Here if hemagglutination does not occur, the presence of antibodies is indicated.

Radioimmunoassay (RIA)

The RIA is a highly sensitive test that uses radioactive materials to detect small amounts of antigens and determine the quantitative amount of antigen in tissues, body fluids, or blood. Its primary use is in detecting hepatitis B antigens in blood collected for transfusion (Chapter 35). Although a very useful test, it does suffer from certain disadvantages: it is complex, requires expensive equipment, and uses radioactive materials. Specially equipped laboratories are usually required to run this test.

Enzyme-Linked Immunosorbant Assay (ELISA)

The ELISA test is nearly as sensitive as the RIA test, but it does not require radioactive materials and can be done with less elaborate equipment. It can be used to measure the amounts of either antigens or antibodies in a test sample. The procedure for detecting antibodies is shown in Figure 13-6. Here known antigen is absorbed onto the wall of wells in special plastic plates. Then serum to be tested for antibodies is added to the wells. If specific antibodies are present, they will attach to the absorbed antigen; the wells are then rinsed to remove all components of the serum except the

---

Figure 13-4   Complement [▬] fixation test using a known antigen [⟨✛⟩] to test serum for the presence of antibodies [⋏] against this Ag. This test shows the response of serum samples with and without specific Ab. The indicator phase of this test uses sheep red blood cells (SRBC). When complement becomes fixed in the test phase, it is then not available to form a complex with and cause lysis of the SRBC in the indicator phase of the test. Thus no lysis means the test is positive for the presence of antibodies in the original serum.

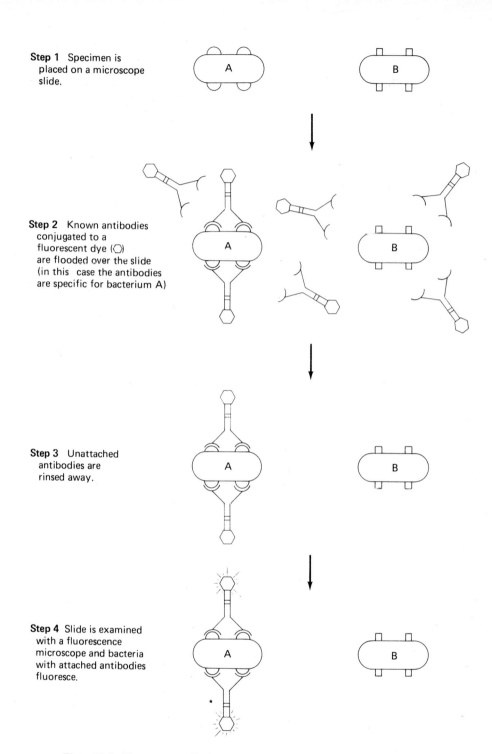

Step 1 Specimen is placed on a microscope slide.

Step 2 Known antibodies conjugated to a fluorescent dye (◯) are flooded over the slide (in this case the antibodies are specific for bacterium A)

Step 3 Unattached antibodies are rinsed away.

Step 4 Slide is examined with a fluorescence microscope and bacteria with attached antibodies fluoresce.

Figure 13-5 Fluorescent antibody procedure for identification of a bacterium in a clinical specimen.

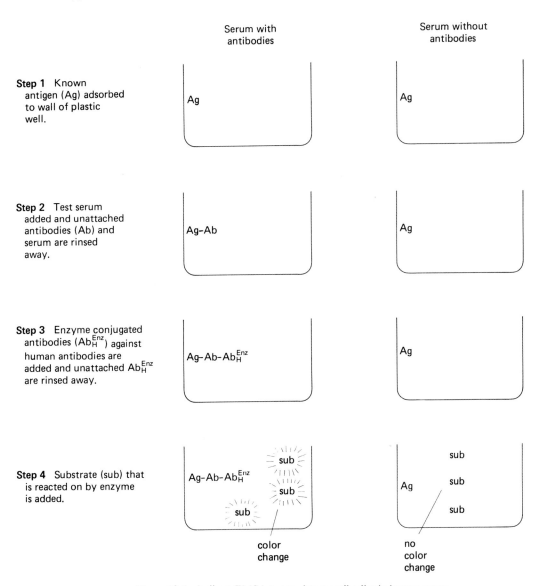

Figure 13-6   Indirect ELISA test to detect antibodies in human serum.

attached antibodies. If the test serum is from humans, the next step would be to add specially prepared antibodies against human gamma globulin; these antibodies are produced in an animal like a goat or rabbit. The antihuman antibodies are conjugated to an enzyme. These conjugated antibodies will react with the human antibodies that are attached to the absorbed antigen. The wells are again rinsed to remove any unattached enzyme-conjugated antibodies. Next, a substrate is added that will be acted on by the enzyme in such a way that a color is produced. The intensity of the color can be measured by a spectrophotometer or, less accurately, by the eye and is proportional to the amount of antibody that attached to the antigen. When all reagents are prepared, the ELISA test can be carried out in less than one hour. This test is very useful in applications where a rapid detection of antigens or antibodies is needed and it is adaptable to most routine serologic tests.

MONOCLONAL ANTIBODIES

Monoclonal antibodies are preparations of antibodies that are all specific for the same antigenic determinant. Such pure antibody preparations have many useful applications in various areas of medicine and research. It is not possible to produce preparations of pure antibodies in intact animals, for animals are invariably exposed to a variety of antigens and most antigens contain a variety of antigenic determinants. Thus their serum will always contain a mixture of antibodies. Monoclonal antibodies are produced by cells growing in test tube (in vitro) cultures, using a unique procedure developed in the mid-1970s at Britain's Medical Research Council by Milstein and Köhler. These researchers were able to fuse two types of cells together into a single cell called a *hybridoma*. The hybridoma cells are able to express properties of both parent cells. The two cells used to make monoclonal antibodies are a mouse tumor cell, called a *myeloma cell*, and an activated B cell from the spleen of an immunized mouse. The myeloma cell has the ability to grow indefinitely in a test tube but is not able to produce specific antibodies. The activated B cell can produce specific antibodies against a single antigenic determinant but cannot grow in a test tube; however, the myeloma-B cell hybridoma is able to grow indefinitely in test tubes and to produce antibodies. Once a hybridoma that is secreting antibodies against a known antigen is produced, massive cultures of this cell can be propagated and will, in turn, produce large amounts of the pure or monoclonal antibody. Often it is necessary to screen many hybridoma cells to find the one that is producing the desired specific antibody (Figure 13-7).

Because of their specificity for a single antigenic determinant, reactions between monoclonal antibodies and antigens are much more precise than those produced from the antisera of intact animals. Thus monoclonal antibodies are widely used in diagnostic kits to identify isolated microorganisms or detect antigens. Monoclonal antibodies are also useful for specific antiserum therapy against infectious diseases, toxins, and possibly some forms of cancer. In some applications, monoclonal antibodies are attached to specific drugs; when injected into a patient, the antibodies specifically attach to the pathogen or target tissue, which concentrates the effect of the drug against the target and minimizes its effect on normal tissues. Monoclonal antibodies are used in research work in which specific identification of components can be made by immune reactions. They are also used as "handles" to pluck a given substance specifically out of a mixture of chemicals. Today monoclonal antibody procedures are being applied in many areas of medicine, research, and industry and represent a highly useful new technology.

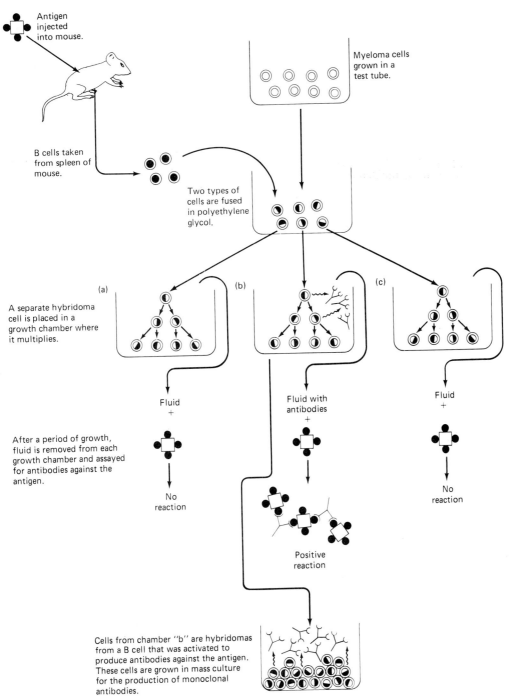

Antigen injected into mouse.

Myeloma cells grown in a test tube.

B cells taken from spleen of mouse.

Two types of cells are fused in polyethylene glycol.

(a)

(b)

(c)

A separate hybridoma cell is placed in a growth chamber where it multiplies.

After a period of growth, fluid is removed from each growth chamber and assayed for antibodies against the antigen.

Fluid +

Fluid with antibodies +

Fluid +

No reaction

No reaction

Positive reaction

Cells from chamber "b" are hybridomas from a B cell that was activated to produce antibodies against the antigen. These cells are grown in mass culture for the production of monoclonal antibodies.

Figure 13-7 A schematic outline of a method used to produce monoclonal antibodies.

SUMMARY

1. Several types of immunity are known and can generally be classified as either active or passive forms of immunity. Active immunity is the result of the individual's own production of antibody whereas passive immunity is based on the receipt of antibody produced by some other human or animal.

2. Numerous types of vaccine can be used to stimulate active immunity in humans. These vaccines depend on the presence of complete antigens found in the normal unaltered pathogen. The degree of immunity and the length of the immune state depend on the kind of vaccine used and the type of immunity made available.

3. The presence of antibody is determined by laboratory procedures known collectively as serology. There are many serologic tests. These tests are useful in determining the degree of immunity maintained by an individual. They are also helpful in determining the presence or absence of some disease states.

Introduction to Infectious Diseases

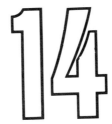

The various defense mechanisms of the host were described in preceding chapters. When functioning properly, these mechanisms are important in determining the outcome of the interactions between pathogenic microorganisms and the host. Some mechanisms that allow certain microorganisms to overcome or circumvent these defense mechanisms and then cause tissue damage are discussed in this chapter. The methods used to determine if a specific microbe is the cause of a disease are also discussed and an introduction to the methods used here for presenting the various infectious diseases of humans is given.

MICROBIAL PATHOGENICITY AND VIRULENCE

A great majority of the microorganisms found in nature are unable to grow in the human body and so cannot produce disease; they are the saprophytic microbes. Some microbes, however, possess mechanisms that enable them to produce disease; they are the pathogens. Some microbes cause diseases indirectly by producing toxins (poisons). These toxins may be in foods that are eaten by the host. Most microbial diseases are categorized as *communicable*, or *infectious*, which means that the microbe itself must be transmitted to the host. The source of the microbe may be another host or some nonliving reservoir. In order to be a successful pathogen of a communicable disease, a microorganism must be able to:

1. Survive passage from one host to another or from the reservoir to the host

2. Attach to or penetrate into the host's tissues
3. Withstand for a period of time the host's defense mechanisms
4. Induce damage to or malfunction of the host's tissues

Microbial *pathogenicity* (the disease-producing capabilities of a microbe) is a result of the functioning of one or more of the mechanisms discussed in the following pages. Microbes that vary in their ability to cause disease exist. Those with strong capabilities are highly virulent whereas those with weak capabilities are pathogens of low virulence.

In some cases, the mechanisms of pathogenicity and virulence possessed by a pathogen are well characterized; at other times the processes by which a microbe causes disease are not well understood. The known and postulated general mechanisms of pathogenicity and virulence are discussed next. Table 14-1 lists the bacterial virulence factors commonly found in organisms causing infectious disease.

Attachment

In order to infect a host, most microbes must first attach to a specific receptor site on a tissue of the host. Most microbes that lack the chemical groups that take part in this specific attachment are flushed or otherwise expelled from the body. This specificity, which is also called *trophism*, is determined by traits of both the host and the pathogen. The specificity of receptor sites may vary from organ to organ within the body of the host and from one host species to another. Thus one infectious disease may involve only specific tissues or organs of the body whereas another disease may involve different tissues. Similarly, some animal species are highly susceptible to a given pathogen whereas another species is completely refractory to that same pathogen. The significance of specific attachment sites for the initiation of viral infections has been

TABLE 14-1 SOME BACTERIAL VIRULENCE FACTORS

Virulence factor	Characteristics	Bacteria or example
Toxin	Endotoxin, lipopolysaccharide gram-negative cell wall, heat-stable, pyogenic	Gram-negative bacteria
	Exotoxin, polypeptide, antigenic highly toxic, toxoids formed	Diphtheria toxin Staphylococcal enterotoxin Tetanus neurotoxin
Enzyme	Protein, specific activity	Collagenase-Clostridium Coagulase-Staphylococci Hyaluronidase-Streptococci
Capsule	Polysaccharide or polypeptide, antiphagocytic	*Haemophilus influenzae* *Streptococcus pneumoniae* *Bacillus anthracis*
Pili/Fimbriae	Attachment to host cells	*Neisseria gonorrhoeae*

recognized for many years. Today it is recognized that specific tissue attachment is also important for the initiation of many bacterial infections.

Circumventing Defense Mechanisms

Various mechanisms present in some bacteria increase their survival time in the host. One such mechanism is the ability to decrease the rate at which pathogens are phagocytized. Many bacteria possess *capsules* that block the attachment of the bacterial cell to the phagocytic cell and thus interfere with phagocytosis; some pathogenic strains of staphylococci and streptococci secrete a substance called *leukocidin* that kills white blood cells before they can phagocytize the bacteria. Certain microbes are readily phagocytized but are able to withstand the destructive mechanisms functioning in nonstimulated macrophages. These microbes survive and may continue to multiply while inside the phagocyte. They may also be transported by the phagocyte to other tissues while being protected from antibodies and other antimicrobial substances in the body fluids.

An enzyme called *hyaluronidase* that breaks down hyaluronic acid is secreted by some pathogens and may aid the spread of the bacteria between cells of a tissue. Hyaluronic acid is a substance that binds host cells together. Some bacteria possess enzymes called *fibrinolysins* that dissolve the fibrin clots that form part of the barrier of the inflammatory response. Such bacteria are less readily contained by the inflammatory reaction.

Most strains of *Staphylococcus aureus* possess a surface protein called *protein A*. Protein A interacts with the constant region of IgG molecules that points the reactive variable ends of the antibody molecules away from the bacterium, thereby minimizing the effects of antibody immunity against staphylococci.

Induction of Tissue Damage or Malfunction

Inflammation

Certain bacteria stimulate vigorous inflammatory responses that, in turn, alter the function of or destroy the normal host tissues. *Streptococcus pneumoniae*, for example, a major cause of bacterial pneumonia, induces an acute inflammatory response in the lungs that results in a rapid accumulation of fluid exudate. These fluids interfere with the normal functions of the lungs. The tubercle bacillus induces a strong cell-mediated immune response that results in the formation of nodules of scar tissue and eventually causes the destruction of normal lung tissue.

Enzymes

Various enzymes secreted by certain pathogenic bacteria are thought to contribute to the disease process by destroying tissues. *Collagenase* and *lecithinase* are enzymes produced by the bacteria that cause gas gangrene. These enzymes break down tissue fibers and cell membranes and probably contribute to the cell destruction associated with gangrene. *Hemolysins* are enzymes that destroy red blood cells. They are produced by several different pathogenic bacteria. Their direct contribution, if any, to pathogenicity is not known, however. *Lipases* and *nucleases* are bacterial enzymes that break down fats and nucleic acids; their roles, if any, in disease processes are not known.

Toxins

Some microbes produce toxins that are important mechanisms in the production of diseases. There are two general categories of toxins, *exotoxins* and *endotoxins*. Exotoxins are usually secreted from the bacterial cell into the surrounding medium. Endotoxins are part of the cell wall and only small amounts may escape into surrounding fluids from living bacteria. Greater amounts are released only when the bacteria die and their cell walls disintegrate. The two types of toxins differ markedly in potency and functions.

Exotoxins are proteins and are extremely powerful. The botulism food-poisoning toxin is the most powerful chemical toxin known. It has been estimated that 1 mg of purified tetanus toxin could kill 100 million mice. The action of exotoxins on the host is highly specific, often involving a single essential chemical reaction in the host's tissues. Examples of this specificity are the botulism and tetanus toxins that specifically interfere with the transmission of nerve impulses and the diphtheria toxin that specifically inhibits protein synthesis by preventing the elongation of the polypeptide chain during the process of translation. The actions of the exotoxins are covered in greater detail later in this text when the specific toxin diseases are discussed. The exotoxins can be converted into toxoids that are used as vaccines to stimulate specific antitoxin immunity against the toxin. These antitoxins readily neutralize the toxins and play an important role in recovery, treatment, and immunity against diseases caused by exotoxins. Fortunately, most exotoxins are readily destroyed by heat, an important factor in reducing the number of outbreaks of food poisoning.

Endotoxins possess characteristics that differ considerably from those of the exotoxins. Endotoxins are less potent and larger amounts are needed to induce disease symptoms. Their effects on the host are general and produce such clinical signs and symptoms as fever, diarrhea, and circulatory disturbances, including shock. Endotoxins are composed of complexes of proteins, polysaccharides, and phospholipids. They cannot be converted into toxoids and are highly resistant to inactivation by heat. The endotoxins are found primarily in the cell walls of gram-negative bacteria whereas exotoxins are produced by both gram-positive and gram-negative bacteria.

Exotoxins can cause disease even when the producing bacterium is restricted to a relatively superficial tissue, such as mucosal epithelium. Or, as in the case of food poisoning, exotoxin production may occur remote from the host. In contrast, endotoxins generally affect the host when they are released following the death and destruction of large numbers of gram-negative bacilli that may be infecting the tis-

TABLE 14-2 COMPARISON OF CHARACTERISTICS
OF EXOTOXINS AND ENDOTOXINS

Characteristics	Exotoxins	Endotoxins
Potency	High	Low
Effects on cells	Specific	Nonspecific
Stability to heat	Labile (inactivated at 60° to 80° C)	Stable (resists 120° C for 1 hr)
Forms toxoids	Yes	No
Composition	Proteins	Protein lipopolysaccharide complexes

sues. Endotoxins undoubtedly contribute significantly to the pathogenesis of many diseases caused by gram-negative bacteria. It is possible to produce some disease symptoms in a host by injecting endotoxins. Occasionally endotoxin-contaminated intravenous fluids have inadvertently been infused into a patient, resulting in serious reactions, including shock. This situation can even occur in fluids that have been sterilized in an autoclave, for endotoxins are not readily destroyed by heat. Exotoxin and endotoxin characteristics are summarized in Table 14-2.

DETERMINING THE ETIOLOGIC AGENT

The mere presence of a microorganism in a lesion or diseased tissue is not sufficient to prove that this microbe is the cause (the etiologic agent) of the disease. This problem was recognized early in the study of infectious diseases by Robert Koch, who developed criteria to be used to incriminate a suspected microbe as the etiologic agent of a given disease. These criteria, known as *Koch's postulates*, are as follows:

1. The suspected microorganism must be found routinely in hosts with the disease.
2. The microorganism must be isolated from the host and grown in pure culture.
3. When microbes from the pure culture are inoculated into a healthy susceptible host, they must be able to cause the same disease.
4. The microorganism must next be recovered from the experimentally infected host.

Koch's postulates have served as useful criteria in establishing the etiologic agents of many more distinct infectious diseases. Nevertheless, the etiological role of certain microbes in many more subtle diseases—particularly those caused by the synergistic reaction of several microbes or factors and those produced in compromised hosts by opportunist microbes—has not been as readily demonstrated by these criteria.

A STUDY OF INFECTIOUS DISEASES

The following chapters present an overall view of many diseases of humans that are caused by microorganisms. The various diseases are discussed according to the taxonomic categories of the causative microorganism. It is felt that this approach provides a concise coverage of the subject. Diseases caused by bacteria are described first, followed by fungal, protozoal, and viral diseases. The section on bacterial diseases starts with diseases caused by the gram-positive cocci, followed by the diseases caused by gram-negative cocci, spirochetes, acid-fast bacilli, and gram-positive and gram-negative bacilli. DNA-containing viruses appear first in the section on viral diseases and are followed by the RNA-containing viruses. In the following discussions of infectious diseases emphasis is given to the clinical characteristics, mechanisms of disease production (pathogenesis), and modes of transmission, treatment, and prevention—that is, those concepts of greatest concern to paramedical personnel who are directly involved in patient care. Less emphasis is given to the detailed methods used by microbiologists in the diagnostic laboratory.

Each of the following chapters covers the diseases caused by a single genus or by a group of related microorganisms. The coverage of most diseases includes the following general sections:

1. *Causative microbe.* This section contains a brief description of some general morphological and physiological properties of the microorganisms, along with information on classification when appropriate.

2. *Pathogenesis and clinical diseases.* This section includes a discussion of the mechanisms whereby the microbe is able to cause diseases and the types of clinical diseases resulting from the infection.

3. *Transmission and epidemiology.* In this section the mode of transmission and the relationship of various factors in influencing the distribution and frequency of diseases in various human populations are discussed.

4. *Diagnosis.* This section describes the general procedures used to identify a given disease in a patient.

5. *Treatment.* The responses of the infection to the various chemotherapeutic agents, antitoxins, or other medications are discussed here.

6. *Prevention and control.* This section describes the various methods used to prevent or reduce the amount of contact with infectious agents. The use of vaccines and preventative (prophylactic) treatments where applicable is also discussed.

7. *Clinical notes.* Following the discussion of many diseases, a report on an actual occurrence of that disease is given. These reports are taken from the U.S. Department of Health, Education and Welfare/Public Health Service publication called the *Morbidity and Mortality Weekly Report* (MMWR). This document is published weekly by the Centers for Disease Control (CDC) in Atlanta, Georgia. Along with the selected case reports, MMWR gives a weekly update

on the rate of various diseases in the different states. The clinical notes presented in this textbook were selected to demonstrate current problems encountered with infectious diseases. They are also selected to help amplify and show applications of some concepts related to the epidemiology, treatment, diagnosis, or control of these diseases. In some cases, the reports have been modified from the original in order to make them more understandable to the introductory student or simply to reduce their length.

SUMMARY

1. Characteristics that endow a microorganism with virulence and facilitate its survival in the host, leading to pathogenicity, are those characteristics that permit the organism to withstand the host defenses, maintain residence in the host, and produce factors damaging to host tissue.
2. Bacterial virulence factors include the production of exotoxins, endotoxins, and enzymes. These substances circumvent the host defense mechanisms and produce tissue damage, resulting in disease.
3. The application of Koch's postulates has resulted in the determination of the etiology of infectious diseases.

Staphylococci

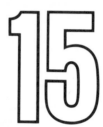

Pathogenic staphylococci are frequently present on the skin or mucous membranes of humans. Generally they act as opportunists, causing infections in damaged tissues. Hospital-acquired staphylococcal diseases are recognized as a major problem and the prevention and control of these infections depend on the combined efforts of all hospital personnel.

STAPHYLOCOCCAL DISEASES

Bacteria

The spherical-shaped bacterium called *Staphylococcus aureus* is the causative agent of a wide variety of human infections. Many strains, with varying degrees of virulence, exist and are frequently carried on the skin, in the nose, and around the rectum of healthy persons. These bacterial cells usually occur in grapelike clusters, a characteristic that provided the basis for their name (*staphyle* in Greek means a bunch of grapes). This bacterium is gram positive and nonspore forming and some strains have notable capsules. Blood agar is the medium generally used for its isolation from infected tissues; however, most common media will support its growth. *S. aureus* produces round, raised, opaque colonies that usually have a golden-yellow (aureus) color. The morphology of staphylococci is shown in Figure 15-1. *S. aureus* are differentiated from other staphylococci by their ability to clot plasma; this is caused by the secretion of an enzyme called *coagulase*. Staphylococci that do not secrete coagulase

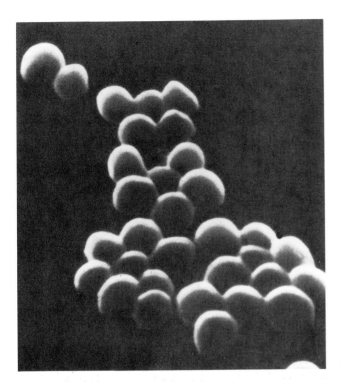

Figure 15-1 Scanning electron micrograph of a staphylococcus showing the characteristic cluster arrangement (magnification 8000×). (A. S. Klainer and I Gies, *Agents of Bacterial Disease.* Harper & Row: Hagerstown, MD, 1973. Figure 12a, p. 18.)

are of very low virulence and are currently classified into several species. The most ubiquitous coagulase negative species is *S. epidermidis* that is a common contaminant on human skin.

Several features contribute to the difficulty often encountered in controlling and treating staphylococcal infections. First, *S. aureus* is widespread, being found on the tissues of many healthy individuals (from 30 to 50% of the population at any given time). Secondly, it is very stable, surviving for months when dried in pus or other body fluids, and it is more resistant to common disinfectants than most other vegetative bacteria. Also, genetic traits are readily transferred between strains of *S. aureus* by plasmids and phages (Chapter 5), which has led to the emergence of many strains that are resistant to commonly used antibiotics.

Pathogenesis and Clinical Diseases

Although most strains of *S. aureus* are of relatively low virulence and usually harmless when restricted to the superficial layers of intact skin, they are often able to cause infection once they gain entry into damaged skin or deeper body tissues. The pathogenicity of *S. aureus* appears to be associated with the production of various enzymes and toxins and includes such substances as hemolysins, coagulase, leukocidin, hyaluronidase, and a fibrinolysin. Some *S. aureus* secrete a toxin called *exfoliatin* that causes the peeling of superficial skin layers of infected persons. About 50% of the strains of *S. aureus* may secrete enterotoxins that cause acute intestinal symptoms (food poisoning) when ingested in contaminated foods. The presence of protein A on virulent staphylococci may protect them from antibodies. The sites of the major staphylococcal infections of humans are shown in Figure 15-2.

Superficial infections
Even though staphylococci are able to infect all tissues of the body, the most common infections are of the superficial tissues. *S. aureus* is a common cause of boils, carbuncles, impetigo (Figure 15-3), and infections of surgical or accidental wounds and burns. Characteristically these infections form an abscess; a localized lesion with a cavity of destroyed (necrotic) tissue filled with pus (suppuration). Scar tissue forms on healing.

Systemic infections
Various forms of trauma resulting around a superficial abscess, such as squeezing a boil, may force large numbers of staphylococci into the blood where they are carried to many tissues of the body. If this situation occurs, the body's natural defenses may not be able to cope with the bacteria and abscesses may develop in various tissues. The presence of bacteria in the blood is called bacteremia or, more commonly, blood poisoning. *S. aureus* may settle in the lungs to cause pneumonia or in the pelvis of the kidneys to cause pyelonephritis. In young children the staphylococci have a tendency to infect the bone, causing osteomyelitis. When staphylococci infect the heart chambers or valves, the disease is called endocarditis. When they infect the meningeal tissues that line the central nervous system, it is called meningitis, and so on.

Toxic-shock syndrome and scalded skin syndrome
Toxic-shock syndrome usually begins suddenly with high fever, vomiting, and diarrhea. In some cases, sore throat, headache, muscle aches, shock, kidney failure, and a red skin rash may be seen. Death may result without prompt supportive treatment. This syndrome was first recognized when a sharp increase in the number of cases was reported in the late 1970s and 1980. Intensive epidemiologic studies demonstrated that most cases occurred in females during their menstrual period and that most were associated with the use of superabsorbent tampons. Staphylococci that produced exfoliatin were found in high concentrations in the vaginal canal of affected females. It is now theorized that the introduction of superabsorbent tampons in the late 1970s created a condition in a small percentage of users that permitted the excessive growth of exfoliatin-producing staphylococci. Once this association was recognized, the use of such tampons was discouraged and the number of cases of toxic-shock syndrome greatly decreased (Figure 15-4). The organisms involved are characteristic of other staphylococci but are also noted to have slower growth rates and to produce small

A Tissues where *S. Aureus*
   are often found but do not
   normally cause disease

Diseases that may be caused by
S. Aureus are:
B Pimples and impetigo
C Boils and carbuncles
   on any surface area
D Wound infections and
   abscesses
E Spread to lymph nodes and to
   blood (septicemia), resulting
   in widespread seeding
F Osteomyelitis
G Endocarditis
H Meningitis
I Enteritis and enterotoxin
   (food poisoning)
J Nephritis
K Respiratory infections:
   Pharyngitis
   Laryngitis
   Bronchitis
   Pneumonia

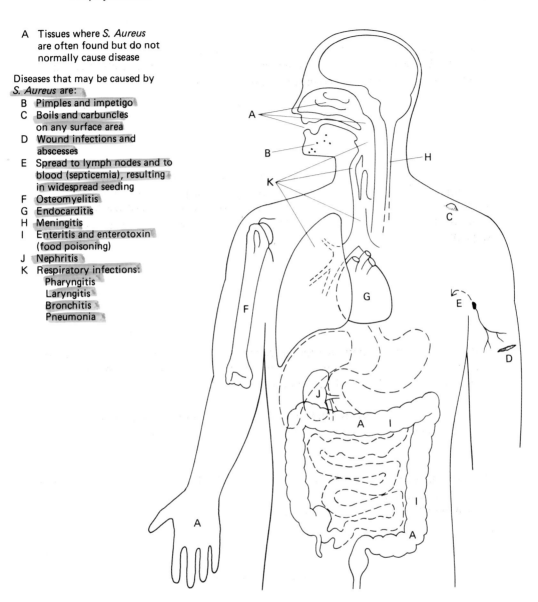

Figure 15-2 The sites of the major staphylococcal infections of humans.

colonies. Infections of infants or young children with exfoliatin-producing strains of *S. aureus* may cause a condition termed *scalded skin syndrome*. Wide areas of skin become denuded and have the appearance of scalded skin; this syndrome may be fatal.

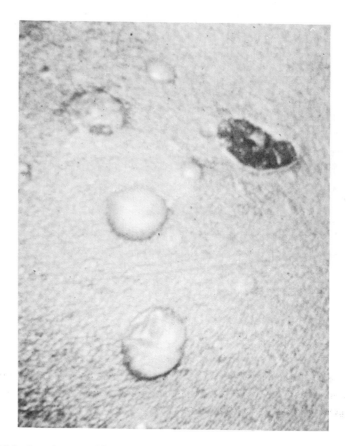

Figure 15-3 Impetigo caused by a staphylococcus. This is an infection of the skin most often occurring in children. (Centers for Disease Control, Atlanta)

S. epidermidis may cause minor skin abscesses and in compromised surgical patients with implanted prosthetic devices (artificial body parts) it may cause troublesome infections.

Food poisoning

This is not an infection but an intoxication resulting from the ingestion of food containing preformed staphylococcal enterotoxin. During the preparation of foods it is very easy for the food handler to seed the food with staphylococci from his nose or from a skin lesion. If this food is not properly cooled and refrigerated at 4°C, the staphylococci may multiply and release enterotoxin. Enough enterotoxin may be produced in 2 to 6 hours to cause severe symptoms. Foods that are not cooked after preparation—for example, potato salads and cream pies—are common sources of this type of food poisoning. This toxin is fairly stable to heat and is not destroyed in

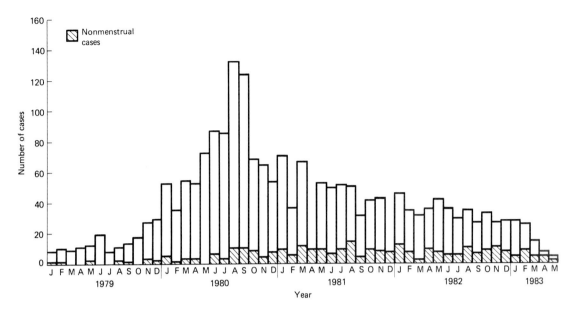

Figure 15-4 Reported cases of toxic-shock syndrome in the United States, 1979 to mid-1983.

foods that are cooked at moderate temperatures after the toxin has been formed. Such symptoms as severe nausea, vomiting, abdominal pain, diarrhea, and prostration may begin to occur as early as 2 hours after ingesting the toxin. Complete recovery generally occurs within a day or two.

Transmission and Epidemiology

Because humans are intermittent carriers of *S. aureus*, sources of infections are often difficult to determine. In many cases, the source may be autogenous; that is, it originates with the patient. A burn on the hand, for example, could become infected from bacteria carried on the patient's own skin or in his nose. Spreading from person to person may occur by direct or indirect contact. Medical personnel who work with patients with staphylococcal infections must use good aseptic procedures to avoid transmitting staphylococci to other patients. Nurses or physicians who are carriers or who have skin lesions may unwittingly infect patients. Care must be taken that the hands of medical personnel or that contaminated instruments do not spread *S. aureus* from one patient to another.

Because many strains of staphylococci are widespread, specific identification methods are needed to distinguish between strains when tracing the route of transmission of an infection. A laboratory procedure called *phage typing* is used to make this distinction (Figure 15-5). Phages are viruses that attack and destroy only specific host

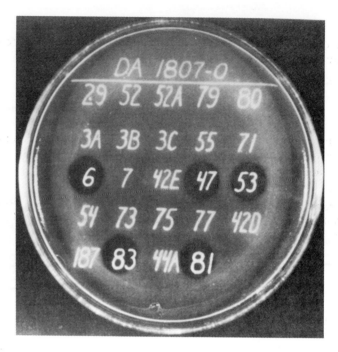

Figure 15-5 Phage typing of *Staphylococcus aureus*. The agar plate was first inoculated with a pure culture of *S. aureus* so as to form a complete layer of bacteria. A suspension of each test phage was dropped on its designated location (indicated by number). Clearing resulted where the phage destroyed the bacterium. In this example, the test bacterium was susceptible to phages 6, 47, 53, 81, and 83. (Centers for Disease Control, Atlanta)

strains of bacteria (Chapter 31). By using a series of staphylococcal phages against the staphylococci isolated from a given environment, it is possible to determine which staphylococci are identical to or different from the strain isolated from a lesion or from foods because different strains have different patterns of resistance and susceptibility to different phages used. (See following clinical notes.)

Diagnosis

Diagnosis is generally based on the isolation of *S. aureus* from a lesion. *S. aureus* on blood agar plates will produce a zone of hemolysis around its typically golden-yellow colony. The pathogenic strains of *S. aureus* are coagulase positive. These characteristics of *S. aureus*, along with its ability to ferment mannitol, are used to differentiate it from the ever-present *S. epidermidis*. Some *S. aureus* produce white colonies; thus colony pigmentation is not a dependable characteristic for identifying this bacterium.

Treatment

More than any other bacterium, the *S. aureus* has the ability to develop resistance against chemotherapeutic agents. During the 1950s most hospitals and hospital personnel became colonized with strains that had developed resistance to penicillin. New antibiotics have since been developed and are still relatively effective. Emergence of resistant strains against these new antibiotics has been slowed by avoiding abuses in antibiotic therapy (see Chapter 9). When treating staphylococcal infections, the most effective antimicrobial agents should first be determined by sensitivity testing and then vigorously administered until the infection is cured.

Abscesses should be drained, when possible, to remove inflammatory debris that may block the diffusion of antimicrobial agents to the site of the bacteria. Also, drainage may remove an environmental niche where the staphylococci are in a metabolically inactive stage and would thus not be affected by the chemotherapeutic agent.

Control and Prevention

Most individuals seem to develop antibodies against staphylococci early in life. These antibodies may contribute substantially to the resistance that most healthy individuals have against this bacterium; however, in injured tissues or in compromised patients this immunity is often not sufficient to prevent infection. No successful vaccines are available against *S. aureus*.

Prevention of staphylococcal infection is primarily a function of good aseptic techniques in hospitals and clinics where both infectious and susceptible patients congregate. Methods must be used to minimize the spread of microorganisms in critical areas. First, patients with open infected wounds should be isolated. Secondly, personnel who work in critical areas, such as operating rooms or newborn nurseries, should be screened to determine if they are carriers of drug-resistant strains. Those who are carriers should be restricted from these areas until their condition is cleared up. Any type of infected lesion on hospital personnel should be promptly treated and precaution should be taken to protect patients from infection from this source.

The newborn nursery presents special problems in that about 90% of infants become carriers of *S. aureus* during the first 10 days of life. It is important that they do not become colonized with the virulent drug-resistant strains prevalent in hospitals. Skin disinfectants, especially hexachlorophene, are useful in decreasing the staphylococcal carrier rate in infants. The practice of immersing (bathing) newborns in hexachlorophene solutions has been discontinued to reduce the chance of any toxic reaction (p. 118), but discrete washing of the skin with this disinfectant is appropriate and effective. In some cases, it has been beneficial to colonize infants on purpose with a nonvirulent strain of *S. aureus*. This step seems to interfere with subsequent colonization by virulent strains.

Air-handling systems should be designed to carry patient-generated airborne bacteria away from other patients or hospital personnel and to prevent any recirculation of these microorganisms to other areas of the hospital.

Staphylococcus aureus Bacteremia

An analysis of the 140 reports of bacteremia due to *Staphylococcus aureus* received in the first three months of 1975, by the public health laboratory in Great Britain, illustrates both the severity of the infection (16% of the reports concerned patients who died) and the variety of clinical conditions with which it is associated. The infections were distributed among all age groups, and the greatest number of patients, 26, presented with fever of unknown origin, of clinical septicemia with no apparent source of infection; such patients appear to be at particular risk since 7 (27%) died. Twenty-two (16%) of the patients were children and no deaths were reported. A further 20 patients (14%)—7 of whom were children—had septic arthritis; one of these patients, a 65-year-old man, died.

Infected blood clots in blood vessels resulted in bacteremia in 16 patients, of whom 11 had infected intravenous catheter sites and 4 were heroin addicts. The 13 postoperative cases were mostly secondary to surgical wound infection and included 1 fatality. Staphylococcal infection was believed to have contributed to the 3 reported deaths among 11 patients with cancer or other serious debilitating illness. Bacteremia was secondary to staphylococcal pneumonia in 12 patients; the severity of this condition is reflected in the death of 7 of the 10 patients for whom the outcome was reported. Endocarditis was reported in 8 patients, 3 of whom died; 1 of the 8 patients had an aortic valve prosthesis, but the remaining patients had infections apparently unrelated to cardiac surgery (*MMWR 24*:268, 1975).

Staphylococcal Food Poisoning on a Cruise Ship

In February 1983, an outbreak of staphylococcal food poisoning occurred on a Caribbean cruise ship sailing from the United States. The probable source was cream pastries served during two separate meals.

The overall attack rate of acute gastroenteritis on board, estimated from the 56 passengers who responded to a 10% systematic survey of the 715 passengers, was 32%. Ninety-four percent of patients filling out questionnaires complained of nausea and/or vomiting, 82% reported diarrhea, and 60% reported abdominal cramps. Symptoms usually subsided within 12 hours, although 36% of patients indicated illness lasted at least 2 days. The incubation period ranged from 1 to 8 hours (median 5 hours).

When plotted by time of onset, the number of cases peaked twice, corresponding to meals served 2 days apart. Forty-six (95.8%) of 48 patients and 20 (58.8%) of 34 well passengers ate the cream pastry served for dessert on the evening of February

22 ($p < 0.001$). Seven (70%) of 10 patients and 4 (13.5%) of 30 controls ate a similar pastry item for lunch on February 24 ($p < 0.001$).

Staphylococcus aureus, phage type 85/+, was isolated from the stools of 5 (38.4%) of 13 patients cultured and from none of 9 controls. The same staphylococcal phage type was grown from a perirectal swab, an anterior nares culture, and a swab of a forearm lesion from 3 of the 7 crew members who made pastry. Pastries from the implicated meals were not available for culture because the pastry kitchen routinely disposed of leftovers.

Investigation of the ship's pastry kitchen did not reveal any improper food handling in the preparation of the pastry items. Refrigeration temperatures were adequate, and the food handlers were free of pustular skin lesions. However, because the pastry was prepared in large quantities in several steps by a number of food handlers, opportunities could have existed for the introduction of staphylococci into the pastry, with adequate time for incubation of the enterotoxin.

Editorial note: Although *Staphylococcus* remains the second most common etiologic agent (after *Salmonella*) in foodborne outbreaks in the United States, this is the first well-documented outbreak of staphylococcal food poisoning on a cruise ship sailing from the United States. This outbreak emphasizes the importance of extreme care in adequately refrigerating perishable food items prepared in large kitchens. The elaboration of staphylococcal enterotoxin requires incubation at temperatures above 6.7°C (44°F). The investigation also shows the value of phage typing to support epidemiologic evidence on the probable source of an outbreak, despite the inability to culture the implicated food item (*MMWR 32*:294, 1983).

SUMMARY

1. Staphylococci are ubiquitous gram-positive cocci not infrequently associated with infections of both humans and animals.

2. Of the several species of Staphylococcus, *S. aureus* is the most virulent and most commonly isolated from human infections. This organism is typical of other pyogenic cocci in that infections are characterized by the production of pus.

3. Numerous disease conditions may occur due to the staphylococci, ranging from food poisoning through osteomyelitis and pneumonia to the relatively recently described toxic shock syndrome. Treatment of many of these infections requires surgical intervention along with aggressive antibiotic therapy.

Streptococci

16

Both pathogenic and nonpathogenic species of streptococci are found associated with humans and animals. The pathogenic species produce a wide variety of toxins and cause a wide variety of lesions and diseases. Historically some streptococcal diseases have been among the most serious diseases of humans. Fortunately, these bacteria are easily destroyed by chemotherapeutic agents. And even though streptococcal infections are still common, today their impact on illness and death is only a small fraction of what it was prior to the 1930s.

Bacteria

Streptococci are gram-positive, coccal-shaped bacteria that usually appear in chains of various lengths. These bacteria are moderately resistant to environmental factors; that is, they may remain living for days to weeks after being expelled from the body. Streptococci are readily killed by common disinfectants and are highly susceptible to a wide range of chemotherapeutic agents, including penicillin. They have not developed widespread resistance to penicillin. Bacterial species of the genus *Streptococcus* are widespread in nature and are part of the normal bacterial flora of the skin, nose, mouth, and mucosal surfaces (including the gut) of humans and animals. It is often difficult to distinguish clearly between many streptococcal species, which has made a precise classification of these bacteria difficult. Streptococci grow well on blood agar plates and many species secrete hemolysins (enzymes that dissolve RBC) that produce different patterns of hemolytic zones around the colonies. These hemolytic patterns are used to make a preliminary identification of streptococcal groups. A clear zone

212

TABLE 16-1 NONGROUP A STREPTOCOCCI THAT CAUSE
DISEASE IN HUMANS

Organisms	Diseases
Group B streptococci	Neonatal meningitis, sepsis
Streptococcus groups C, G	Occasional wound infection, possible rare pharyngitis
Group D—enterococci	Urinary tract infection, bacteremia endocarditis
Viridans streptococci	Endocarditis, rare meningitis or cystitis
Streptococcus pneumoniae	Pneumonia, wound infections, sepsis meningitis

surrounding the colony is called *beta*-hemolysis. A zone with an opaque greenish color is called *alpha*-hemolysis. Some species produce no hemolysis.

The most usable classification system, the Lancefield system, uses differences in carbohydrate antigens located in the cell wall. Under this system streptococci have been divided into 18 major groups, designated A through R. The most important streptococcal infections of humans are caused by the species *Streptococcus pyogenes*, which are mostly of Lancefield group A. Group A can be further subdivided into some 80 types based on differences in an antigen called the *M-protein.* This "M-protein" is important, for it is responsible for virulence; antibodies formed against it give protection to the host. The other groups or categories of streptococci include some species that are also associated with human infections and are listed in Table 16-1. The major emphasis of this chapter is on the diseases caused by *S. pyogenes* with a brief summary of diseases caused by some other streptococci. A bacterium previously called *Diplococcus pneumoniae* has been reclassified as a streptococcus and is now called *Streptococcus pneumoniae*; this bacterium is a major cause of pneumonia and is discussed separately in Chapter 17.

DISEASES CAUSED BY STREPTOCOCCUS PYOGENES

Pathogenesis and Clinical Diseases

Various extracellular and intracellular substances produced by *S. pyogenes* contribute to their ability to withstand the body's defense mechanisms and cause tissue damage. Several more prominent substances and their effects are as follows:

1. *Capsule*, which helps retard phagocytosis
2. "M-protein," which both retards phagocytosis and helps the bacteria adhere to mucosal epithelium
3. *Erythrogenic toxin*, which produces the fever and rash associated with scarlet fever
4. *Streptolysin O* and *streptolysin S*, two separate hemolysins that lysis red blood cells and damage various host cells

5. *Streptokinase*, a fibrinolysin that digests fibrin in the inflammatory barrier

6. *Hyaluronidase*, the spreading factor

In addition, various other cellular substances may also contribute to the pathogenicity and/or virulence of *S. pyogenes*.

The major types of clinical conditions associated with group A streptococci are shown in Figure 16-1 and are discussed next.

Sore throat (pharyngitis)

This disease, referred to as "strep throat," is very common. Children up to 15 years of age average about one infection per year. Each subsequent infection is caused by a different type, for antibody immunity will generally offer protection against repeated infections with the same type for some time. This infection is often mild, but strains vary in virulence and infections with highly virulent bacteria may cause a severe sore throat with fever, headache, swollen cervical lymph nodes, and pussy (purulent) ex-

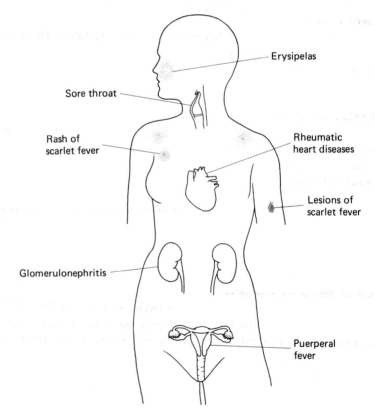

Figure 16-1 Some of the prominent clinical diseases associated with group A streptococcal infections.

udate in the throat. Infections in older children and adults tend to be milder and less frequent, due in part to the antibody immunity that has developed against many strains encountered in earlier childhood. The infection may also spread from the throat directly into the lungs to cause pneumonia or may penetrate into the pleural cavity, causing severe inflammation (pleuritis).

Scarlet fever

Scarlet fever is basically an extension of the sore throat and may result simply from the production of erythrogenic toxin by the streptococci. This toxin diffuses into the blood and is carried to the skin, where it causes a diffuse reddish rash. The more virulent erythrogenic toxin-producing strains are quite invasive and are able to spread through the lymphatic system and into the blood. They may then be carried throughout the body, resulting in infections of the joints, bones, endocardium, skin, and so on. This form of scarlet fever is quite severe and was a common cause of death in the era before penicillin.

Puerperal fever

This disease, also known as childbed fever, is an infection of the uterus that occurs in women shortly after childbirth (postpartum). The streptococci often spread from the inflamed uterus to the blood and the resulting widespread infection may cause death.

Infections of the skin

The *S. pyogenes*, like *Staphylococcus aureus*, are able to cause lesions on the skin where prior injuries, such as insect bites, wounds, and burns, have occurred. Impetigo is commonly caused by streptococci and erysipelas is a specific type of streptococcal skin lesion. Erysipelas usually occurs on the face and probably starts from streptococci coming from the throat or nose and entering a skin abrasion. The lesion spreads outward, causing marked reddening (erythema) and swelling (edema) of the skin with a sharply defined advancing edge. Recovery usually takes a week or longer if no treatment is given. This infection has a tendency in some persons to reoccur periodically at the same site for several years.

Poststreptococcal diseases

The poststreptococcal diseases are *glomerulonephritis* and *rheumatic fever*, which have their onset from 1 to 4 weeks after an acute streptococcal infection. Today these two diseases are the most serious problems associated with streptococcal infections. From 1 to 4% of the children in the United States develop rheumatic fever. In spite of much research, the mechanisms and pathogenesis of these diseases are not well understood. Some evidence indicates that they are immune complex diseases, which means that there is an interaction between antibodies and tissue-associated antigens, which, in turn, induces an inflammatory response. The inflammatory response results in the formation of scar tissue, which replaces some of the normal body tissue. The anti-

bodies involved in these two diseases are those produced in response to the streptococcal infection.

Glomerulonephritis involves the basement (filtering) membrane of the glo-
meruli of the kidneys. The inflammation and scarring of these membranes may result
in severe kidney malfunctions and, in some cases, death. This disease is most commonly induced by a single streptococcal type—type 12 of group A—and may result
following infection of the skin or other tissues. Other types may occasionally cause
this disease. Primary infections with type 12 streptococci are infrequent and only a
small percentage (1 to 15%) of those infected develop glomerulonephritis. About 80
to 90% of the cases undergo slow spontaneous healing whereas the others develop a
chronic form of the disease. Recurrent attacks are rare.

Rheumatic fever may develop as a sequela in from 1 to 4% of acute streptococcal infections of the respiratory tract only and may be caused by almost any one of the
group A strains. Rheumatic fever usually develops in children 5 to 15 years of age.
Some signs and symptoms are fever, malaise, inflamed and aching joints (arthritis),
subcutaneous lesions, and heart lesions. These complications may occur alone or in
various combinations. However, about half the cases may be mild and go undiagnosed. Injury to the heart (rheumatic heart disease) is the most serious effect of
rheumatic fever and currently is the most common cause of permanent heart valve
damage in children. Subsequent infections with group A streptococci may aggravate
and cause recurrences of this disease. Because many different strains of streptococci
cause this disease, persons who have had one attack must guard against reinfection
with any streptococcus.

Transmission and Epidemiology

The various strains of S. pyogenes are widespread in humans, many of whom are
asymptomatic carriers. These bacteria are found in the respiratory tract, mouth, intestines, or on the skin of about 5% of the general population in the summer and
around 10% in the winter. The carrier rate is generally higher in children between 1
and 15 years of age. Because of this high carrier rate, streptococci are readily transmitted when large numbers of persons share common environments.

Persons with acute infections are an obvious source of infection and transmission can readily occur from these individuals via respiratory droplets or by direct or
indirect contact. When highly virulent strains are carried into elementary schools,
sharp outbreaks of pharyngitis and scarlet fever may occur. Due to the accumulative
buildup of antibodies to many different types, outbreaks among adults are less likely.

Diagnosis

Diagnosis of a streptococcal infection is based on both clinical and laboratory findings. The basic laboratory procedure is to swab material from the site of infection
onto a blood agar plate. Colonies producing the beta-hemolytic reaction are further
studied to see if they are group A S. pyogenes.

Staphylococcal infections may be difficult to distinguish from some streptococcal infections, particularly skin lesions, and staphylococci also produce hemolysin. To differentiate between the two types of bacteria, a catalase test is used. This test is done by placing a small amount of growth from a colony in hydrogen peroxide; if the enzyme catalase is present, bubbles of oxygen are released. Staphylococci are positive for catalase and streptococci are negative. The *S. pyogenes* can be distinguished from other streptococci by placing a paper disk containing a low concentration of the antibiotic bacitracin on a freshly swabbed agar plate; *S. pyogenes* will be inhibited whereas the other streptococci will not.

Glomerulonephritis and rheumatic fever are primarily diagnosed on clinical findings. Because they follow a severe streptococcal infection, the patient should be expected to have a high antibody titer to the streptolysin O antigen. An antistreptolysin O (ASO) test is used to measure this antibody titer; a high titer indicates a recent streptococcal infection.

Treatment

The beta-hemolytic streptococci are highly susceptible to most antimicrobial agents. Penicillin is still highly effective and is the antibiotic of choice. Other antibiotics can be used in patients who are allergic to penicillin. Erythromycin is generally recommended. Because streptococci tend to develop resistance to tetracyclines and sulfa drugs, these agents should not be used.

Penicillin therapy will usually produce a rapid cure of most acute infections. Treatment should be started as soon as possible in order to reduce the chance of the subsequent development of rheumatic fever. Prompt diagnosis and treatment are particularly important in children, for they have the greatest predisposition to rheumatic fever. Early treatment is also important in helping to reduce the chance of transmitting the infection. Moreover, therapy can be used to try to clear streptococci from known carriers; this factor is particularly important for medical personnel who work with highly susceptible patients.

Control and Prevention

Vaccines are not available for the preceding streptococcal diseases; and because of the large numbers of serotypes, the development of vaccines is considered unfeasible.

The best control measure is to use basic medical procedures to prevent the transmission of infection. Individuals with a known infection should be isolated; for instance, a child with pharyngitis should not attend school or an infected patient in a hospital should be isolated from other patients. Medical personnel have a special responsibility to follow standard aseptic procedures to avoid transmitting these organisms between patients. Care should be used in delivery rooms and in working with recently delivered mothers to prevent transmission to their highly susceptible uterine tissues. A major uncontrollable parameter remains the carrier of *S. pyogenes* who may unwittingly transmit this infection.

The best means to prevent rheumatic fever and glomerulonephritis involves early diagnosis and treatment of children who have acute streptococcal infections. The recurrence of rheumatic fever is prevented by prophylactic (preventative) penicillin treatment—that is, daily doses of penicillin. Often persons who received severe heart damage from the first attack of rheumatic fever must be given penicillin therapy for years or for their lifetime. In many of these cases, it is often difficult to resolve the balance between benefits and abuses of such long-term penicillin therapy.

OTHER STREPTOCOCCAL INFECTIONS

Group B
These streptococci are commonly found in the genital and intestinal tracts of normal persons. They are also widely found in the vagina of pregnant women. Thus infants frequently become colonized at birth and about 0.5 to 1% of these colonized newborn infants develop pneumonia, septicemia, and/or meningitis from these group B streptococci. Group B streptococci may also cause urinary tract infections, ear infection, or wound infections in patients of all ages.

Group C
Occasionally species of group C streptococci have been implicated as the cause of such infections as impetigo, abscesses, and pneumonia.

Group D
An estimated 20% of the cases of bacterial endocarditis and 10% of urinary tract infections are caused by group D streptococci.

Viridans group
At least 10 species of non-beta-hemolytic streptococci are designated as viridans streptococci. They are the primary cause of 50 to 70% of all cases of bacterial endocarditis and are frequently isolated from patients with deep wound infections, abdominal abscesses, and septicemia. Normally present in the mouth and pharynx, they are thought to be a contributing cause of tooth decay.

CLINICAL NOTES

Hospital Outbreak of Streptococcal Wound Infection

Seven cases of group A beta-hemolytic streptococcal wound infections, six culture-proven and one presumptive, occurred from January 30 to February 15, 1976, among postsurgery patients at a 135-bed community hospital in northern Utah. Five patients had culture-proven wound infections, a sixth had a wound infection with gram-positive cocci in the exudate, and a seventh had culture-proven bacteremia and meningitis. All cases occurred less than 48 hours after surgery.

Initial review of the patients' charts revealed that major surgery was the only experience shared by all. The six culture-confirmed cases were then compared to the 34 other patients who had operations on the same days as the cases. Exposures to one anesthesiologist and to one surgeon were the only factors significantly associated with subsequent infection.

Cultures of throat and anus were obtained from all operating room personnel. The same anesthesiologist was found to carry the epidemic organism; he had asymptomatic anal carriage.

The operating room was closed on February 17. The anesthesiologist withdrew from surgery and was treated with benzathine penicillin. Repeat throat and anal cultures 3 days after initiation of treatment and 10 days after completion were negative. Increased surveillance by infection control committee members revealed no further wound infections or colonization by group A streptococci (*MMWR 25*:141, 1976).

Outbreak of Scarlet Fever: California

An outbreak of scarlet fever and poststreptococcal acute glomerulonephritis (AGN) occurred among residents of Santa Catalina Island, California, from March through July 1977. The epidemic organism, M2T2 SOR+ group A streptococcus, was previously implicated in outbreaks of scarlet fever and AGN occurring in Los Angeles and Mexico City.

Since the end of March, 65 cases of streptococcal pharyngitis (53 of them with scarlet fever) were identified by physician reports and a school survey. Symptoms among all patients with streptococcal disease consisted of fever (in 93%), sore throat (89%), rash or desquamation (82%), vomiting (62%), headache (59%), and enlarged lymph nodes in neck (44%).

Six cases were diagnosed between the end of March and the end of May, but the incidence increased dramatically in June, peaked in the third week, and declined after school recessed June 18. Sporadic cases continued to occur in July; the most recent onset was July 23. Distribution of cases over the 4-month period suggested person-to-person transmission. Except for 7 adults and 10 preschoolers, illness was confined to a single school (grades K-12) but involved only grades K-6; fifth-graders experienced the highest attack rate (14/23, 61%). The teacher in that class was also affected and the attack rate for children sitting at the front of that classroom was higher than for those in the back. The secondary attack rate in family members who did not attend the elementary school or a local preschool was 12.2%.

All cases were screened for signs and symptoms of AGN. Diagnosis showed three definite and three probable cases of nephritis, based on hematuria, cylinduria, and hypocomplementemia. Only one child had symptoms of nephritis; the others were asymptomatic and would not have been identified without screening efforts. Streptococci from 31 to 32 ill persons from whom the isolate was available for typing were identified as belonging to the epidemic strain M2T2 SOR+ group A streptococcus.

The first two cases in the outbreak were in a preschool child and his mother who had recently returned from an area of Mexico in which scarlet fever was prevalent. The organism may have been introduced to the island at this point, although there was ample opportunity for transmission from elsewhere on the mainland (*MMWR 26*:311, 1977).

SUMMARY

1. The genus *Streptococcus* includes a large number of primarily commensalistic bacteria. These organisms are often found as normal flora in both animals and humans. They are gram positive and diseases produced by these organisms are suppurative.

2. The pathogenic streptococci are classified on the basis of a polysaccharide capsular antigen. The group A organisms are of particular concern to humans, although human infections are also caused by members of the other groups, notably groups B and D.

3. The relatively benign disease, streptococcal sore throat, is of importance primarily because of the delayed sequela associated with such infections. Most streptococcal diseases are readily treated with penicillin.

Streptococcus Pneumoniae

17

For many years *Streptococcus pneumoniae* was classed as a separate genus called *Diplococcus*. Research has demonstrated close similarities to the streptococci, however, and so the diplococci were reclassified as a species of the genus *Streptococcus*. They are routinely referred to as pneumococci, for they are the main cause of bacterial pneumonia in adults.

PNEUMOCOCCAL INFECTIONS

Pneumococcal infections rank among the important causes of human illness and death. Before the era of antibiotics pneumococcal pneumonia was the number one cause of death. Even with the use of antibiotics, it is still one of the leading causes of death and the only infectious disease to have the dubious distinction of still being in the "top 10" causes of death in the United States. Pneumococcal pneumonia is a potential threat to every hospital patient or person with compromised defense mechanisms. Medical personnel must be continually alerted to the possible occurrence of this disease in the care of all patients.

Bacterium

S. pneumoniae is a gram-positive coccus that characteristically occurs in pairs or short chains (Figure 17-1). The virulent strains possess a prominent capsule that plays an important role in the pathogenesis of pneumococcal diseases by retarding the rate

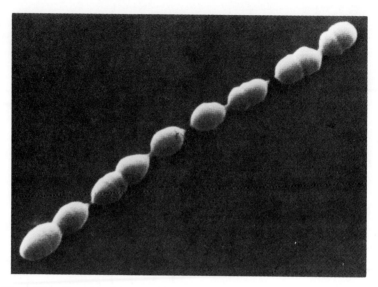

Figure 17-1 Scanning electron micrograph of *Streptococcus pneumoniae* showing the chain arrangement and the tendency to form pairs of cocci (diplococci) (magnification 10,000×). (A. S. Klainer and I Gies, *Agents of Bacterial Disease.* Harper & Row: Hagerstown, MD, 1973. Figure 5-3, p. 69.)

of phagocytosis. It can be cultivated on enriched media supplemented with 5% blood. *S. pneumoniae* produces alpha-type hemolysis, which may cause it to be mistakenly identified as a viridans streptococcus (see p. 218). Pneumococci are generally highly susceptible to penicillin as well as other antibiotics; however, some penicillin-resistant strains are now emerging. They do not survive long outside the body and are readily destroyed by disinfectants. Based on antigenic differences of the capsule, 83 different serotypes have been identified.

Pathogenesis and Clinical Diseases

S. pneumoniae is widespread in the general population. From less than 10 to over 60% of healthy persons may be carrying this bacterium in their respiratory tract. The higher carrier rates are seen during the winter. This bacterium does not possess any apparent enzymes or toxins associated with invasiveness; the major mechanism of virulence is the prominent capsule that impedes phagocytosis. Yet in a healthy active person the macrophages are usually able to control any pneumococci that may enter the lower respiratory tract. Only when the defense mechanisms of a host become suppressed are the pneumococci able to multiply and establish a focus of infection. As the pneumococci begin to multiply, they induce an acute inflammatory reaction with a rapid infiltration of edematous fluid. This fluid nourishes the bacteria, which, in turn, increases their rate of multiplication and stimulates a greater inflow of fluids. The initial accumulation of fluids also impedes phagocytosis and may impede the infiltration of antimicrobial agents into the lesion. The infiltrated fluids may rapidly fill the infected lung (called consolidation) and contain many PMN and RBC. This fluid takes on the characteristics of typical inflammatory exudate. In most less serious cases, the increased number of PMN, along with the macrophages, is able to contain the pneumococci; the infiltrated fluid then disperses and the lung tissue is restored to its original condition without permanent damage. When given early, antibiotics greatly accelerate the recovery process.

In more serious pneumonias the accumulation of fluid continues and spreads from one lobe to another and areas of consolidation develop in which the pneumococci are less susceptible to phagocytosis and antibiotics. Such infections may continue to expand, resulting in the death of the patient. On the other hand, if specific antibodies develop in time, a crisis may be reached, followed by recovery. Many host factors influence the eventual outcome of pneumonia and, perhaps more than in any other disease, the overall health and well-being of the patient play an important role in the outcome.

The pneumococci may spread from the lungs into the pleural cavity or pericardium and cause abscesses in these areas. The infection in the pleural space is called pleurisy. The infection may also spread via the blood or by direct extension to other body tissues. Septicemia, otitis media (infection of middle ear), and meningitis are common outcomes when the pneumococci spread beyond the respiratory tract; currently pneumococci are one of the most frequent causes of these infections in young children.

The symptoms of classical pneumonia begin with the rapid onset of shaking chills and fever between 38.8 and 41.4°C. Severe chest pains are often present. A cough develops and the sputum is pussy and rust colored (contains RBC). The crisis is reached in about 5 to 10 days, in many untreated cases, followed by recovery. Overall the death rate in untreated cases is 30% compared to 5% in treated cases. The outcome is greatly influenced by the age and underlying predisposing conditions of the patient. The stages in the development of pneumococcal pneumonia are outlined in Figure 17-2.

Transmission and Epidemiology

In most cases, the source of infection is endogenous—that is, from the pneumococci already present in the respiratory tract. Person-to-person transmission of the pneumococci readily occurs, but the disease only results in those with predisposing conditions. The common predisposing factors are viral infections of the respiratory tract (Figure 17-3), physical injury to the respiratory tract from inhaling toxic or irritating substances, including anesthetic gases, prolonged immobilization in bed, which may result in accumulation of fluids in the lungs, alcoholism, increasing age, diabetes, immunodeficiency diseases, or immunosuppression, and so on.

Pneumonia is most often seen in infants, elderly persons, alcoholics, or persons with chronic diseases. An estimated 500,000 persons in the United States will contract pneumonia each year and about 50,000 deaths will result. The seasonal variations and

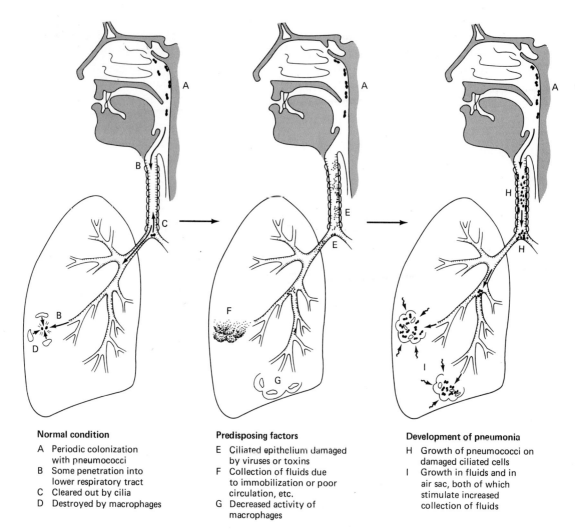

Normal condition

A   Periodic colonization
    with pneumococci
B   Some penetration into
    lower respiratory tract
C   Cleared out by cilia
D   Destroyed by macrophages

Predisposing factors

E   Ciliated epithelium damaged
    by viruses or toxins
F   Collection of fluids due
    to immobilization or poor
    circulation, etc.
G   Decreased activity of
    macrophages

Development of pneumonia

H   Growth of pneumococci on
    damaged ciliated cells
I   Growth in fluids and in
    air sac, both of which
    stimulate increased
    collection of fluids

Figure 17-2   Predisposition to and the development of pneumococcal pneumonia.

increased number of cases of all types of pneumonia occurring during influenza epidemics are shown in Figure 17-4.

About 75% of the pneumonia in adults is caused by only 9 of the 83 different pneumococcal serotypes. More pneumonia is seen in the winter and generally parallels the incidence of viral respiratory infections.

Diagnosis

Typical cases are usually diagnosed on the basis of physical examination and lung x rays. Laboratory diagnosis entails demonstrating the pneumococci in the sputum

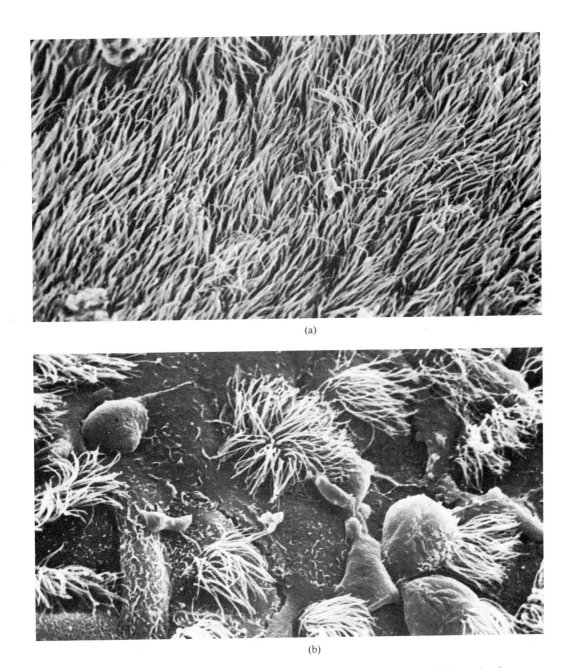

(a)

(b)

Figure 17-3 (a) Scanning electron micrograph of normal ciliated epithelium showing a continuous protective blanket of cilia. (b) Ciliated epithelium damaged by a viral infection which renders the respiratory tract much more susceptible to secondary bacterial infections. (S. E. Reed and A. Boyd, *Inf. Imm. 6*:68–76, Figures 1 and 4, with permission from ASM)

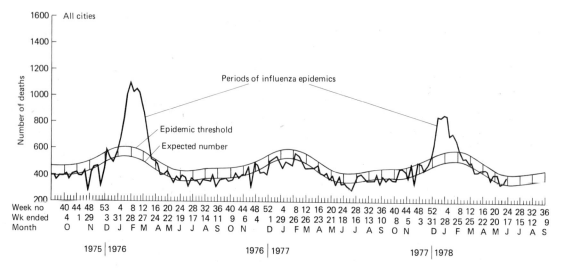

Figure 17-4 The reported number of deaths from pneumonia in 121 selected cities in the United States, September 1975 to June 1978. The sharp increases result from persons being predisposed to pneumonia as a result of influenzal infections (*MMWR 27*:422, 1978).

by direct microscopic examination and by culturing on artificial media. If specific antiserum is added to a suspension of a pneumococcus, it will cause the bacterial capsules to become visible. This reaction is called the *quellung reaction* and is useful in determining the specific pneumonococcal serotype. Differentiation of the pneumococci from viridans streptococci is often necessary, for they produce the same reaction on blood agar plates. The pneumococci are distinguished from the viridans streptococci by their bile solubility. For this test, pneumococci are added to solutions containing bile salts and the cells dissolve whereas in a similar test the "viridans" cells do not dissolve. Alternatively, the optochin disk test may be used; here a paper disk containing a chemical called optochin is placed on an agar plate that has been seeded with the test bacterium. Optochin inhibits the growth of pneumococci but not of viridans streptococci.

Various serologic tests are available to detect the presence of pneumococcal antibodies or antigens in the serum of the patient.

Treatment

Most pneumococci are still susceptible to penicillin; only occasionally is a resistant strain isolated (see clinical note). Treatment with penicillin should be started as soon as pneumococcal pneumonia is suspected. The longer treatment is delayed, the more difficult it is to cure the disease. The response to penicillin, when initiated early, is often dramatic and bacteria are cleared from the system in a few hours. The effects of both sulfa drugs and penicillin on pneumonia helped justify the title of "wonder drugs" that was applied to these agents shortly after their discovery. For the first time in history the number one killer of humans could often be cured with relative ease and rapidity. When penicillin cannot be used because of allergic reactions, some broad-spectrum antibiotics are appropriate.

Prevention and Control

Good nursing and medical management practices are effective in minimizing or preventing the development of pneumonia in compromised hospital patients. Prophylactic treatment with penicillin might be warranted in high-risk patients with viral respiratory diseases or other conditions that might predispose the tissues to pneumococcal infections. Even though pneumonia is often caused by endogenous bacteria, exogenous transmission may also be important in a hospital environment and compromised patients should be isolated from pneumonia patients in particular. In extreme cases, such as highly immunosuppressed organ transplant patients, protective isolation from all persons is necessary. Elective surgery should not be performed on a person with a respiratory infection. Hospitalized or confined patients should be required to sit up and get out of bed periodically, if possible, to prevent the pooling of fluids in the lungs. Maintaining good circulation and healthy "dry" lungs is the best preventative measure against pneumococcal pneumonia.

Before the development of effective antibiotics, vaccines against pneumonia were used with some effect. Because of the increased death rates from pneumonia in elderly persons and compromised patients in recent years, plus the difficulty of treating pneumonia in many of these persons, renewed interest in antipneumonia vaccines has been stimulated. A pneumococcal vaccine was licensed in the United States in 1978. This vaccine contained the capsular antigens from 14 of the most commonly encountered serotypes of pneumococci. In 1983 the vaccine was expanded to include antigens from 23 serotypes. Early studies have indicated that this vaccine greatly reduces the incidence of pneumonia. It is recommended for young children and elderly persons or others with health conditions that would predispose them to pneumonia.

CLINICAL NOTE

Multiply-Resistant Pneumococcus: Denver, Colorado

In November 1980, a multiply-resistant strain of *Streptococcus pneumoniae*, serotype 6B, was isolated from the cerebrospinal fluid (CSF) of an 11-month-old infant with meningitis. The isolate was found to be resistant to penicillin G, chloramphenicol, and tetracycline; this is the first instance reported in the United States of a pneumococcus resistant to all 3 drugs.

The minimum inhibitory concentration (MIC) for penicillin G was 1 μg/ml; for chloramphenicol, 16 μg/ml; and for tetracycline, 16 μg/ml. The organism was sensitive to rifampin, and the child, who had responded poorly to penicillin, recovered after treatment with ampicillin, chloramphenicol, and rifampin.

Since the child had regularly attended a day-care center with approximately 55 other children, a survey was conducted at the day-care center to detect carriage of the resistant isolate. Throat cultures from 4 of 14 children (29%) in the toddler room (under age 2 years) were positive for the multiply-resistant pneumococcus (MRP); in the preschool area, 4 of 37 children (11%) and 1 of 10 adult employees (10%) were positive. One-hundred and twenty-five children and staff members in 6 other day-care centers in the metropolitan area had negative throat cultures for MRP. To date, no other cases of invasive disease with this MRP have been recognized.

Editorial note: The first report of penicillin-resistant pneumococci appeared in 1967. Since then, relatively resistant and resistant strains have been reported from many parts of the world. The prevalence of relative resistance reported in clinical isolates has varied from 1% to as high as 16%, but most studies show a prevalence of approximately 2%.

In 1977, multiply-resistant pneumococci appeared in South Africa, and since then have been recognized in the United Kingdom, Australia, New Guinea, and the United States. This report of penicillin-resistant pneumococci and other reports describing relative penicillin resistance in the United States emphasize the need to screen all clinically significant pneumococcal isolates for penicillin sensitivity (*MMWR 30*:197, 1981).

SUMMARY

Streptococcus pneumoniae has historically been of primary importance as a human disease agent. It is still a common cause of serious pneumonia, particularly in compromised patients. Therapy with penicillin has greatly reduced the fear of this organism and a multivalent vaccine that greatly reduces the incidence of this disease is now available.

Neisseria

Bacteria

Bacteria of the genus *Neisseria* are gram-negative cocci that usually appear in pairs (Figure 18-1). Two species are important pathogens of humans: *N. meningitidis,* which commonly causes spinal meningitis, and *N. gonorrhoeae,* the cause of gonorrhea. Although these two species are similar in their structural and physiological makeup, the diseases they cause are clinically quite different and will be discussed separately.

The *Neisseria* are readily inactivated by exposure to drying, chilling, sunlight, acids, and alkalies. They can be cultivated on laboratory media if special care is taken to prevent inactivation. Growth occurs best on blood or chocolate agar (a medium enriched with blood and heated, which turns the blood a chocolate color). The two species can be differentiated on the basis of sugar fermentation tests. Most *N. meningitidis* strains produce apparent capsules whereas *N. gonorrhoeae* strains produce very slight capsules. Fimbriae are present on *N. gonorrhoeae.* Even though the *Neisseria* possess typical gram-negative-type cell walls, they are susceptible to penicillin. *N. meningitidis* is commonly referred to as the meningococcus and the *N. gonorrhoeae* as the gonococcus.

MENINGOCOCCAL INFECTIONS

Pathogenesis and Clinical Diseases

Most meningococcal infections are caused by one of three different serogroups of the *N. meningitidis,* designated A, B, and C. The main mechanisms of pathogenicity and

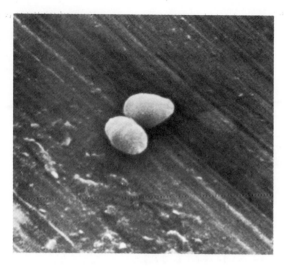

Figure 18-1 Scanning electron micrograph of *Neisseria gonorrhoeae* showing the typical diplococcal arrangement of the "bean-shaped" cocci (magnification 10,000×). (A. S. Klainer and I. Gies, *Agents of Bacterial Disease.* Harper & Row: Hagerstown, MD, 1973. Figure 7-1, p. 83.)

virulence appear to be the capsule that helps retard phagocytosis and an endotoxin in the cell wall that is thought to cause damage to the linings of blood vessels.

The disease spinal meningitis, more specifically called meningococcal meningitis, is a relatively rare outcome of the much more common minor meningococcal infections. The meningococci are widespread in the general population and are readily transmitted via the airborne route. They multiply in the nasopharyngeal area without causing any disease; an infected individual may carry these organisms for many months. Such a carrier state may induce an immune response in the person and cause resistance to the given serogroup with which that person is colonized. This carrier, however, serves as a reservoir from which the bacteria may be transmitted to those who live in close contact with the person. The carrier rate varies in different populations. The rate is 3% in a general population in which no clinical disease is present compared to a rate of 15% to 50% in persons who live or work around patients with clinical meningococcal diseases. The carrier rate in military personnel is generally higher than in other populations.

Once meningococci are colonized in the respiratory membranes, the person may experience mild sore throat and fever. Meningococci may be carried into the lymphatic system and then into the blood. If the host is unable to contain the infection at this point—and no information is available as to how many infected persons progress to this point without symptoms developing—the bacteria become deposited in various tissues, such as skin, meninges, joints, and lungs. In a few days lesions develop in these tissues with the manifestation of signs and symptoms of the disease. In the disseminated infections hemorrhagic lesions may occur in the involved tissue, along with high fever and prostration. Subcutaneous hemorrhagic lesions sometimes occur, giving a spotted appearance. The most often recognized form of the disseminated disease is spinal meningitis, which results from inflammation of the meninges. Spinal meningitis is accompanied by various neurologic symptoms; the death rate in untreated cases is about 85%. With treatment, however, the overall death rate is 10 to 15%. Disseminated meningococcal disease may also occur without meningitis and has a high death rate as well.

The presence of specific antibodies in the serum offers protection against the disseminated disease but apparently does not clear up the carrier stage in the nasopharyngeal tissues. Most adults have acquired antibody immunity against meningococci due to previous subclinical infections whereas most infants have passive immunity during the first months of life. The pathogenesis of this disease is outlined in Figure 18-2.

Transmission and Epidemiology

Transmission of meningococci is usually via the airborne route; because of the large number of carriers in the general population, transmission may occur at any time. Transmission is more efficient from a person with a clinical infection, however, and a significantly higher number of cases occur in a patient's household contacts than in the general population.

Children are frequently exposed early in life and a higher incidence of disseminated disease is seen in the 6- to 24-month age range. This represents the period between loss of passive immunity and acquisition of active immunity. For less obvious reasons, the next age group that is most susceptible are the 10- to 20-year-olds. More than two-thirds of all cases occur in persons under 20 years of age. Many of these outbreaks have been associated with military recruits. The higher number of cases in military recruits probably results from close contact in barracks and the increased exposure due to the high carrier rate in military personnel.

Sporadic cases are seen in most areas; however, epidemics do occur periodically in some geographic areas. The sporadic cases run about 3 per 100,000 in the general population per year whereas the rates during an epidemic may increase to several hundred per 100,000 per year.

Diagnosis

Direct microscopic examination of infected tissues or fluids may reveal the presence of the meningococci and provide a rapid diagnosis. Inoculation onto appropriate nutrient agar is also used to demonstrate the presence of meningococci.

Treatment

Intravenous administration of large doses of penicillin is the most effective treatment. Broad-spectrum antibiotics may be used in penicillin-allergic patients. The sulfonamides are effective if resistant strains are not causing the disease. Currently about one-half the isolates are resistant to the sulfonamides. Treatment is much more effective if started early in the infection. If spinal meningitis is suspected in a young child, immediate treatment is essential, for the disease may progress rapidly and lead

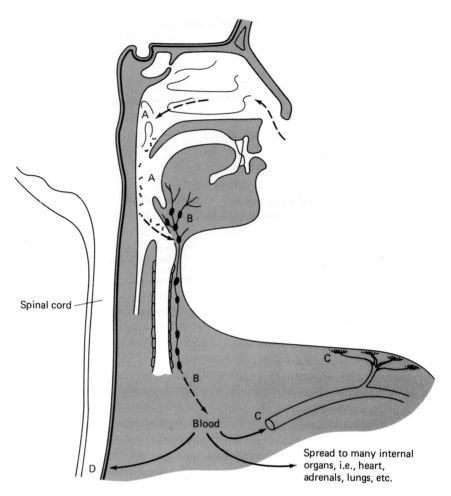

Spinal cord

Blood

Spread to many internal
organs, i.e., heart,
adrenals, lungs, etc.

Figure 18-2   The pathogenesis of meningococcal infections. Stages of infection: A. Bacteria may be implanted in the nasopharynx. This phase of the infection is often asymptomatic, but in some cases may cause a sore throat. B. Bacteria may pass into the blood stream via the lymphatic system. C. Septicemia with inflammation of blood vessels and areas of hemorrhaging in the skin. Much of the damage is caused by endotoxins. The disease may range from mild to rapidly fatal. D. Meningitis, with headache, fever, and signs of meningeal irritation (rash may or may not be present).

to death or permanent neurologic damage within less than 24 hours after the onset of severe symptoms.

Prevention and Control

Vaccines have been developed against serogroups A and C. These vaccines use purified capsular antigens and a single dose produces a good antibody response. Since

1971, over 500,000 military recruits have been vaccinated with serogroup C vaccine and 62,000 Egyptian schoolchildren have been vaccinated with serogroup A vaccine. No serious adverse reactions have occurred in those vaccinated and serogroup C meningococcal meningitis has been virtually eliminated in military recruit populations. Before 1971 serogroup C was frequently the cause of meningitis in military recruits. Vaccines have been used in some cities where outbreaks of meningococcal meningitis occurred, but their use in civilian populations is still being evaluated. These vaccines do not seem to be effective in children under 2 years of age. The vaccine might also be used along with antibiotics in the prophylactic treatment of household contacts of meningococcal disease.

Household contacts and hospital personnel who are exposed to clinical cases should be given prophylactic doses of the antibiotic rifampin to reduce the chance of secondary cases occurring. Meningococcal patients in the hospital should be kept in isolation. Even though the risk to hospital personnel is low, the following clinical notes illustrate the need for precaution in working with patients with meningococcal disease.

CLINICAL NOTE

Hospital-Acquired Meningococcemia

In February 1978 a nurse developed meningococcemia 3 days after assisting in the emergency room evaluation of a patient with meningococcemia and meningitis.

The index patient was a 25-year-old man who was seen in the emergency room with fever, malaise, myalgia, and a headache of 24-hour duration. A diagnostic lumbar puncture in the emergency room was unsuccessful because of the patient's lack of cooperation. He was taken to the postoperative recovery room, where he was given inhalation anesthesia and intubated; a lumbar puncture was then performed. The patient vomited several times in the emergency room and during intubation. Hospital personnel assisting with the anesthesia and lumbar puncture did not wear masks or follow other isolation precautions.

The patient's cerebrospinal fluid (CSF) had a protein level of 767 mg/dl, a glucose of 6 mg/dl, and a white blood cell count (WBC) of 20,7000/mm^3 with 98% neutrophils. Gram stain of the smear showed multiple gram-negative diplococci that were both extracellular and intracellular. No pneumonia was seen on the chest x ray. Cultures of the blood and spinal fluid grew *Neisseria meningitidis,* subsequently identified as a sulfonamide-susceptible group B strain. Following diagnosis of the patient's disease, approximately 6 hours after his admission to the emergency room, he was placed in isolation.

Before he was placed in isolation, 24 medical personnel (physicians, nurses, orderlies, and others) had contact with the patient. These persons were informed of their possible exposure to meningococcal disease. Those with intimate contact with the patient were advised to take rifampin prophylactically for 2 days; 3 nurses and 2 orderlies received prophylaxis.

Three days after the index patient was admitted to the hospital a 39-year-old nurse developed headache, fever, and malaise. She had assisted with the intubation and suctioning of nasopharyngeal secretions from the index case at the time of his diagnostic lumbar puncture. Two days after onset of her symptoms she presented herself for examination and was noted to have scattered petechial lesions on her arms and legs. Her WBC was 17,400/mm^3 with 87% neutrophils. Lumbar puncture showed normal CSF; blood cultures were not obtained. Over the next several days she developed a more severe headache, more petechiae, and joint pains. Six days after her initial symptoms, she was admitted to the hospital and isolated with a presumptive diagnosis of meningococcemia. A repeat lumbar puncture was performed and revealed a WBC of 25mm/^{3}, mostly neutrophils, normal glucose and protein concentrations, and negative-gram stain and culture. A blood culture, however, grew group B *N. meningitidis* susceptible to sulfonamides.

On careful questioning, the nurse recalled that she had exposure to the nasopharyngeal secretions from the index patient, but afterward she had not received antibiotic prophylaxis. She had no other known contacts with persons with meningococcal disease or colonization and at the time of these two cases no other cases of meningococcal disease were occurring in the community.

Transmission of *N. meningiditis* to hospital personnel caring for a patient with meningococcemia or meningitis is rare and has been reported only when there is extensive contact with the infected individual. To minimize the risk of transmission of meningococcal infection to hospital personnel, a patient who has a disease compatible with meningococcal infection should be placed in respiratory isolation when the diagnosis is first suspected. Personnel who have had intimate contact with the patient's respiratory tract secretions should be given rifampin as chemoprophylaxis or a sulfonamide if the strain of *N. meningitidis* is known to be sensitive to sulfonamides (*MMWR 27*:358, 1978).

GONORRHEA

The virulent strains of gonococci possess fimbriae that are able to adhere to the epithelial cells of mucous membranes of the host. This attachment prevents the bacteria from being flushed out of the vagina or urethra by normal body secretions. The term *gonorrhea* was introduced by the ancient physician Galen; it means the "flow of seed" and refers to the flow of pus from the urethra of infected persons. Diseases that may have been gonorrhea were described in ancient medical writings. By the thirteenth century gonorrhea was recognized as a sexually transmitted disease. Not until many years later, however, was a clear distinction made between gonorrhea and syphilis, for the two diseases often occurred simultaneously in the same person (see Chapter 1).

Gonorrhea is among the most prevalent of the classical venereal diseases—or the sexually transmitted diseases as they are now called—and is the most frequent reportable disease in the United States. Gonorrhea usually responds well to penicillin therapy; in fact, the availability of this drug in the 1940s made people believe that gonorrhea could be controlled or eliminated. Nevertheless, the liberalized sexual attitude of the 1960s–1970s, together with the development and use of oral contraceptives, caused a marked upsurge in the number of cases of gonorrhea. At present, a worldwide pandemic of gonorrhea is occurring. Currently penicillin-resistant strains are widespread, a factor that may impede further control of this disease.

Pathogenesis and Clinical Diseases

The patterns of gonorrhea vary somewhat among the male, female, and the newborn. Therefore the clinical diseases are discussed separately for each group.

Gonorrhea in the male

The gonococci are usually deposited in the lower portion of the urethra during sexual intercourse. The bacteria attach to the surface cells of the urethra. The growing gonococci induce an acute inflammatory response in 2 to 8 days that may be accompanied by fever, a pussy discharge, and pain during urination. In most cases, the male experiences definite symptoms when infected. The infection may spread by direct extension along the ducts of the genitourinary tract with accompanying inflammation. The inflammation may close the urethra and prevent urination in 1% of the cases. The infection may also spread to the vas deferens (sperm ducts) and cause scarring and closure of this duct, which then results in infertility of the patient. In some cases, the bacteria spread into the blood and are carried to various internal organs or bone joints, where inflammation may develop.

Gonorrhea in the female

Infection usually results from gonococci transmitted during sexual intercourse. The ensuing infection is of the cervix and often remains at a low level; in up to 80% of the infected females it is asymptomatic. Those patients with signs of the disease experience vaginal discharge, fever, a burning sensation, and abdominal pain. The abdominal pains are normally associated with spread of the infection to the fallopian tubes, a serious condition known as *salpingitis*. This form of gonorrhea may induce scarring with closure of the fallopian tubes that results in loss of fertility. The fallopian tubes are also predisposed to secondary infections by other bacteria. Further extension of the infection into the lower abdomen occurs in 10% of the women with gonorrhea and is called *pelvic inflammatory disease*. The duration of the asymptomatic infections is not known, but some evidence indicates that the infection may persist for months. Women using oral contraceptives are thought to be more susceptible to gonorrhea due to changes in the pH of the vaginal mucosa induced by birth control pills. The gonorrhea may spread into the blood and be carried to other organs in a small percentage of infected females.

Rectal gonorrhea is seen in about half the infected females and is common in homosexual males.

Gonorrhea in children

Persons of all ages are susceptible to gonorrhea. The most common form of child-hood gonorrhea is seen as an eye infection (gonococcal ophthalmia neonatorum) of the newborn. Contamination takes place during passage through the birth canal of a mother who has gonorrhea. If not treated, severe inflammation of the eyes may result. Before routine disinfection of the eyes of newborns was required, gonococcal ophthalmia was the major cause of blindness in children.

Transmission and Epidemiology

Gonorrhea in adults is almost always transmitted by sexual contact. Increases and decreases in disease rates are directly related to major social changes associated with war or liberalized attitudes toward sex. The reported cases of gonorrhea are shown in Figure 18-3. Since the early 1960s, the rate of gonorrhea has increased steadily in most parts of the world and is now considered of epidemic proportions. Most cases of gonorrhea are seen in the ages and social groups that are most sexually active. The highest rate of disease is seen in the 15- to 30-year-age groups with a peak rate in the 20- to 24-year-age groups. High rates are also seen in such subpopulations as divorced persons and homosexuals. Over a million cases of gonorrhea are officially reported in the United States each year, but the actual number is thought to be three or four times greater.

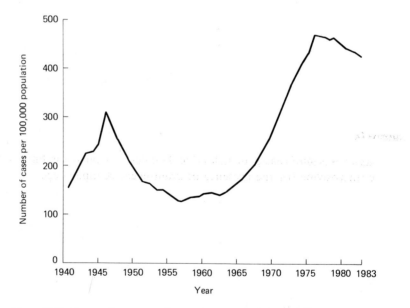

Figure 18-3   Reported case rates of gonorrhea per year in U.S. civilians, 1941–1983. The leveling-off of reported cases since 1975 is thought to be a result of increased government control program initiated in 1973 (modified from CDC annual summaries).

TABLE 18-1 LOCATIONS WITH IDENTIFIED STRAINS OF β-LACTAMASE-
PRODUCING *NEISSERIA GONORRHOEAE* THROUGH MAY 1981[a]

Africa	Americas	East Asia	Europe	South East Asia
Morocco	Canada	Philippines	France	Indonesia
Ghana	United States	Hong Kong	Belgium	Singapore
Mali	Mexico	Taiwan	Netherlands	Malaysia
Nigeria	Panama	Guam	United Kingdom	Thailand
Central African	Argentina	Japan	West Germany	India
Republic	Colombia	Republic of Korea	Denmark	Sri Lanka
Gabon		New Zealand	Poland	
Zaire		New Hebrides	Switzerland	
Madagascar		Australia	Sweden	
Zambia			Norway	
Senegal			Finland	

[a]Information obtained through WHO Epidemiological Surveillance System; adapted from PAHO
Epidemiologic Bulletin.

Generally immunity to gonorrhea infection does not develop and a person may be infected over and over again. The probability of a male becoming infected after sexual intercourse with an infected female is about 20%. The probability of the female contracting the disease from an infected male is thought to be greater; however, it is not as well determined because many females contract asymptomatic infections that go undetected.

Penicillin-resistant strains of gonococci have now developed. These strains carry a plasmid that directs the formation of the enzyme β-lactamase (penicillinase) that is able to inactivate penicillin G, ampicillin, and cephalosporins. The impact of these strains on the epidemiology of gonorrhea could be of great significance (Table 18-1, Figure 18-4).

Diagnosis

Diagnosis is much easier in males than females. The pussy discharge is examined with the microscope for the presence of gram-negative diplococci; if positive, the diagnosis is confirmed (Figure 18-5). If the microscopic test is negative, an attempt should be made to isolate the gonococcus on a culture medium to provide a positive diagnosis. It is much more difficult to observe gonococci microscopically in smears of exudate from infected females and this procedure is of little diagnostic value in women. Cultures should be obtained from the cervix and anal canal and, if possible, inoculated directly onto a selective agar medium for gonococci, such as modified Thayer-Martin medium. If the specimen must be transported to the laboratory, special handling methods are required to prevent the inactivation of these delicate microorganisms. Because the diagnosis of asymptomatic infections in females is often difficult, there is currently a great need for a simple reliable test to detect these infections. Serologic tests are not well developed and are of limited value at present.

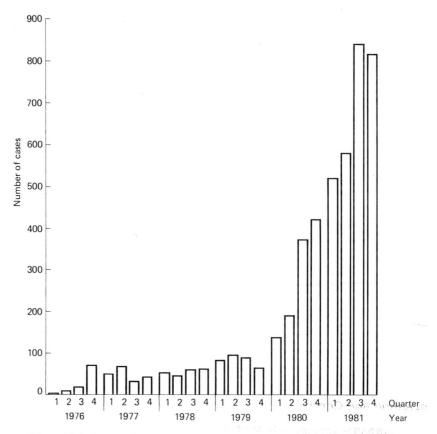

Figure 18-4 Reported cases, by quarter, of gonorrhea caused by penicillinase-producing *N. gonorrhoeae* in the United States, 1976 to 1981. The number of cases of gonorrhea caused by penicillin-resistant strains appear to be increasing (modified from CDC annual summaries).

Treatment

Penicillin is still the drug of choice. Over the years gonococci have developed increased resistance to penicillin and currently a single injection of 4.8 million units is needed for most cures. Treatment with penicillin is usually dramatic and since the 1940s has functioned as a so-called wonder drug in curing gonorrhea. But in 1976 a strain of gonococci that is completely resistant to penicillin developed. Persons with this resistant strain or who are sensitive to penicillin can be cured with various other recommended treatment schedules (Table 18-2). The broad-spectrum antibiotics needed to treat the cases of gonorrhea caused by penicillin-resistant strains often have adverse side effects and are significantly more expensive than penicillin. Should the penicillin-resistant strains become widespread, the treatment and control of gonorrhea would become much more difficult and expensive than it has been during the past 30 years.

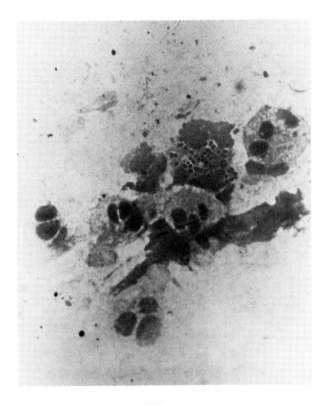

Figure 18-5 Optical micrograph of pus from a patient with gonorrhea showing a phagocytic cell (PMN) filled with gonococci (magnification 900×). (A. S. Klainer and I. Gies, *Agents of Bacterial Disease.* Harper & Row: Hagerstown, MD, 1973. Figure 7-3, p. 86.)

Prevention and Control

No vaccines are currently available, although experimental data are being gathered for vaccine use. Gonorrhea in the newborn is prevented by irrigating the eyes with a 1% solution of silver nitrate. This procedure is required by law in all states and has almost eliminated gonococcal ophthalmia in the newborn. Penicillin is sometimes used in place of silver nitrate; however, because of the emergence of penicillin-resist-

TABLE 18-2 RECOMMENDED THERAPY FOR GONORRHEA

Infection	Primary therapy	Alternative therapy
Uncomplicated gonorrhea	Penicillin (4.8 million units)	Tetracycline (2.5 g/day)
Penicillin resistant gonorrhea	Spectinomycin (2 g intramuscularly)	Cefoxitin with probenecid or Sulfamethoxazole/ trimethoprine (9 tablets/day)
Spectinomycin resistant gonorrhea	Cefoxitin with probenecid (2 g and 1 g intramuscularly)	Cefotaxime (1 g intramuscularly)

ant gonococci, it might be best always to use silver nitrate. If a pregnant female has gonorrhea, she should be treated before delivery to further reduce the hazard to the newborn infant.

Gonorrhea in adults is preventable: avoid exposure to the disease. Still, history has clearly demonstrated that prevention will not be accomplished by this means. The risk of exposure can be reduced by using such devices as condoms. Reporting cases of gonorrhea to public health officials is helpful in that it aids in finding and treating persons who might be serving as sources of infection. Numerous educational activities have been tried at various age levels in attempts to reduce the incidence of gonorrhea. But the increasing rate of gonorrheal infections shows that these programs have had limited success.

CLINICAL NOTE

Antibiotic-Resistant *Neisseria gonorrhoeae*: United States

During October through December 1977 the Centers for Disease Control in Atlanta, Georgia, received three resistant gonococcal isolates from two patients in different geographical areas of the United States. All three isolates had exceptionally high values for the minimum inhibitory concentration (MIC) of both penicillin and tetracycline.

The first patient was a 19-year-old man with gonococcal urethral discharge who was treated in a local hospital with penicillin capsules on September 7, 1977. Ten days later he was seen in the local venereal disease clinic because of the same symptoms. A gram stain of urethral discharge was positive for *Neisseria gonorrhoeae* and he was treated with oral ampicillin, 3.5 g, and probenecid, 1.0 g. A culture taken at the time was positive for *N. gonorrhoeae;* a disk diffusion test for penicillin resistance was positive. The patient was lost to followup.

The second patient, a 19-year-old woman, was referred to a local clinic because she was a contact to a confirmed case of gonorrhea. She gave a history of vaginal discharge for 3 days. In addition, she had been treated 1 year with oral tetracycline, 250 mg per day, for acne. Throat and endocervical cultures were positive for *N. gonorrhoeae.* The endocervical isolate was resistant on penicillin disc-testing. The patient was treated with spectinomycin, 2 g, and followup cultures were negative (*MMWR* 27:121, 1978).

SUMMARY

1. The gram-negative diplococcal *Neisseria* include two species of major clinical significance: *N. meningitidis,* the etiologic agent of epidemic meningitis, and *N. gonorrhoeae,* the causative agent of gonorrhea.

2. *N. meningitidis* is often found as normal body flora and yet is responsible for a fulmanent infection that causes rapid mortality in its victims. The balance between a normal flora and disease due to this organism is not well understood.
3. Gonorrhea has become such a common disease that it is literally a household word. The epidemic state of this disease and the ease with which it is generally treated belie its potential for producing life-threatening infections.

Spirochetes

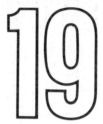

The spirochetes are members of a family called *Spirochaetaceae* that includes long, slender, coiled, motile microorganisms (Figure 19-1). Three genera of spirochetes contain species that are able to cause diseases in humans, the most important being syphilis, which results from the bacterium *Treponema pallidum*. Other syphilislike diseases called yaws, pinta, and bejel are caused by bacteria closely related to the syphilis spirochete. Two less common diseases, relapsing fever and leptospirosis, are produced by spirochetes of the genera *Borrelia* and *Leptospira*, respectively.

SYPHILIS

Bacterium

T. pallidum is a slender, spiraled organism with a length of 5 to 20 μm. The width is 0.2 to 0.5 μm, which makes observation with a standard bright-field microscope difficult. The treponemas are highly motile and move through fluid in a twisting motion. When a fresh, wet, mounted specimen is viewed with a dark-field microscope, the motile spirochetes are easily seen. *T. pallidum* has not been grown on any artificial culture media. Humans are the only natural host; monkeys and rabbits, however, can be experimentally infected. The testes and skin of rabbits support the growth of some syphilis spirochetes and are used to grow these bacteria for experimental use and diagnostic tests.

    T. pallidum is quite fragile and only lives for a short period when shed from the body. It is readily killed by disinfectants and is highly susceptible to penicillin and

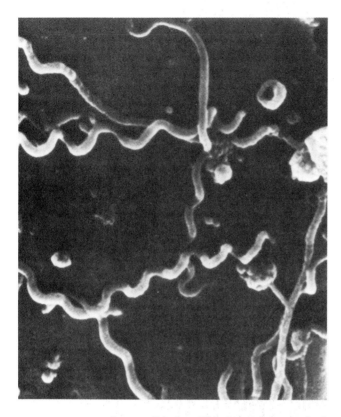

Figure 19-1   Scanning electron micrograph of the syphilis spirochete *T. pallidum* growing in rabbit testicular cells (N. S. Hayes, K. E. Muse, A. M. Collier, and J. B. Baseman, *Inf. Imm. 17*:174–186, Figure 3c, with permission from ASM).

many other antibiotics. This bacterium can be kept alive and motile for up to 2 weeks if stored at 25°C under anaerobic conditions in a special medium.

Pathogenesis and Clinical Disease

Syphilis is a disease that, when untreated, may go through several stages over an extended period of time with varying clinical manifestations. The stages of syphilis in adults are primary, secondary, latent, and tertiary (Figure 19-2). Congenital syphilis also occurs. Antibodies form against the syphilis organisms, but in many cases do not offer protection to the host. Because clinical signs may be confused with other diseases, syphilis has been referred to as the mimicker of other diseases.

Primary syphilis

The treponemal spirochetes are deposited on the mucosal membranes or skin by direct contact. Contact is almost always sexual. Medical personnel treating or examining syphilitic lesions without proper barrier protection can also become infected, however. Treponema seem able to penetrate the mucosal tissues or gain entry through small lesions in the skin. The bacteria begin to multiply at the site of entry and are also carried to the adjacent lymph nodes and eventually to the blood, where they

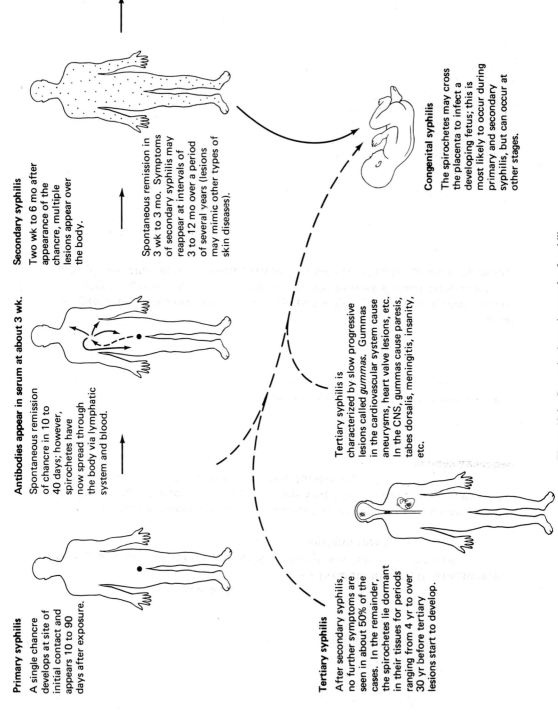

Primary syphilis

A single chancre develops at site of initial contact and appears 10 to 90 days after exposure.

Antibodies appear in serum at about 3 wk.

Spontaneous remission of chancre in 10 to 40 days; however, spirochetes have now spread through the body via lymphatic system and blood.

Secondary syphilis

Two wk to 6 mo after appearance of the chancre, multiple lesions appear over the body.

Spontaneous remission in 3 wk to 3 mo. Symptoms of secondary syphilis may reappear at intervals of 3 to 12 mo over a period of several years (lesions may mimic other types of skin diseases).

Tertiary syphilis

After secondary syphilis, no further symptoms are seen in about 50% of the cases. In the remainder, the spirochetes lie dormant in their tissues for periods ranging from 4 yr to over 30 yr before tertiary lesions start to develop.

Tertiary syphilis is characterized by slow progressive lesions called *gummas*. Gummas in the cardiovascular system cause aneurysms, heart valve lesions, etc. In the CNS, gummas cause paresis, tabes dorsalis, meningitis, insanity, etc.

Congenital syphilis

The spirochetes may cross the placenta to infect a developing fetus; this is most likely to occur during primary and secondary syphilis, but can occur at other stages.

Figure 19-2   Stages in the pathogenesis of syphilis.

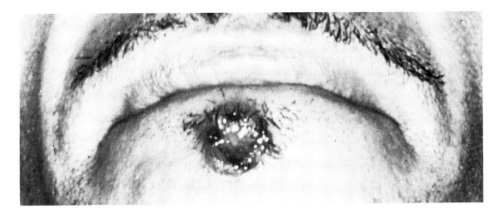

Figure 19-3 Primary syphilis with a chancre on the lower lip. (Centers for Disease Control, Atlanta)

spread throughout the body. As a rule, after 10 to 30 days, but in some cases up to 90 days, a primary lesion appears at the site of infection, which is usually genital. This lesion, called a *chancre*, is shallow and ulcerative, has a firm base, and is relatively painless. A chancre may reach more than 1 cm in diameter and is teeming with spirochetes (Figure 19-3). In some patients, often women, the chancre goes unnoticed due to its location in the deeper passages of the genital tract. The adjacent lymph nodes are usually swollen.

The chancre spontaneously disappears within 3 to 6 weeks and so a naive patient may mistakenly believe that the disease is cured. The patient may then be without symptoms for a period ranging from 2 weeks to 6 months before the manifestation of secondary syphilis.

Secondary syphilis

The spirochetes that spread through the body from the primary site of entry become deposited in many tissues, where they slowly multiply. Secondary syphilis is usually characterized by the appearance of a generalized rash and lesions over the body (Figure 19-4). The lesions on the skin and mucous membranes may contain large numbers of spirochetes and are highly infectious. The patient may also experience such symptoms as headaches, fever, and sore throat. Lesions may also be present in bones, the central nervous system, or other organs. The skin lesions may be quite prominent; in earlier days this stage of the disease was called "great pox" to distinguish it from another common disease with smaller lesions—that is, smallpox. The secondary stage gradually subsides. Complete recovery may be slow with some signs remaining for several years. Any one of the following conditions may occur from this phase of the disease:

1. Complete remission with no further manifestations of the disease. This occurs in about 40 to 50% of untreated patients.

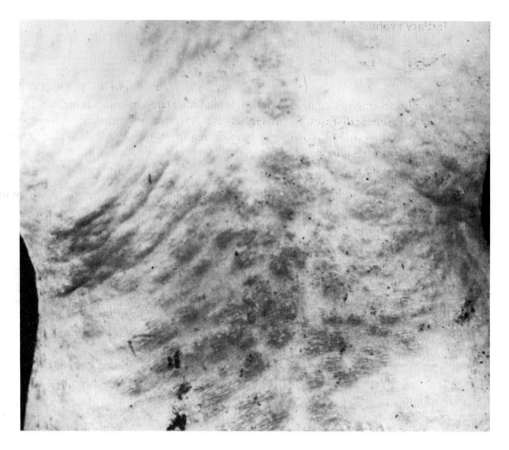

Figure 19-4   Secondary syphilis with rash-type lesions on the back. (Centers for Disease Control, Atlanta)

2. Recurrence of secondary lesions, often in modified forms. This may occur at 3- to 12-month intervals over the next several years. These recurring lesions may mimic other types of skin diseases.
3. Progression first into latent and then into tertiary syphilis.

Latent syphilis

This is the period following secondary syphilis. The first four years are referred to as the early latent and the subsequent period as the late latent. No symptoms of the disease are present during the late latent period, but high levels of antibodies are in the serum. About half the patients who progress to the late latent phase have no further symptoms of syphilis. The others progress to the tertiary stage of the disease.

Tertiary syphilis

Signs of tertiary syphilis may appear any time from 4 to over 30 years following the secondary stage. Lesions, called *gummas* (Figure 19-5), develop in various tissues of the body and may be due to a hypersensitivity reaction to the small number of spirochetes that have persisted in the body. Lesions may develop in the central nervous system, resulting in late neurosyphilis, which may cause mental changes or resemble other neurologic diseases. Neurosyphilis is a major cause of insanity. The cardiovascular system is often involved, a common manifestation being the development of aneurysms in the aorta.

Congenital syphilis

T. pallidum readily passes the placental barrier and a pregnant syphilitic woman may transmit the infection to the developing fetus. Congenital infection almost always occurs when the expectant mother has primary syphilis, about 90% of the time if she has secondary syphilis, and around 30% of the time during latent syphilis. The fetus does not develop signs of congenital syphilis until the second trimester. The spirochetes become disseminated throughout the fetus and about 25% die *in utero*, resulting in a spontaneous abortion or stillbirth. Over half the syphilitic infants who are alive at birth show marked signs of the disease. Many die shortly after birth. Others may have marked congenital defects and some may appear normal at birth but de-

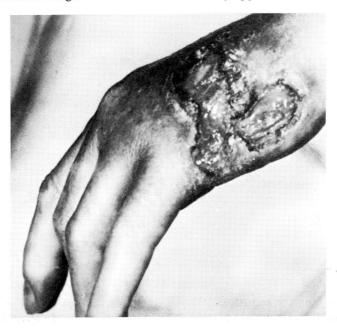

Figure 19-5 Tertiary syphilis with an ulcerative gumma on the hand. (Centers for Disease Control, Atlanta)

velop symptoms at later periods. The manifestations of congenital syphilis are variable but include such signs as skin lesions, enlarged spleens, anemia, pneumonia, eye damage, neurologic symptoms, mental retardation, and deformed bones, teeth, and cartilaginous tissues.

Transmission and Epidemiology

Generally transmission is by sexual contact and persons most likely to contract this disease are those who have multiple sexual contacts. The epidemiologic patterns of primary and secondary syphilis are very similar to those seen with gonorrhea; that is, most cases occur in sexually active young adults. The rate of increase in number of cases has not been as great in recent years as for gonorrhea (Figure 19-6), however. Overall about 1 case of syphilis is reported to every 20 to 30 cases of gonorrhea. Moreover, the number of cases of tertiary syphilis has not been increasing as rapidly as in the past. Perhaps it is an indication that many persons with primary and secondary diseases are being treated and so avoiding further progression of the disease.

Diagnosis

The appearance of a primary chancre or secondary lesions is suggestive of syphilis; these signs, however, may be confused with lesions or skin rashes caused by allergies or other infections. Beginning students tend to confuse the terms chancre and canker. Canker sores are common small ulcerations of the mucous membrane of the mouth

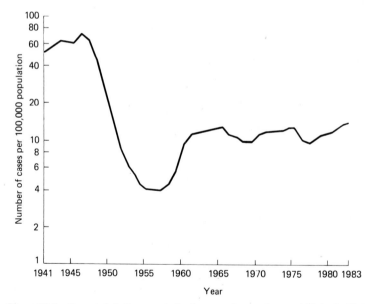

Figure 19-6 Reported civilian cases of primary and secondary syphilis in the United States, 1941–1983. Syphilis is the third most frequently reported communicable disease in the United States. Reported cases of primary and secondary syphilis totaled 32,163 for 1983 (modified from CDC annual summaries).

that may result from allergies to foods or other factors. They are not related to syphilis. Some small chancres in the mouth, however, may resemble a canker sore and may be diagnostically significant in a sexually active person. Diagnosis is first made by demonstrating the presence of the spirochetes in exudate from the lesion and then by serological tests.

Direct dark-field microscopic examination of exudate from primary or secondary lesions often demonstrates the presence of the motile syphilis spirochete (Figure 19-7). The exudate can also be fixed to a slide and stained with a specific fluorescent-labeled antibody for examination with a fluorescence microscope.

Various serological tests have been used over the past 70 years to detect syphilis antibodies. Antibodies appear several weeks after the primary lesion develops and remain in those persons who continue to harbor the spirochetes on through the latent and tertiary stages. The serological tests for syphilis, often referred to as STS, are perhaps the most widely used of all serologic tests. They are often required when applying for marriage licenses, for some types of employment, entrance into a military service, and as part of prenatal examinations. About 40 million such tests are run each year in the United States.

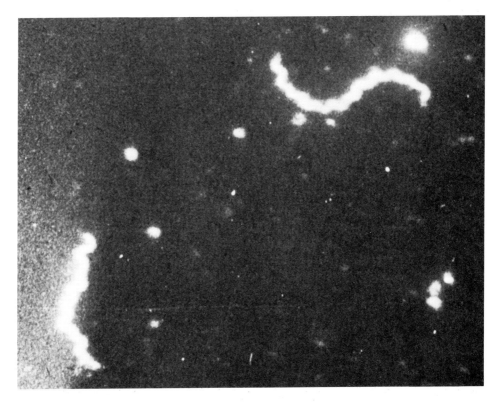

Figure 19-7 *Treponema pallidum* from a syphilitic lesion as observed with a dark-field microscope. (Centers for Disease Control, Atlanta)

Two general types of serologic tests are used (Table 19-1). The first detects a nonspecific antibody, called *reagin,* that reacts with antigens from several sources and is produced by some diseases other than syphilis. Among others, reagin reacts with a cardiolipin antigen that is extracted from beef hearts. Because the cardiolipin antigen is inexpensive, it is used in routine screening tests for syphilis. Flocculation tests, the chief tests used today, consist of adding the cardiolipin antigen to the test serum. Of these, the most used test is called the VDRL (Venereal Disease Research Laboratories) test and is positive when the cardiolipin forms into fine aggregates or floccules. For many years the screening tests consisted of the Wasserman or Kolmer complement fixation tests, which use the cardiolipin antigen. They are seldom used today. Persons with a number of other diseases, such as hepatitis, diabetes, and malaria, or other chronic diseases may give a positive reaction to these screening tests for syphilis; such reactions are called *biological false positives.* All sera that are positive in the screening tests must be retested to confirm the results with a more specific serologic test that detects antibodies specific for *T. pallidum.* One such specific test, called the *Treponema pallidum immobilization* (TPI) test, uses the suspension of live motile syphilis spirochetes. The test serum is mixed with the spirochetes; if specific antibodies are present, the motion of the spirochetes stops. Because it is difficult to maintain a supply of living syphilis spirochetes, a second test has been developed that uses killed *T. pallidum* and is replacing the TPI tests. It is the fluorescent treponemal antibody (FTA) test. The FTA test uses freeze-dried *T. pallidum* that are fixed to a glass slide. The test serum is added; if specific antibodies are present, they react with the *T. pallidum.* To determine if this reaction has taken place, the slide is rinsed to remove any unattached antibodies and then covered with fluorescent-labeled antibodies against human gamma globulin. If the test is positive, the spirochete-fluorescent antibody complex fluoresces when examined under a fluorescence microscope.

Treatment

Penicillin is highly effective in treating syphilis and there is no evidence that resistant strains of *T. pallidum* are developing. Persons allergic to penicillin can be treated with erythromycin and tetracyclines. To treat primary or secondary syphilis successfully, penicillin must be maintained continuously in the system for 7 to 10 days. In the later stages of the disease penicillin therapy should continue for at least 21 days. Treatment of syphilis at any stage before the onset of tertiary disease will block further progression of the disease. Treatment of pregnant syphilitic women early in pregnancy usually prevents congenital disease. Treatment later in pregnancy clears the infection in the fetus and prevents the occurrence of further tissue damage. Infants suspected of having congenital syphilis should receive treatment as soon as possible.

Prevention and Control

No vaccine is available. One widely used procedure to limit the spread of syphilis is to follow up and treat all persons who have had sexual contact with known syphilitic patients. This procedure, however, is often limited by a lack of public health person-

TABLE 19-1   SEROLOGIC TESTS FOR SYPHILIS (STS)

Nontreponemal tests	Use
Flocculation Tests	
VDRL (Venereal Disease Research Laboratory)	Screen and Diagnosis
Reagin Tests	
PCT (plasmacrit)	Screen
USR (Untreated Serum Reagin)	Screen
RPR (Rapid Plasma Reagin)	Screen and Diagnosis
Complement fixation Tests	
Kolmer or Wasserman (Complement fixation)	Rarely Available

Treponemal tests	
Immobilization	
TPI (Treponema pallidum immobilization)	Diagnosis-Research
Immunofluorescence	
FTA–ABS (Fluorescent treponemal antibody absorption)	Diagnosis and Screen
Hemmagglutination	
TPHA (Treponema pallidum Hemagglutination Assay)	Screen and Diagnosis

nel and operating funds. In addition, educational programs try to help people understand the mode of transmission, recognize symptoms, and how to receive treatment. Routine serologic tests are able to detect some infected people. This factor is of prime importance in reducing the threat of congenital syphilis. Restricting one's sexual contact to a marriage partner is the most effective means of preventing syphilis and other sexually transmitted diseases.

OTHER TREPONEMAL INFECTIONS

Three similar clinical diseases called yaws, pinta, and bejel result from treponemal spirochetes that are generally indistinguishable from *T. pallidum*. These diseases occur in people living under conditions of poor hygiene in the tropics or the Mideast. Transmission occurs by direct contact, not necessarily sexual, and primary infection usually happens in young children. Primary, secondary, and tertiary symptoms are seen. The exact relationship of these diseases to syphilis is not clear. It has been theorized that syphilis may have evolved from these diseases or vice versa.

Yaws, pinta, and bejel are readily cured by penicillin. Infection rates decrease significantly when improvements are made in personal hygiene and living conditions.

RELAPSING FEVER

Sporadic cases of relapsing fever in humans are caused by spirochetes of the genus *Borrelia*. Various species of *Borrelia* are carried by ticks and lice. Infection is transmitted to humans when they become infested and bitten by the insect vector. Tick-borne relapsing fever is seen occasionally in campers, for instance, who may spend time in tick-infested areas. The louse-borne disease is seen in persons living in poverty or under crowded impoverished conditions associated with wars or other calamities.

The clinical disease is characterized by a sudden onset with accompanying fever, headache, and muscle pain. A rash may be seen in some patients. The infection may involve many tissues of the body. The first episode lasts 3 to 7 days; a relapse occurs after an interval of 1 to 2 weeks. This cycle may be repeated several times. Treatment is with broad-spectrum antibiotics and the disease is prevented by avoiding exposure to ticks and lice.

CLINICAL NOTE

Tick-borne Relapsing Fever: Colorado

Three cases of tick-borne relapsing fever were reported to the Colorado State Health Department during the late summer of 1977. The last case occurred in a 10-year-old Girl Scout from Denver, who spent 6 days (August 11–16) at a ranch about 8 miles west of Deckers, Colorado. During this time she slept on a mattress in a wooden-floored tent with 3 other girls. A total of 24 girls and 4 counselors were similarly housed in the immediate area. The patient reported an "insect bite" on the third day of camp and first became ill 6 days later on August 19 with a fever that lasted 4 days. A second recurrence of fever on August 30 prompted the taking of a thick blood smear, which showed the presence of spirochetes and confirmed the diagnosis of tick-borne relapsing fever. The patient was treated with tetracycline and showed immediate improvement.

No other illnesses occurred in the group or were reported from other Girl Scout units camping during July and August. The elevated platform tents used by Girl Scout campers were not conducive to rodent infestation. The general area has many natural harborages for chipmunks, however, and several nests, removed from decaying tree stumps within the camp, contained fleas and mites.

Editorial note: Although ticks were not found in association with this case, the vector probably was *Ornithodorus hermsi*, a nest tick of chipmunks and pine squirrels. No other relapsing fever vector is known to occur in the coniferous forest biome in North America.

The fact that no ticks were present in the rodent nests collected is not surprising. Normally *O. hermsi* ticks remain in the nest, where all life functions are accomplished and where the ticks can feed on their rodent hosts. If the rodent resident does not return, ticks eventually disperse from the nest in search of a blood meal. This dispersion could lead them to a human rather than a rodent host, although ticks do not prefer a host-parasite relationship involving humans; so it tends to be of short duration (*MMWR 26*:357, 1977).

LEPTOSPIROSIS

One species of the genus *Leptospira*—*L. interrogans*—is a pathogen found in a wide variety of wild and domestic animals. Among other tissues, the kidneys of the animals become infected and the leptospira are shed in the urine.

Humans become infected by direct or indirect contact with the urine from infected animals or with animal tissues. Leptospirosis is most often seen in persons who are frequently exposed to animals, such as veterinarians, farmers, abattoir workers, persons living in rodent-infested housing, and dog owners. Infections have also occurred from contact with contaminated water.

The portal entry to the leptospira is probably through the mucosa or breaks in the skin. The organisms spread through the blood and usually the kidneys become infected; other tissues are infected as well. A wide variety of symptoms may be seen. Less than 100 cases of human leptospirosis are confirmed by laboratory diagnosis each year in the United States, although it is thought that many more cases do occur but are not specifically diagnosed. It is possible both to isolate this spirochete on artificial media and to measure specific antibodies by various serologic tests. Isolation, however, is difficult and is infrequently accomplished.

Vaccines are used in veterinary medicine and are available to persons in high-risk occupations. Penicillin, streptomycin, and tetracyclines are effective if used early in the disease but are generally not effective if given after about four days of illness.

CLINICAL NOTE

Leptospirosis: Tennessee

The first reported common-source outbreak of *Leptospira interrogans* in the United States occurred in Tennessee in August 1975.

An onset of illness struck 7 children, 4 males and 3 females, ranging in age from 11 to 16 years, in the period of August 1 to 10. It was characterized by fever, headache, nausea, and/or vomiting, chills, myalgias, and abdominal pain. Hospitalization was needed in 5 of the 7 cases; diagnoses included acute viral gastroenteritis, shigellosis, aseptic meningitis, and fever of unknown origin. The patient with the last diagnosis underwent laparotomy because of suspected appendicitis. A patient was treated as an outpatient for gastroenteritis and another did not consult a physician. The median duration of illness was 14 days and the mean hospital stay of the hospitalized patients was 6.6 days.

All 7 patients had serologic evidence of recent infection with *Leptospira interrogans*. Urine for culture was obtained from 6 patients 16 to 25 days after onset of illness; all were negative for leptospires.

All 7 patients had swum in a local creek in the month preceding their illness. No other common source could be identified. A case-control study showed a definite association between acquiring leptospirosis and swimming in the creek. A question-naire and serologic survey of 91 other people who had swum in the creek during the summer of 1975 failed to detect any additional cases.

Samples of the creek water taken for culture and for animal inoculation 4 weeks after the outbreak did not yield the organism. Serum specimens were obtained from 50 cattle in five of seven herds pastured along the creek, but serologic testing did not implicate any herd. Wildlife was also considered as a possible source of contamination. Limited trapping was unsuccessful; no wild animals were obtained for testing. Because of the prominent gastrointestinal illness and because of failure to incriminate a bacterial pathogen, the outbreak was initially believed to have a viral etiology. Leptospirosis was considered only after the initial epidemiologic investigation incriminated swimming in the stream as the only common factor shared by all 7 patients (*MMWR* 25:84, 1976).

SUMMARY

1. The spirochete of greatest medical concern is *Treponema pallidum*, the causative agent in syphilis. This disease occurs in several distinct stages with the last stage responsible for the most serious pathology. It is a classic example of a sexually transmitted disease, although other means of transmission occur. No vaccine is available for control, but the disease responds well to antibiotic therapy.

2. Other spirochetial diseases, although relatively uncommon in the United States, can be severe and include such exotic-sounding names as leptospirosis, yaws, pinta, and relapsing fever.

Bacillus and Clostridium

20

Bacteria of the genera *Bacillus* and *Clostridium* are large, gram-positive, spore-forming bacilli (Figure 20-1). Species of both genera are widespread in nature and most are saprophytes. The most significant pathogen of the genus *Bacillus* is *Bacillus anthracis*, the causative agent of anthrax. The species *B. cercus* causes food poisoning if it grows in unrefrigerated food, where it produces enterotoxins. Species of the genus *Clostridium* are found in the intestinal tract of most animals and in the soil. They are obligate anaerobes and the pathogenic strains produce powerful exotoxins. The common diseases caused by the clostridia are tetanus, food poisoning, cellulitis, and gas gangrene.

ANTHRAX

Anthrax is primarily a disease of animals. During the developmental years of medical microbiology anthrax was a frequently encountered disease in sheep and cattle. Because of the relatively large size and definite shape of the bacillus, plus the availability of experimental animals, anthrax served as an excellent model for the study of infectious diseases. Many important discoveries regarding the germ theory of disease and immunity resulted from investigations of anthrax (see Chapter 1).

Bacterium

B. anthracis is a large, aerobic, gram-positive bacillus 5 to 10 μm long and 1 to 3 μm wide. The spores are highly resistant and may remain viable on animal products or in the soil for years. This bacterium is easily grown on laboratory media.

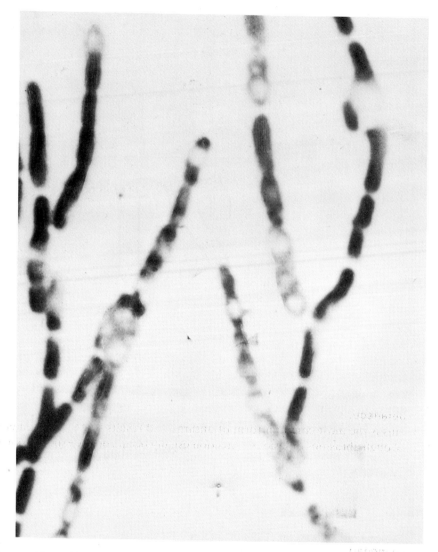

Figure 20-1 Micrograph of *Bacillus anthracis* showing endospores. (Centers for Disease Control, Atlanta)

Pathogenesis and Clinical Disease

The spores of *B. anthracis* enter the body either through abrasions of the skin or by inhalation or ingestion. The virulent strains possess a capsule around the vegetative cell that retards phagocytosis and a toxin is produced that causes the signs and symptoms of the disease. The three main clinical forms of anthrax are shown in Figure 20-2.

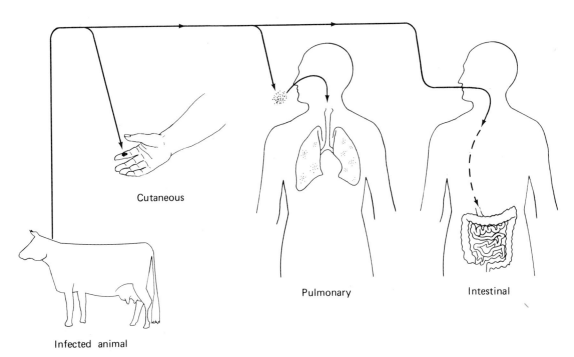

Figure 20-2   Three forms of anthrax that might be contracted by exposure to infected animal products.

Cutaneous

This is the most common form of anthrax and results when spores enter the tissues through abrasions or lesions. Infection usually occurs on the exposed skin surface. A local lesion develops that rarely contains pus, but it is swollen, hemorrhagic, and forms a black scab (Figure 20-3). If the infection remains localized, death rates are low. The infection spreads to the blood in about 5% of the cases and this generalized infection is often fatal.

Pulmonary

This form of anthrax, which results from inhalation of the spores, is seen in persons who handle contaminated animal products and is sometimes referred to as "wool-sorters' disease." The onset is sudden, with high fever and respiratory distress. Death usually results in untreated cases.

Intestinal

Intestinal anthrax is rare and results from eating contaminated meat. Severe enteritis results and mortality rates are high.

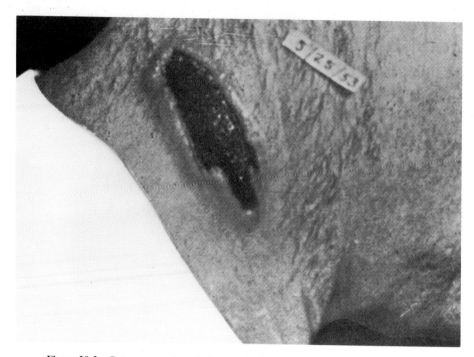

Figure 20-3 Cutaneous anthrax lesion on the neck, fifteenth day of disease. The patient had worked with air-dried goat skins from Africa. (Armed Forces Institute of Pathology, AFIP MIS #75-4203-9)

Transmission and Epidemiology

Transmission among animals usually occurs from the ingestion of spores. Anthrax spores may remain viable for 20 to 30 years or longer in a pasture contaminated by the remains of animals dying of anthrax. At present, relatively few cases of anthrax occur in animals in the United States. It is still found in animals in certain countries, however, and this presents a hazard to persons living in those countries who come in contact with contaminated animal products. Since the 1950s outbreaks in the United States have resulted from contact with contaminated hides covering bongo drums, infected pig bristles used in shaving brushes, goats' hair used in weaving, and similar items, all imported from foreign countries. Overall the risk of contracting anthrax in the United States is slight, an average of only two cases per year being reported in the past 10 years. Public health personnel should be aware of the threat of anthrax and be able to recognize the possible sources of infection.

Treatment and Control

Anthrax can be successfully treated with penicillin or broad-spectrum antibiotics. Vaccines are available to control the disease in animals and humans of high risk. Carcasses of diseased animals should be buried deep in the soil or burned to prevent the spread of spores. Gas sterilization or radiation may be used to decontaminate hides, wool, and related animal products.

CLINICAL NOTE

Anthrax: California

The first known anthrax case involving a home craftsman working with yarn occurred in January 1976 in a 32-year-old man who operated a home-weaving business in California. The patient died. *Bacillus anthracis* was isolated from some yarns used by the patient.

The contaminated yarn, obtained from a distributor in Los Angeles, was imported from Pakistan. A second distributor in New York imported materials from the same source. The distributors voluntarily recalled the yarn, according to the Consumer Product Safety Commission.

The patient developed inhalation anthrax on January 17, with fever and symptoms of an upper respiratory infection. He became acutely ill on January 21 and was hospitalized that day with a complaint of fever, chills, pharyngitis, headache, nausea, anorexia, and pleurisy. Admission examination revealed a 38.8°C fever, decreased breath sounds on the left side, spasticity of the left lower and upper extremities, unresponsiveness to simple commands, and a disconjugate gaze. The pleural fluid and a peripheral blood smear contained large gram-positive bacilli.

Despite intravenous aqueous penicillin (5 million units every 6 hours), intramuscular streptomycin (500 mg every 12 hours), and intensive supportive therapy, the patient died 28 hours after admission. *Bacillus anthracis* was isolated from both clinical and autopsy specimens.

The patient was a self-employed weaver who frequently worked with a variety of imported yarns. He had not traveled outside the local community for at least 2 weeks prior to the onset of his illness and had no probable source of infection other than his work materials.

Yarn from both distributors was obtained and cultured. *Bacillus anthracis* was recovered from various animal-origin yarns obtained from each. The contaminated products, sold in 4-oz skeins or balls, included camel hair, goat hair, or sheeps' wool in varying combinations. Commonly sold in plastic bags, the yarn was most often used in such handicrafts as wall hangings and macrame objects (*MMWR 25:33*, 1976).

TETANUS

Bacterium

Clostridium tetani, the causative agent of tetanus, is a large gram-positive, spore-forming, motile, obligate anaerobic bacillus. It can be grown on blood agar or media containing meat. Various strains exist, but all produce the same exotoxin.

Pathogenesis and Clinical Disease

Because of the wide distribution of C. *tetani*, wounds are often contaminated with its spores. Yet the disease of tetanus does not develop in a great majority of cases. The condition of the wound must be such that an anaerobic environment exists and some dead tissue is present. These conditions allow spores to germinate, bacteria to proliferate, toxin to be produced, and block the body's defense mechanisms. Such conditions are often seen in puncture wounds produced, for instance, by nails or splinters. Yet other types of wounds or conditions resulting in tissue damage may also offer a suitable environment. One frequently encountered form of tetanus occurring in underdeveloped countries is tetanus of the umbilicus of infants born at home and treated with unsterile instruments.

The tetanus toxin is extremely potent; a small amount is able to cause the disease. Still, the growth of C. *tetani* per se causes no tissue damage. Usually signs and symptoms of the disease begin to occur 4 to 10 days after injury and are entirely the result of the toxin spreading through the body. The toxin specifically affects the synaptic junction of the nerves by preventing the inhibition or erasing of nerve impulses once they have crossed the synaptic junction. The nerve continues to send impulses, a condition that results in spasmotic contractions (tetany) of the involved muscles. Early symptoms are muscle stiffness with the muscles of the jaw often developing spasms first. This condition gives the disease its common name of *lockjaw*. As the disease progresses, spasms develop in other muscles. The spasms may be brief, but they can occur frequently and cause great pain and exhaustion. In some cases, the spasms may be powerful enough to cause bones to break. Respiratory complications are common and death rates high, especially in young children and elderly persons. In nonfatal cases, recovery takes several weeks but is usually complete.

Transmission and Epidemiology

Transmission and epidemiology of tetanus do not follow the pattern seen in many infectious diseases where the microbes are passed from host to host. Some situations are conducive to the development of tetanus, however. Soils or materials in contact with animal wastes are usually heavily contaminated with C. *tetani* and offer excellent sources of infection. Before the development of an effective vaccine, tetanus often resulted from wounds received in wars. Hundreds of thousands of cases of tetanus occurred during the Civil War, but only 12 cases were reported among U.S. troops during World War II. About 100 cases per year are reported in the United States, 40% of which result in death. The numbers of reported cases in this country are shown in Figure 20-4. Large numbers of cases still occur in some underdeveloped tropical countries.

Diagnosis

Diagnosis is made on the basis of the clinical disease. C. *tetani* is a common contaminant of wounds and may be found in patients who do not develop tetanus. Therefore the isolation of the bacterium from a patient may not be diagnostic.

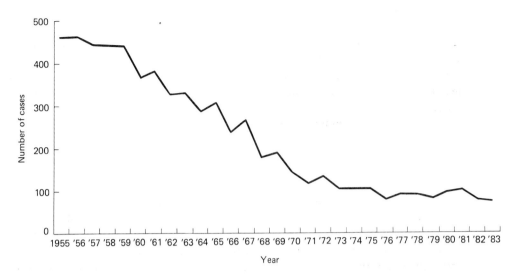

Figure 20-4 Reported cases of tetanus by year in the United States, 1955–1983 (modified from CDC annual summaries).

Treatment

As soon as clinical tetanus is suspected, steps should be taken to neutralize the existing toxin and prevent the formation of new toxin. Antitoxin, produced in humans, should be administered immediately. The wounds should be debrided to remove dead tissues or foreign bodies and large doses of penicillin or tetracycline should be given to prevent further growth of the bacterium. If muscular spasms occur, antispasmatic drugs should be used and respiration should be maintained by a positive pressure-breathing apparatus if necessary.

Prevention and Control

At present, the major involvement with *C. tetanus* by most medical personnel in developed countries concerns the prevention of this disease. Prevention through immunization has been extremely effective.

Immunization with tetanus toxoid should begin with infants 1 to 3 months old. The toxoid is usually given in combination with diphtheria toxoid and pertussis vaccine as the DPT vaccine. Three doses of DPT should be given several weeks apart. A booster dose should then be given 1 and 4 years later. After the age of 7, a booster should be given every 10 years. During the accident-prone years most young children are repeatedly given booster doses with each new injury, a practice that is both unnecessary and unwise. Parents should keep an immunization record for their children so that such unnecessary immunizations can be avoided. When a person suffers an injury that is likely to result in tetanus and that person has no history of immunization, passive immunization with human antitoxin should be given as temporary protection. It should be followed by active immunization with the toxoid.

Neonatal umbilical cord tetanus can be prevented by actively immunizing pregnant females who have no history of previous immunizations. The newborn infant will then have natural passive immunity at the time of birth, which should reduce the chance of developing umbilical cord tetanus.

CLINICAL NOTE

Neonatal Tetanus: Illinois

On May 6, 1975, a midwife delivered a male infant at home in a town across the Mexican border from Laredo, Texas. She reportedly cut the infant's umbilical cord with unsterilized scissors, tied it with a piece of string, and applied olive oil to the umbilical stump. The infant was adopted on the day of birth by a family from Chicago and appeared to be well until the third day of life when, enroute to Chicago, he became irritable and ate poorly. When 5 days old, he could no longer nurse from a bottle. He was unable to open his mouth when crying and had several trembling spells associated with rigid flexion of his arms and extension of his legs. During these spells his head was kept in a neutral position; he perspired noticeably and was cyanotic. Each spell lasted approximately 10 minutes and occurred every 3 to 4 hours. The symptoms worsened and on the sixth day the infant was taken to the University of Chicago's Wyler Children's Hospital.

On admission it was noted that he had risus sardonicus (a grinning expression produced by spasms), opisthotonus (difficulty in opening mouth), trismus (spasms with head and neck bent backward), and a temperature of 39.5°C. His umbilicus was inflamed and exuded a yellow purulent discharge. Laboratory evaluations at that time included a negative cerebrospinal fluid (CSF) examination and a normal serum calcium level. Gram stain of the umbilical discharge showed a mixed flora, including some large gram-positive rods, which were thought by some observers to be compatible with *Clostridium tetani*; however, cultures grew only microaerophilic streptococci, peptostreptococci, and bacteroides. Neonatal tetanus was diagnosed on clinical grounds and the infant was given 1000 units of human tetanus immune globulin intramuscularly; antibiotic therapy with penicillin and gentamicin was begun. To control the muscle spasms, phenobarbitol and chlorpromazine were given and the infant was then rehydrated and maintained by continuous intravenous infusion.

Episodes of muscle spasm and periods of restricted respirations and cyanosis gradually decreased over the first two days of hospitalization; by the third day the infant could tolerate feeding and the administration of a sedative via a nasogastric tube. Gentamicin was discontinued on the third hospital day when admission blood and CSF cultures proved negative. Hypothermia of 35°C, noted on the fourth hospital day, was attributed to chlorpromazine and diazapam was substituted for chlorpromazine and phenobarbitol to control muscle spasms. The infant's temperature returned to normal and the intensity of the muscle spasms decreased. But increasing tolerance to diazapam developed and the dose was increased over the next week to 10 mg/kg/day; for several days chlorpromazine was also given again in small doses. Penicillin was discontinued on the twelfth hospital day. On or about the thirteenth hospital day the tendency to have spasms began to decrease, and by the nineteenth day no symptoms related to tetanus toxin were discernible. On the twentieth hospital day bottle feedings were begun. Medications were gradually decreased as symptoms subsided and were discontinued by the thirty-fourth day with no apparent residual (*MMWR 24*:313, 1975).

BOTULISM FOOD POISONING

Bacterium

C. botulinum is a large, gram-positive, anaerobic bacillus that produces an exotoxin that causes food poisoning. Its spores are among the most heat resistant and are able to withstand temperatures of 100°C for several hours. These spores will survive in heat-processed foods if the temperature does not reach the required level. Growth can occur in a wide variety of culture media as well as many types of food. Seven serotypes, based on the antigenic characteristic of the exotoxin, have been identified and are designated A through G. Cases due to type G have not been reported in humans.

Pathogenesis and Clinical Disease

In most cases, botulism results from the ingestion of preformed toxin produced during the growth of *C. botulinum* in foods. Botulinum toxin is one of the most powerful known toxins and extremely small amounts are able to cause illness or death in humans.

The toxin, generally type A, B, E, or F, is absorbed primarily from the small intestine, passes into the blood, and is carried to the peripheral nerves where it specifically reacts at the muscle-nerve junction. The toxin produces complete paralysis of the nerve impulse by preventing the release of acetylcholine. Death results from the paralysis of respiratory functions. Symptoms may appear as soon as 12 to 36 hours after ingesting contaminated food or may take as long as 8 days to appear. The first symptoms are often weakness and dizziness. Double vision (diplopa), difficulty in speaking (dipphonia) and swallowing (dysphagia), and dilated pupils usually occur. Some abdominal distress may be experienced. Fever is rare. Muscle weakness develops, leading to paralysis as the disease progresses. When paralysis of respiratory muscles occurs, death results. The mortality rate varies between 20 and 70% and is influenced by the amount and serotype of toxin consumed as well as the time between ingestion and the initiation of antitoxin therapy.

In 1976 it was discovered that *C. botulinum* could grow in the intestines of infants and produce enough toxin to cause serious illness. The spore may be in various infant foods, but honey has been implicated in several cases. Not all infants appear to be susceptible and at present it is not known just which conditions allow the intestinal tracts of some infants to support the growth of *C. botulinum*. Signs of the disease in these patients may start with constipation, followed by weakness and then paralysis of the muscles of the head and neck. Paralysis may proceed to the arms and legs with death resulting from paralysis of the respiratory muscles. In cases that progress slowly, medical treatment can be applied in time to save the infant. In rapidly developing cases, death may result before significant signs are noted. Such death may be included under the sudden infant death syndrome (sudden crib death), a problem that has long baffled medical investigators. It is now suspected that at least a percentage of sudden infant deaths is a result of infectious botulism.

Occasionally *C. botulinum* grows in contaminated wounds where toxins are produced that diffuse into the blood and cause typical signs and symptoms of botulism poisoning.

C. botulinum is able to grow in various environmental niches, such as animal feed, carcasses of dead animals or invertebrates, and sediments in lakes or ponds. Outbreaks of botulism poisoning occur when these contaminated materials are eaten by domestic or wild animals or birds. Under certain conditions outbreaks of botulism have occurred in wild ducks, resulting in the death of hundreds of thousands of the birds. Such wildlife epidemics are commonly due to botulinum toxin types C and D.

Transmission and Epidemiology

The *C. botulinum* spores are often present on food. Production of botulinum toxin results when the microorganism grows in an anaerobic environment in foods stored at room temperature. Alkaline foods favor the growth of *C. botulinum* and the development of the exotoxin.

Because botulism is a poisoning rather than an infectious disease, transmission from person to person does not occur. Circumscribed outbreaks, however, may result when a toxin-containing food is eaten by a number of people. Transmission of botulism generally involves home-canned foods; then the disease usually occurs only among family members. Outbreaks from improperly sterilized commercially canned food are quite rare. With commercially canned food, only four deaths from botulism poisoning have resulted in the United States in the past 45 years whereas during this time more than 775 billion cans of food have been eaten. Yet the threat of botulism is always present and continued monitoring of food-processing procedures and foods is needed to maintain this remarkable safety record. In general, from 20 to 30 cases a year are reported in the United States. Nevertheless, in 1977 several significant outbreaks of botulism food poisoning resulted when restaurants illegally used home-canned sauces and relishes and the total number of cases for that year increased to 114 (Figure 20-5).

Diagnosis

Time is important in dealing with botulism food poisoning; so a preliminary diagnosis must often be made on the basis of clinical and epidemiological evidence. A diagnosis based on clinical appearance is often difficult, for early symptoms are eas-

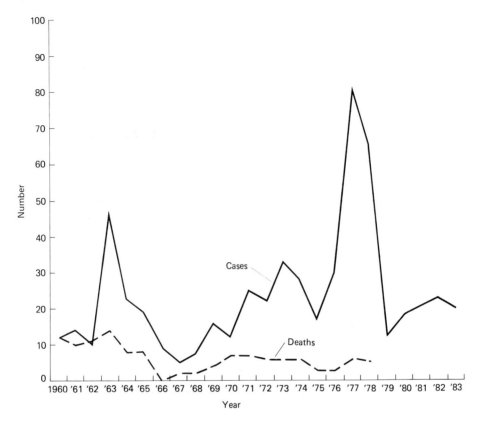

Figure 20-5 Reported cases and deaths from food-borne botulism by year in the United States, 1960–1983. All cases in 1980 were associated with home-canned or home-processed foods (modified from CDC annual summaries).

ily confused with other diseases. Furthermore, few physicians have personally seen patients with botulism and so would not easily recognize the symptoms. When isolated cases occur, there is little reason to suspect botulism. When botulism is suspected, serum, stool, and gastric-washing specimens should be collected and suspected foods obtained. The presence of toxin in these materials can be detected by injecting extracts into mice.

Treatment

Once botulism is suspected, antitoxin should be given as soon as possible. Because any one of three or four different toxin serotypes may cause the disease, a polyvalent antitoxin is used. The antitoxin will not reverse the effects of toxin already affecting the nerves but will neutralize any circulating toxin. Supportive care, particularly in maintaining respiratory functions, is very important.

Prevention and Control

Proper procedures in preparing home-canned foods—that is, using pressure cookers to ensure destruction of spores—are the most important preventative measures. Before being served, home-canned foods should be boiled for several minutes to destroy any toxin that might be present.

Immunization with toxoids is effective but seldom used due to the rarity of botulism in the general public. With the current awareness of infant botulism—and if further research shows it to be a widespread problem—it might be desirable to vaccinate pregnant females so that passive immunity is present in the infant during the early months of life when it is most susceptible to this form of the disease.

CLINICAL NOTES

Follow-up on Infant Botulism: United States, January 1978

Infant botulism, a disease apparently resulting from intraintestinal toxin production by *Clostridium botulinum,* was first recognized as a distinct clinical entity in late 1976. Since then, cases have been identified with increasing frequency (1, retrospectively, in 1975, 15 in 1976, 42 in 1977) and have been reported to the Centers for Disease Control from 15 states throughout the country: California (37), Pennsylvania (4), Utah (4), Washington (2), and (1 each) Arizona, Colorado, Montana, Nevada, New Jersey, New York, North Dakota, Oregon, Tennessee, Texas, and Wisconsin. Cases have occurred most frequently in the fall months, particularly in the past year; however, increased physician awareness may have accounted for this observation.

All patients identified thus far have had sufficient neuromuscular paralysis to require hospitalization. Constipation was the first symptom of illness in most cases, but frequently it was initially overlooked. A spectrum in the severity of symptoms has been noted. Some infants showed only lethargy, mild weakness, and slowed feeding whereas others became acutely ill with obvious feeding difficulty, severe generalized weakness, and hypotonia over a 1- to 3-day period, which, in some cases, progressed to respiratory insufficiency. A California and a Utah infant died following respiratory arrest.

Polyvalent antitoxin was administered to the first patient (1975) because the case was thought to be food-borne botulism. However, subsequent patients who received meticulous supportive care that focused on their nutritional and respiratory needs have been successfully managed.

In general, affected infants were the product of a normal gestation and delivery. They had no congenital abnormalities and were healthy until onset of illness. Of the 58 patients, 33 (57%) were males. The median age at onset was 10 weeks, the range 3 to 26 weeks.

No source of ingestible preformed botulinal toxin has been identified for any infant; neither did the patients share any exposure to a common food. Cases have occurred in exclusively breast-fed and exclusively formula-fed infants, although most infants had some exposure to food items other than milk. A potential source of *C. botulinum* spores, however, has been identified for 6 cases. Vacuum cleaner dust from the home of an infant with type A illness was found to contain *C. botulinum* type A whereas soil from the yard of an infant with type B illness yielded type B organisms. Three opened jars of honey taken from the homes of 3 infants with type B botulism who had been fed honey and water were found to contain type B organisms. Similarly, an unopened jar of honey of the same brand as that fed to an infant with type A illness was shown to harbor type A organisms. In contrast, *C. botulinum* was not found in 17 other commercial honey specimens, in 1 specimen from a private beekeeper, or in over 100 other foods tested, including cereals, baby food, formula, and breast milks; however, testing of foods and other potential sources of spores has not been done for all cases.

Editorial note: The identification of 57 of the 58 cases in only 24 months in 15 states located throughout the United States indicates that infant botulism occurs more commonly than previously realized. In California, Pennsylvania, and Utah some hospitals and physicians diagnosed subsequent cases shortly after identifying their first case. If cases are evenly distributed in the country, then by a conservative estimate at least 250 cases needing hospitalization may be occurring annually. Furthermore, because botulinal spores are found worldwide, there is no reason to suppose that cases are limited to the United States. Failure to identify cases in other countries may be explained by lack of physician awareness and limited laboratory facilities. Intensive case-finding is needed to provide sufficient data to elucidate the actual incidence, full clinical spectrum, mode of transmission, and other risk factors associated with this toxigenic disease.

Indications for the use of botulinal antitoxin or oral antibiotics in the therapy of infant botulism are at present uncertain. It is not known whether administration of either will ameliorate the disease, shorten hospitalization, or diminish the risk of serious complications (*MMWR 27*:17, 1978).

Botulism and Commercial Pot Pie: California

On August 3, 1982, a 56-year-old woman residing in Los Angeles County, California, developed diplopia (double vision), weakness, difficulty breathing, and chest pain. She had respiratory arrest on admission to the hospital but was intubated, resuscitated, and placed in intensive care. Examination showed complete bilateral ptosis (drooping of eyelids), paralysis of eye muscles, facial weakness, and lack of reflexes. Cerebrospinal fluid was normal except for increased glucose. She had a past history of seizure disorder, diabetes mellitus, and organic brain syndrome. An infectious-disease consultant thought her subsequent fever was due to pneumonia secondary to aspiration, and he suspected botulism as the underlying cause of her illness.

The patient lived with her husband and grown son who both prepared meals for her and attempted a strict diet in consideration of her diabetes. When asked about the patient's food history before onset of illness, the husband and son named no likely suspects for botulism. No home-preserved foods had been served, and, with one exception, she had not eaten other foods that were not freshly prepared for her or were not also consumed by her husband and son. The exception was a commercial beef pot pie, which was accidently mishandled, then consumed by the patient one day before illness began.

The son had prepared the pot pie for an earlier evening meal. The frozen pie was baked in an oven for 40 to 45 minutes. As he was about to serve it to his mother, his father came home with some freshly cooked hamburgers just purchased at a take-out restaurant. The pot pie was put aside on an unrefrigerated shelf. Two and one-half days later, the son came home and found his mother had just consumed this pot pie without reheating it.

An uneaten portion of the pot pie, still in its metal plate, was retrieved by the family members. Type A botulism toxin was found in this pie by a mouse-inoculation test performed at a U.S. Department of Agriculture laboratory in Beltsville, Maryland, and type A toxin was also demonstrated in the patient's serum by the state's Microbial Disease Laboratory.

Editorial note: This is the third case of botulism associated with commercial pot pies reported from California; one other episode (involving two clinically diagnosed patients) was reported from Minnesota in 1960. Mishandling of the pot pies occurred in three of these episodes, and mishandling was also suspected in the fourth. The known mishandlings consisted of leaving the baked pot pie in the oven with the pilot light on, thereby maintaining "incubator" temperatures overnight. The pies were then eaten with no (or insufficient) reheating to destroy toxin. Or, as in the present case, the baked pie sat out at room temperature for over 2 days during hot weather—conditions that also could simulate an incubator.

In these situations, it is suspected that the original baking killed competing organisms in the pies and eliminated much of the oxygen. The heat-resistant, anaerobic *Clostridium botulinum*, which was evidently present and can be found in many fresh, frozen, and other food products, was then presumably able to germinate and produce toxin under the crust during storage at warm, incubator-like temperatures. Products such as pot pies should be kept frozen before heating and ideally should be served hot after the first cooking. If any such product is to be saved, it should be quickly refrigerated, then reheated to hot temperatures. This would minimize any risk of botulinal poisoning (*MMWR* 32:39, 1983).

CELLULITIS AND GAS GANGRENE

Bacteria

Various different species of the genus *Clostridium* are able to grow in damaged body tissue. These bacteria may release toxins and enzymes that produce further tissue damage to the surrounding healthy tissue. *C. perfringens* is the most frequently involved species. These clostridia are common inhabitants of the intestinal tracts of humans and animals and are found both on clothing and in the soil. *C. novyi* and *C. septicum,* along with other clostridia, are less commonly involved.

Pathogenesis and Clinical Disease

Numerous toxins and enzymes produced by clostridia are able to destroy tissues, particularly muscle fibers and connective tissues. Many wounds that occur in wartime or from accidents become contaminated with various clostridia. When a niche of devitalized (dead or dying) tissue or foreign debris exists in a wound, it may create an anaerobic area in which the clostridia can proliferate. As the toxins and enzymes of the growing clostridia are released, the tissues adjacent to the wound are devitalized and the supply of oxygenated blood is stopped. This situation creates an expanded anaerobic area into which the clostridia can grow; the result is a further production of toxins, which again extends the area of tissue damage. Phagocytic cells of the host are essentially helpless against this infection, for the bacteria are sequestered in dead tissue out of reach of the defense mechanisms of the host.

Several forms of clostridial wound infections occur. A condition called *anaerobic cellulitis* is less severe than gas gangrene (myonecrosis) and does not involve the muscles. The infection spreads through subcutaneous tissues and between muscles. Gas is produced by the bacteria causing distention of the tissues. Myonecrosis is a more severe form of the infection with toxic destruction of adjacent muscle tissues and an ever-widening expansion of the lesion. The swollen tissues have a dark yellowish discoloration and produce a foul-smelling, dark fluid exudate. Gas is formed by the bacteria, causing some distention of the subcutaneous tissues and considerable pain. Symptoms of gas gangrene begin to appear 12 to 72 hours following injury. Along with the local tissue involvement, a generalized toxic reaction may be seen in the patient. Death results without proper treatment. Gas gangrene may develop in the uterus after mechanically induced abortion and is seen more frequently following illegal abortions induced by nonmedical practitioners. Rapidly developing gas gangrene may occur in any section of the bowel that is deprived of a normal blood supply.

Transmission and Epidemiology

As with the other clostridial diseases, person-to-person transmission is not a factor in the epidemiology. Disease results when host tissues are altered so that they allow the growth of the clostridia. Gas gangrene is a serious threat to persons with traumatic injuries, bowel obstructions, bowel surgery, reduced blood supply to given tissues, and so on. Elderly persons with poor circulation are prime candidates for this type of infection. Gas gangrene is a major problem in battlefield wounds when treatment is delayed.

Diagnosis

Laboratory diagnosis is difficult and early diagnosis is made on clinical grounds.

Treatment

Removal of dead tissue from the wound is the first step in treatment. Penicillin or other antibiotics, along with antitoxins, should be given and are helpful if all dead tissue is removed. In many cases of gas gangrene, the spread of the infection cannot be stopped unless all infected tissue is removed; this often requires amputation of the involved limb. Hyperbaric oxygen (chambers of oxygen gas under 3 atmosphere of pressure to increase the amount of O_2 in the tissues) has been used with some limited beneficial effects in treating these anaerobic infections.

Prevention and Control

Prompt cleaning and surgical debridement of wounds constitute the most important preventative measure. The rapid evacuation to field hospitals by helicopter of military personnel wounded during combat has greatly reduced the incidence of gas gangrene associated with battlefield wounds. Antibiotic treatment may help prevent the development of clostridial infection in wounds.

OTHER CLOSTRIDIAL DISEASES

Food Poisoning

C. perfringens, a common cause of food poisoning, is most often associated with meats. The spores may survive the normal cooking process. The spores germinate as the meat cools and within a few hours at warm temperatures massive numbers of bacteria develop. The ingested bacteria grow in the intestines and release toxins that cause diarrhea, cramps, and abdominal pain. Onset is 8 to 20 hours after ingestion of contaminated meat and symptoms last about one day. Deaths do not result.

Pseudomembranous Colitis

A potentially serious form of diarrhea following some antibiotic treatments is caused by *C. difficile*. This bacterium is a normal inhabitant of the intestinal tract but is not able to compete with the normal bacterial flora. When antibiotic treatments reduce the normal bacterial flora, *C. difficile* is able to proliferate rapidly and secrete toxins. These toxins cause fluids to collect in the bowel and damage the cells of the bowel. The first symptoms are abdominal pain with watery diarrhea. Mixtures of fibrin, mucus, and white blood cells accumulate in patches on the mucosa of the colon. These patches are called *pseudomembranes* (false membranes) and are the basis of the name *pseudomembranous colitis*. About one-third of the patients with this disease die, possibly from combined effects of both the primary disease for which they were being treated and the antibiotic-induced colitis.

SUMMARY

1. The genus *Bacillus* and the genus *Clostridium* represent genera containing gram-positive, spore-forming rods. These organisms are ubiquitous throughout nature and are responsible for a relatively small number of serious human infections.

2. *Bacillus anthracis* is aerobic and only the disease anthrax is of major importance. This disease, though rare in the United States, is a serious, often life-threatening one acquired by associating with infected animals or contaminated animal by-products.

3. Diseases due to clostridia include tetanus, gas gangrene, and botulism. These are serious infections requiring medical assistance. Usually the diseases are acquired through an injury that then becomes contaminated with the disease-causing organisms. Botulism generally results from the ingestion of contaminated foods. Control of these organisms is difficult because of the presence of the endospores produced by both the *Clostridium* and *Bacillus* species.

Corynebacterium

Several species of corynebacteria are found in humans and animals. The once widespread and serious disease of diphtheria is the major disease caused by corynebacteria.

DIPHTHERIA

Diphtheria is a disease caused by an exotoxin that is released by some strains of the bacterium *Corynebacterium diphtheriae*. The ability of a given strain of *C. diphtheriae* to produce the exotoxin is determined by the presence of a lysogenic bacteriophage. As discussed in Chapters 5 and 32, some bacteriophages have the ability to insert their DNA into the DNA molecule of the host bacterium, a process called *lysogeny*. The gene that directs the production of the diphtheria toxin is carried by the bacteriophage and is therefore produced only by those *C. diphtheriae* that contain the bacteriophage genes.

Early research on diphtheria, during the latter 20 years of the 1800s, led to the discovery of bacterial exotoxins and demonstrated that such toxins are the cause of some bacterial diseases. This research also led to the development of methods for treating toxic diseases with antitoxins.

Bacterium

C. diphtheriae (Figure 21-1) is a narrow, 1.0- to 1.5-μm, gram-positive bacillus that may range in length up to 5 μm. When prepared on slides for staining, the cells are

272

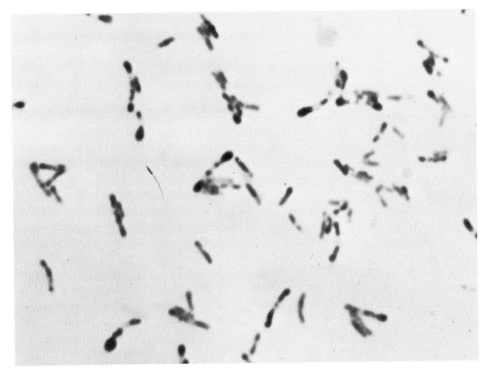

Figure 21-1 Micrograph of *Corynebacterium diphtheriae*. (Centers for Disease Control, Atlanta)

often oriented in palisades or in V and L shaped arrangements. When mixed together, such cellular arrangements are said to give the appearance of Chinese letters. The cells are pleomorphic (multiple shaped), often with bulging at one end that gives a club shape (*Coryne* = club). They may also contain accumulations of phosphates (metachromatic granules) that stain differently from the other cell materials and give a beaded appearance. Although these bacteria can be cultivated on a variety of media, in diagnostic laboratories they are grown on a selective medium containing tellurite salts. Reduction of the tellurite causes these bacteria to produce gray or black colonies. Using this procedure, three different types of *C. diphtheriae*—gravis, mitis, and intermedius—are determined. All three types, however, produce the same toxin and clinical disease. *C. diphtheriae* is more resistant to drying than many vegetative bacteria and may remain viable for as long as 3 to 4 months in dried respiratory exudates.

Pathogenesis and Clinical Disease

Both toxin-producing and non-toxin-producing strains of *C. diphtheriae* can adhere to and colonize the mucosal tissue of the upper respiratory tract. Humans are the only natural host. Transmission is primarily from person to person by airborne drop-lets. The disease results entirely from the effects of the exotoxin. The toxin specifi-cally adheres to and is initially absorbed into cells around the growing *C. diphtheriae*. The toxin inhibits protein synthesis of the affected cells and no structural damage is seen until the lack of newly synthesized proteins causes the death of the cells. As the dead host cells accumulate, an inflammatory response is induced. The bacteria con-tinue to produce toxin, which causes the lesion to expand. An incubation period of several days to one week is required before the patient begins to experience clinical symptoms of diphtheria. Lesions, which usually appear first in the tonsillar-pharyn-geal area, are characterized by patches of a thick fibrinous exudate containing many entrapped host cells and bacteria. The layer of exudate, called a *pseudomembrane*, adheres firmly to the epithelial surfaces. As the disease progresses, the pseudomem-brane may spread upward into nasopharyngeal tissues and downward into the larynx and trachea. In severe cases, obstruction of the airway may occur, resulting in suffo-cation of the patient. It is sometimes necessary to maintain breathing by inserting a tube in the trachea. The lesions remain superficial and rarely do the bacteria invade deeper tissues. Besides the formation of the pseudomembrane and a sore throat, the patient experiences fever, malaise, and enlarged regional lymph nodes, resulting in swelling of the neck. The term "bull-neck" is sometimes used to refer to this condi-

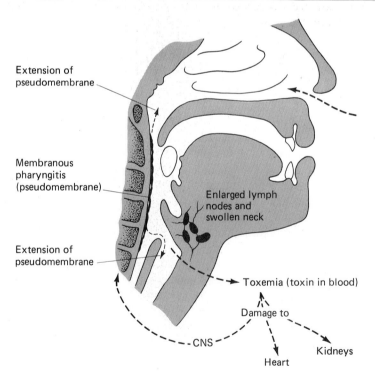

Figure 21-2 Pathogenesis of diphtheria.

tion. The exotoxin is also absorbed into the blood and carried to various internal organs where cell destruction may occur. The most frequent and serious damage occurs to the heart and central nervous system (CNS) with death often resulting from damage to the heart. The disease may linger for many weeks and, due to damage to the CNS, varying levels of paralysis may occur after 5 weeks. Aspects of the pathogenesis of diphtheria are shown in Figure 21-2. Before methods of treating or preventing this disease were available, diphtheria was a major killer disease of children. Persons recovering from the natural disease, however, have lifelong immunity.

When poor sanitation exists, primary or secondary diphtherial lesions may occur on the skin (Figure 21-3). The toxin is also produced in these lesions, however, and patients experience an illness similar to pharyngeal diphtheria.

Transmission and Epidemiology

Recovery from diphtheria does not necessarily eliminate the *C. diphtheriae* from the throat; many patients remain healthy carriers for prolonged periods. The epidemiology of diphtheria was greatly altered during the past several generations in countries where widespread immunization had been practiced. This practice also greatly reduced the number of healthy carriers. At present, only a few hundred cases of diphtheria occur each year in the United States, many in children coming from lower socioeconomic groups. Some cases also occur in older persons who were vaccinated as children but who lost their artificially acquired immunity (Figure 21-4).

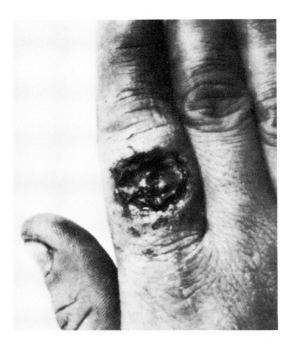

Figure 21-3 Cutaneous diphtherial lesion about 15 days after onset. (Armed Forces Institute of Pathology, AFIP MIS #44 997-1)

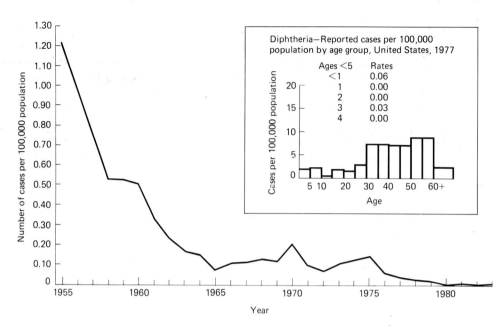

Figure 21-4 Reported case rates of diphtheria in the United States between 1955 and 1983 showing continued decrease in recent years. The insert shows the age distribution of cases occurring in 1977 (adapted from CDC reports).

Diagnosis

The diagnosis of diphtheria is most frequently made on the basis of clinical or serological evidence. Nevertheless, the isolation of toxin-producing C. *diphtheriae* from the throat or lesion provides a positive diagnosis.

Treatment

When diphtheria is suspected, the patient should receive passive immunization with antitoxin. Early antitoxin treatment is necessary in order to be effective because, once the toxin has bound to cell receptors, the reaction cannot be reversed. Penicillin or other effective antibiotics should also be given to stop further growth of C. *diphtheriae* in the throat and to prevent the patient from developing into a carrier. Persons who are asymptomatic carriers can be freed of C. *diphtheriae* by antibiotic treatment.

Prevention and Control

Diphtheria can be prevented and controlled to a large extent by active immunization with a toxoid vaccine. The vaccine is administered during the second or third month of life in combination with vaccines for tetanus and whooping cough (DPT vaccine).

A booster is given a year later and again when the child enters school. Revaccination every 10 years thereafter is also recommended.

Unimmunized persons who may have been exposed to diphtheria can be passively immunized with antitoxin. A procedure called the *Schick test* can be used to determine if a person is susceptible to diphtheria. Here a small amount of diphtheria toxin is injected subcutaneously; if the person has no protective antibodies, an inflammatory reaction occurs at the site of toxin injection. Such a person should then be actively or passively immunized, depending on circumstances.

CLINICAL NOTE

Fatal Diphtheria: Wisconsin

A fatal case of diphtheria was reported to the Wisconsin State Department of Health and Social Services. A 9-year-old unimmunized female developed listlessness and a sore throat on June 30, 1982, ten days after arriving at a camp in Colorado operated by a religious group that does not accept immunizations. On July 6, a physician evaluated the patient for her sore throat; a throat culture was taken and oral penicillin prescribed. The patient was hospitalized on July 8 for persistent sore throat, diminished fluid intake, and gingival bleeding. Laboratory tests revealed a white blood cell count of 26,500/mm^3 with 92% polymorphonuclear cells and a platelet count of 10,000/mm^3. The throat culture obtained July 6 was reported to contain normal flora, group A beta hemolytic streptococci, and large numbers of diphtheroids. The patient was transferred on July 8 to a tertiary care children's hospital.

On admission, she was afebrile and had moderate upper airway obstruction, diffuse ecchymoses (small hemorrhagic spots), bleeding from the nose and gums, prominent swollen cervical lymph nodes, and swelling of the jaw and throat. Initially, the pharynx was poorly visualized due to trismus (spasms with difficulty in opening mouth). On later examination, it revealed severe hemorrhagic and nectrotic tonsillitis; no membrane was observed. Treatment with penicillin G, gentamycin, moxalactam, peritoneal dialysis, and platelet transfusions was instituted. The hospital course was complicated by disseminated intravascular coagulation, cardiac condition abnormalities, and mental confusion. The patient died on July 14. A *Corynebacterium* species isolated from a throat culture obtained July 10 was subsequently confirmed by the Milwaukee Bureau of Laboratories and State Laboratory of Hygiene to be a toxigenic strain of *C. diphtheriae*.

An investigation was undertaken to determine the source of exposure to *C. diphtheriae* and to identify and evaluate the patient's contacts. The camp session had been attended by 108 employees, campers, and counselors from Wisconsin and 12 other states: many were unimmunized. In addition, 119 immediate and extended family members and hospital employees in Wisconsin, who might have had close contact with the patient after onset of illness, were identified. With the aid of state and local health departments and private physicians, 224 of the 227 contacts were evaluated. None reported respiratory illness before or after exposure to the patient, and nasopharyngeal or throat cultures obtained from 218 contacts were negative for *C. diphtheriae* (*MMWR 31*:553, 1982).

SUMMARY

The single, commonly serious infection caused by members of the genus *Corynebacterium* is diphtheria. Diphtheria is caused only by lysogenic strains of the bacterium that produce a powerful exotoxin and is generally held under control by appropriate immunization. The organism is frequently found in the human respiratory tract, but superficial wound infections are also known to result in the disease diphtheria.

Mycobacteria and Related Microorganisms

22

Tuberculosis and leprosy are the major diseases of humans caused by bacteria of the genus *Mycobacterium*. Their impact is difficult to determine, but they would certainly rank among the most devastating of all human diseases. Although modern medical practices and improved living standards have greatly reduced their prevalence in developed nations, both diseases are still major medical problems in many developing countries.

The mycobacteria are distinguished by their acid-fast staining property, which results from the high content of lipids in the cell wall. Such lipids also render these bacteria highly resistant to inactivation by dehydration, disinfectants, and other environmental factors.

TUBERCULOSIS

Bacterium

The species *Mycobacterium tuberculosis*, commonly referred to as the tubercle bacillus, is the major cause of human tuberculosis. It is a non-spore-forming rod measuring about $0.5 \times 3\mu m$. This bacterium can be grown on simple culture media; however, in routine laboratory isolation procedures best results are obtained with a medium containing egg yolk and starch, such as the Lowenstein-Jensen medium. This bacterium is an obligate aerobe and grows slowly. Doubling time is from 12 to 20 hours and several weeks may be required for visible colonies to develop (Figure 22-1). Experimental infections can be produced in a variety of laboratory animals.

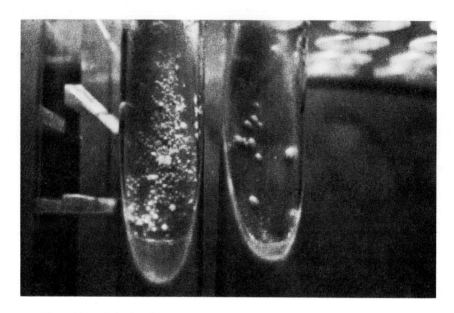

Figure 22-1 Colonies of *Mycobacterium tuberculosis* after several weeks growth on an agar surface. (S. S. Schneierson, *Atlas of Diagnostic Microbiology*, p. 39. Courtesy Abbott Laboratories, Abbott Park, IL.)

Many other species of mycobacteria are found in nature. The species that cause tuberculosis in cattle and birds—that is, *M. bovis* and *M. avium*—may occasionally cause infection in humans. Various mycobacteria have been isolated from persons with a tuberculosislike disease or skin lesions; these bacteria, sometimes referred to as the nontuberculous or atypical mycobacteria, are often associated with diseases in older patients.

Pathogenesis and Clinical Diseases

Tuberculosis is a complex disease that may go unrecognized in the human host for many years. Characteristically, it may be seen in different stages. Humans are readily infected with the tubercle bacilli, but progression of the disease depends on many subtle host factors. In many cases, the bacteria are disposed of with no manifestation of the disease. In most cases, the infection is by the airborne route with the primary infection developing in the lungs; then the disease remains dormant.

To provide a better understanding of the complex nature of tuberculosis, the following discussion divides the disease into various stages, which are shown diagrammatically in Figure 22-2.

Primary tuberculosis

This stage of the disease results when a person becomes infected for the first time. Aerosolized bacteria from a person with active tuberculosis are inhaled by a susceptible contact. Only the bacilli that reach the alveoli are able to cause infection. These

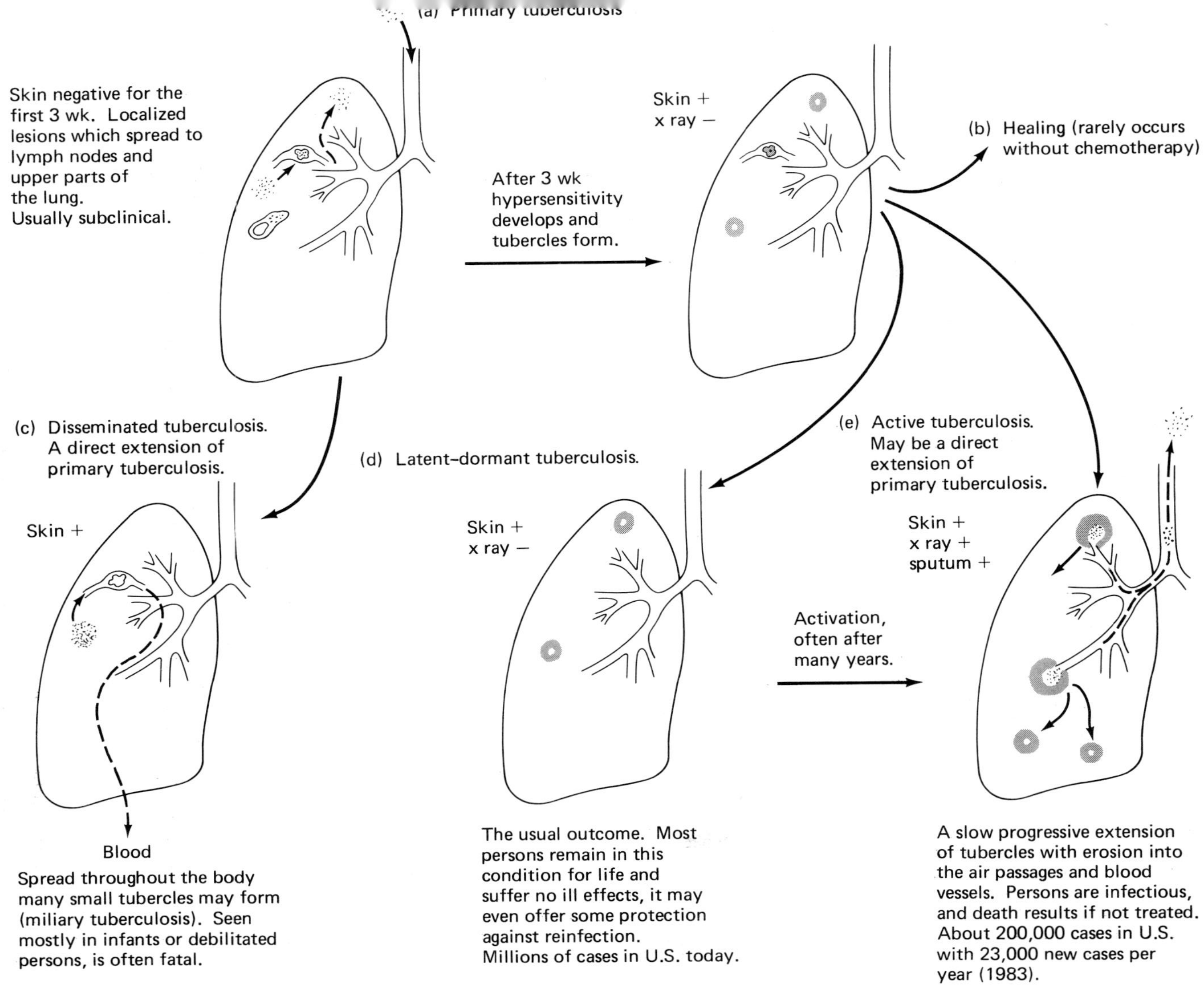

(a) Primary tuberculosis

Skin negative for the first 3 wk. Localized lesions which spread to lymph nodes and upper parts of the lung. Usually subclinical.

After 3 wk hypersensitivity develops and tubercles form.

Skin +
x ray –

(b) Healing (rarely occurs without chemotherapy)

(c) Disseminated tuberculosis. A direct extension of primary tuberculosis.

Skin +

Blood

Spread throughout the body many small tubercles may form (miliary tuberculosis). Seen mostly in infants or debilitated persons, is often fatal.

(d) Latent-dormant tuberculosis.

Skin +
x ray –

The usual outcome. Most persons remain in this condition for life and suffer no ill effects, it may even offer some protection against reinfection. Millions of cases in U.S. today.

Activation, often after many years.

(e) Active tuberculosis. May be a direct extension of primary tuberculosis.

Skin +
x ray +
sputum +

A slow progressive extension of tubercles with erosion into the air passages and blood vessels. Persons are infectious, and death results if not treated. About 200,000 cases in U.S. with 23,000 new cases per year (1983).

Figure 22-2 The most common stages in the pathogenesis of tuberculosis.

bacilli begin to multiply slowly and many are phagocytized by the alveolar macro-phages or neutrophils. During this early phase of the infection the phagocytic cells are generally unable to destroy the bacilli. Consequently, many bacilli are carried by mac-rophages to regional lymph nodes. The defense mechanisms of the host are not fully stimulated during the first few weeks of the infection. Phagocytosis of the bacteria, however, stimulates the development of cell-mediated immunity against the myco-bacterial antigens. A brisk reaction then occurs with activated macrophages concen-trating around the focus of bacterial growth. The growth of the bacilli inside the mac-rophages is slowed and a scar tissue barrier forms around the bacilli. The resulting nodule of scar tissue and white blood cells is called a *tubercle*. At this phase of the disease the patient develops a positive skin reaction, which is a manifestation of cell-mediated immunity against tuberculosis antigens. This process is commonly called "converting" to skin positive. The nodule, in most cases, prevents any further spread of the bacilli and the center of the tubercle provides a niche of dead tissue where the bacilli are protected from the host's defense mechanisms. This primary stage of the disease is usually without clinical symptoms. From this point any one of the following stages may develop.

Healing
The infection may be completely contained and the bacteria destroyed by the primary response. The patient would have experienced no symptoms but would have a posi-tive reaction to the skin test. In persons not receiving adequate chemotherapy it is difficult to determine if this healing does indeed occur.

Disseminated tuberculosis
In a small percentage of persons, mostly young children or immunologically impaired individuals, the infection spreads from the primary site of multiplication into the blood and the bacteria may be seeded throughout the body. In some individuals cellu-lar immunity does not readily develop; without chemotherapy, the bacilli grow in many body tissues and the patient dies. If dissemination occurs and hypersensitivity develops, numerous small tubercles are formed, a condition called *miliary tubercu-losis*. The death rate is high from this type.

Latent-dormant tuberculosis
This stage is the usual outcome of primary pulmonary tuberculosis. During the pri-mary stage secondary foci usually develop around the initial focus and in adjacent lymph nodes. Tubercles are formed around these foci. The bacilli may remain living inside these tubercles for many years or for the lifetime of the infected person. Before chemotherapy was available, a general saying was "Once infected, always infected," when referring to tuberculosis.

During this stage the activated host defense mechanisms prevent the bacilli from spreading to other parts of the body and the environment inside the tubercle protects the bacilli from these same defenses. This "truce" may last for the lifetime of the person or may be "broken" by the influence of various, often not well understood, changes in the physiology of the host. In past years a vast majority of the world's population had latent-dormant tuberculosis. Some estimates place the current number of persons in the United States with latent-dormant tuberculosis at over 20 million; over 50% of the population in many Asiatic countries has this stage of tuberculosis. These persons have an increased resistance to reinfection due to their activated defenses against the tubercule bacilli. It has now been shown, however, that most active cases develop as an extension of this latent infection. So it is not generally considered advantageous to have the latent form of the disease. Persons in the latent-dormant stages remain skin test positive, but the tubercles may not be large enough to be seen by x ray.

Secondary or active adult-type tuberculosis

This stage of tuberculosis may develop as a direct extension of the primary stage in which the initial tubercle formation did not stabilize the infection. But most cases result from a "reawakening" of the dormant lesion. The exact mechanisms associated with this reawakening or activation, often after long periods of dormancy, are not understood. It occurs most often in persons who have had their defense mechanisms compromised—for instance, young adults who become rundown, overworked, malnourished, stressed; elderly persons with general declining health; alcoholics; persons with such diseases as diabetes or silicosis; and those on immunosuppressive therapy. Reported cases of active tuberculosis by race and sex, in 1980, are shown in Figure 22-3.

The previously dormant tubercle begins to expand in size and causes an enlarged central area of dead tissue and debris to form. This material is referred to as *caseous necrosis* (cheesey, dead tissue). The center of the tubercle may become liquified, a situation usually accompanied by an increased proliferation of *M. tuberculosis*. Eventually the expanding tubercle erodes into a bronchial tube and the inner contents are expelled into the airways. At this time the patient begins to expel large

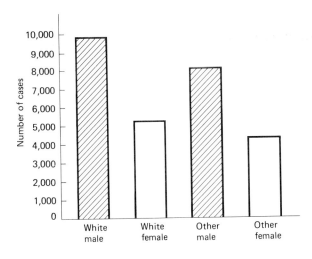

Figure 22-3 Tuberculosis cases by race and sex in the United States, 1980. A total number of 27,749 new cases were reported. Indochinese refugees accounted for approximately 7.8% of the reported cases for 1980 (*CDC Annual Summary,* 1980).

numbers of bacilli from the respiratory tract. The fibrous and calcified walls of the tubercle then form an air-filled cavity where the tubercle bacilli may continue to grow. At this phase of the disease healing or treatment is difficult, for the cavity wall forms a barrier not only against the body's defense mechanisms but also against chemotherapeutic agents. Surgical removal of such cavities is sometimes necessary before chemotherapy can be effective. Without treatment, the tubercular lesion may continue to expand and consume the normal tissue until death results. Earlier tuberculosis was called consumption because of this progressive destruction or consumption of the tissues.

In some cases, the adverse factors that stimulated the "reawakening" of the disease may be removed and the disease may again become stabilized in the dormant stage.

Transmission and Epidemiology

M. tuberculosis is usually found only in humans and large numbers of bacilli may be disseminated by the airborne route from persons with active tuberculosis. A person may unknowingly transmit the bacilli for some time before being aware of having the disease. It is generally felt that prolonged close contact with an infectious person is necessary for successful transmission of this disease. Casual contact with an infectious person, such as passing on a street, would normally not result in transmission. Bovine tuberculosis, caused by *M. bovis*, was a problem at one time because transmission was from cow to humans via contaminated milk. But inspection of cows and pasteurization of milk have almost eliminated this source of infection in the United States and many other countries.

Diagnosis

Diagnosis of tuberculosis occurs in different stages. The first stage is skin testing, which provides a rapid, inexpensive procedure for screening large numbers of persons. The second stage involves chest x rays, and the last stage is the isolation of *M. tuberculosis* from the infected individual.

Skin testing

The highly specific delayed-type hypersensitivity that develops against the tubercule bacilli can be demonstrated by injecting an antigen from the bacillus into the skin (intradermal). This antigen is called *tuberculin* and was originally supplied as *Old Tuberculin* (OT), a crude extract from a broth culture of bacilli. Today a more refined extract called *Purified Protein Derivative* (PPD) is used.

The reference skin test—the *Mantoux* test—uses the intradermal injection of standard amounts of tuberculin. More convenient but slightly less reliable tests have been developed for routine screening programs. One test is a multipuncture procedure using a disposable plastic unit with points covered with liquid tuberculin and firmly pressed into the skin. Another is the "Tine" test, which uses a disposable unit with metal tines that are covered with dried tuberculin and pressed into the skin.

Skin tests are read 48 hours after testing; an area of redness with swelling 10 mm in diameter is considered a strong positive (Figure 22-4). The skin test cannot distinguish clearly between the different stages of tuberculosis, but if someone converts to skin positive, it shows that the person has been exposed to the disease and has progressed at least to the primary stage. Further diagnostic tests are then indicated.

Chest x ray

Routine chest x rays are discouraged. Such examinations are most appropriately used as a followup procedure on those who have converted to skin test positive or to establish the extent of tissue damage in previously diagnosed cases of active or dormant tuberculosis.

Bacteriologic tests

A definite diagnosis of active tuberculosis requires the isolation of *M. tuberculosis* from the patient. The most effective method for obtaining bacterial specimens is the collection of induced sputum samples. The patient inhales a fine aerosol mist that induces deep coughing. The cough carries the sputum and bacilli from the lungs to the mouth. Care should be taken to prevent health care personnel from being exposed to aerosolized bacilli during the collection of induced sputums. Special safety hoods or cubicles are recommended for this procedure (Figure 22-5).

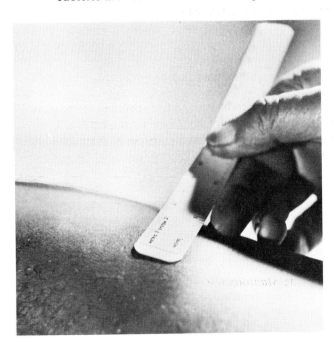

Figure 22-4 A positive Mantoux skin test showing an area of redness and swelling (about 15 mm in diameter) after 48 hours. (Centers for Disease Control, Atlanta)

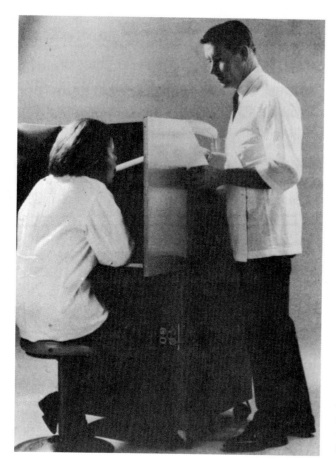

Figure 22-5 A safety hood used during the collection of sputum samples from tuberculosis patients. During the collection process, deep coughing is induced in the patient (seated). All airborne tubercle bacilli expelled by the patient are sucked into this safety hood where they are trapped by filters. The technician (standing) assisting the patient is protected from these airborne bacteria. (Jensen Research Laboratories)

The collected sputum is treated with sodium hydroxide, which kills most microorganisms other than mycobacteria, and an amino acid derivative, *N*-acetylcysteine, which digests the mucus. The bacteria in the sputum are then concentrated by centrifugation and culture plates, as well as slides for microscopic examination, are prepared from the sediment. The presence of acid-fast bacilli gives a rapid provisional diagnosis. The growth of *M. tuberculosis* on the inoculated culture media confirms the diagnosis.

Treatment

The ability to treat tuberculosis successfully with chemotherapeutic agents (Table 22-1) has been the most notable advance in controlling this disease and has led to significant changes regarding tuberculosis patients. No longer is it practical to maintain sanatoria specifically for such patients. The majority can be successfully treated in a relatively short time either in a general hospital that has specific facilities to handle

TABLE 22-1 AGENTS USED TO TREAT TUBERCULOSIS

Major or primary compounds	Minor or secondary compounds
Ethambutol (EMB)	Capreomycin
Isoniazid (INH)	Cycloserine
p-aminosalicylic acid (PAS)	Ethionamide
Rifampin	Kanamycin
Streptomycin	Pyrazinamide
	Thiacetazone
	Viomycin

tuberculosis or at home. Moreover, most patients can be rendered noninfectious and then released from the hospital after some weeks. Generally, however, long-term followup therapy must be carried out on an outpatient basis. An important phase of the hospitalization program concerns the proper motivation and education of patients so that treatment continues through self-medication and return visits to the clinic. The personnel staffing these clinics must be trained to understand the chronic nature of tuberculosis and the need for the patients to return for regular followup appointments.

The antibiotic streptomycin was the first highly effective antituberculosis agent to be developed. Several years later, in the early 1950s, the synthetic compounds isoniazid (INH) and p-aminosalicyate (PAS), were developed. Later the compound ethambutol (EMB) and the antibiotic rifampin were effectively used to treat tuberculosis.

These chemotherapeutic agents are always given in various combinations. Streptomycin, if used, is given by injection, together with one or more of the less toxic INH, PAS, or EMB given orally. Rifampin, combined with INH, is often administered orally throughout the entire treatment period. The time of treatment may vary, depending on the severity of the infection or the patient's reliability in taking the medication properly. The standard regimen has been daily medication for periods of 6 to 24 months. But it has now been determined that under controlled conditions short-course therapy for about 9 months can be effective. If it is difficult to control daily medication, an intermittently supervised high-dose treatment given twice weekly for the conventional time is effective.

Well-regulated programs of administering the antituberculosis drugs are important. Failure to follow prescribed regimens may result in the development of resistant strains of the tubercle bacillus. These strains may lead to infections that cannot be readily treated.

Prevention and Control

The prompt diagnosis of active cases is the most important phase in the control of tuberculosis. Once these individuals have been identified, they can be rendered noninfectious by proper chemotherapy. The next major problem is determining who might have become infected from the index cases. All possible contacts should be investigated, starting with those who shared common environmental air at home or work. The investigation should also extend to those who may have had less extensive contact with the patient. Appropriate diagnostic procedures should be carried out on the contacts, beginning with a history of any prior tuberculosis skin tests, vaccinations, or infections. Skin tests should then be done on all contacts and followup x rays and sputum specimens used if indicated. Contacts showing conversion to positive skin reactions or having other signs of the disease should be placed on prophylactic chemotherapy. It is sometimes advisable to place the more susceptible close contacts, such as young children, on prophylactic chemotherapy even if they show no signs of the disease.

This program of detection and followup has worked quite well in countries with relatively few active cases and with the necessary medical personnel and public health facilities. A vaccine may be advisable in countries where tuberculosis is more prevalent and medical facilities are limited. A live vaccine, containing an attenuated *M. bovis* mutant known as *Bacille Calmette Guerin*, or BCG, has been available since 1923 and induces an increased resistance to tuberculosis but not complete immunity. BCG vaccination has been used in some countries for many years and appears to offer some protection. But this vaccine induces hypersensitivity against the tubercle bacillus and thus renders the tuberculin skin test useless as a diagnostic aid. It is rarely used in countries where the incidence of tuberculosis is low, for it is considered more valuable to have the diagnostic usefulness of the skin test than the moderate protection provided by the vaccine.

CLINICAL NOTE

Tuberculosis: Maryland

Ten cases of active tuberculosis were traced to one source, a 30-year-old man, who was diagnosed as having tuberculosis on September 12, 1974. The patient had been ill for about 7 months, with symptoms that included a productive cough, intermittent fever, night sweats, and weight loss of about 60 pounds.

The patient's tuberculosis was classified as: tuberculosis, pulmonary; microscopy positive (numerous acid-fast bacilli), and culture positive (50 colonies). He was started on three antituberculous drugs. A report of the case was submitted by the hospital nurse epidemiologist to the county health department and an investigation of the patient's contacts began.

All 24 persons identified as household or close contacts of the patient were examined. Of these individuals, 7 were 21 years of age or older. The other 17 ranged in age from 2 to 12 years. One adult and 9 children had negative initial skin tests and remained negative on retesting.

The remaining 14 contacts (6 adults and 8 children) were found to have tuberculous infection as indicated by skin test reactions of 10 mm or more when tested with purified protein derivative (PPD). Primary active tuberculosis was identified in 7 of these 8 children and in 1 adult; 3 of the children were hospitalized. Daily isoniazid (INH) was given to 13 of these contacts and a 2-year-old child was started on INH and p-aminosalicylic acid (PAS). One child (the index patient's daughter) with a 0-mm skin test reaction was started on INH preventive therapy.

It was possible to identify 40 others as casual contacts of the index patient. Of this group, 32 were skin test negative, 5 were positive reactors, and 3 were known positive. Two of the 5 positive reactors were placed on preventive therapy. One friend, who was a negative reactor on initial testing, refused to be retested. He was subsequently hospitalized and diagnosed as having: tuberculosis, pleural; bacteriology pending. He was treated with multiple antituberculosis drugs.

In addition, another casual contact—not included in the original contact study—was diagnosed as having active tuberculosis in 1975.

Moreover, 6 work contacts were examined; 3 were negative skin test reactors and 3 were previously known positives. Contacts who associated with the index patient's children were skin tested, 13 in all (mostly children); all were negative on initial testing and then on retesting.

Because of concern in the small community where the index patient resided, a tuberculin testing program was offered to community residents. As a result, 66 people were tested; 61 were negative reactors and 5 did not return for a reading (*MMWR* 25:93, 1976).

LEPROSY

Bacterium

Mycobacterium leprae is the causative agent of leprosy. This bacterium shares many common characteristics with *M. tuberculosis*: it is an acid-fast bacillus containing large amounts of lipid, induces hypersensitivity, and multiplies slowly. *M. leprae* is found in enormous numbers of certain lesions of infected persons. This feature allowed Hansen in 1874 to make the first reliable causal association between a bacterial agent and a human disease. Leprosy is often referred to as *Hansen's disease*, partly to honor Hansen's discovery and partly to avoid the use of the unpleasant name of leprosy.

Even though this bacterium is found in greater numbers in infected tissues than any other bacterium, it has not been possible to cultivate it on artificial media. Some growth occurs when it is inoculated into the foot pad of a mouse. Today it is known that armadillos are susceptible to this bacillus. Some evidence even suggests that armadillos may be a natural nonhuman host for leprosy. Thus both mice and armadillos are being used in some limited experimental laboratory studies of leprosy.

Pathogenesis and Clinical Disease

Leprosy is probably transmitted from person to person under conditions of poor sanitation and may gain entry via the respiratory tract or skin lesions. The incubation period averages several years but may extend to 20 years. The major growth of the bacilli occurs in the low-temperature body tissues—that is, nose, ears, and the skin of extremities. The leprosy bacilli are easily phagocytized but not destroyed and large numbers are found growing inside macrophages. Nerves are uniquely susceptible to infection; early symptoms of leprosy are often associated with anesthesia (lack of feeling) over an area of the body. The exact mechanism of tissue destruction is not understood but probably results from a combination of neurological damage, massive accumulation of bacilli, and immunologic reactions.

Two forms of leprosy are seen, the *lepromatous* and the *tuberculoid* (Figures 22-6 and 22-7). The lepromatous form is the most severe and is characterized by large nodular lesions. In lepromatous leprosy the immune response is impaired, limiting the formation of granulation (scar) tissue. The tuberculoid form is less severe and is associated with a normal immune response that causes granulation-type lesions; bacilli in the lesions are sparse, tissue damage is less, and response to therapy is better. Forms intermediate between lepromatous and tuberculoid are also seen.

Overall leprosy is a slowly progressing disease that often disfigures and cripples. Death usually results after many years and is commonly associated with secondary infections.

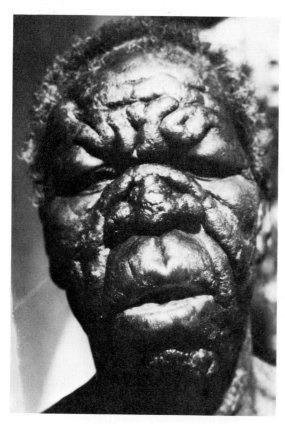

Figure 22-6   A patient with lepromatous leprosy: note the loss of eyebrows and deep furrowing that exaggerates the normal folds of the face. (Courtesy American Leprosy Missions, Bloomfield, N.J. 07003)

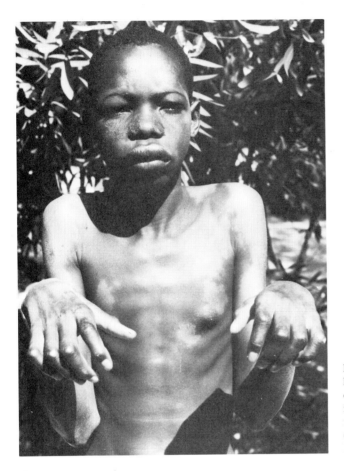

Figure 22-7 A patient with tuberculoid leprosy: note the flat discolored plaques on the shoulder, chest, and hands. Swelling and contraction of the fingers results from inflammation of the nerve fibers. (Courtesy American Leprosy Missions, Bloomfield, N.J. 07003)

Transmission

Leprosy today is generally found in underdeveloped tropical and subtropical areas. Most cases seen in developed countries were contracted—sometimes years earlier—while the person resided in a tropical or subtropical area. Only about 150 cases occur each year in the United States (Figure 22-8). But the disease is still a major problem worldwide. Estimates are that over 20 million people have leprosy and that only 10% are currently under treatment.

From a historical perspective the epidemiology of leprosy offers some unexplainable paradoxes. Early reports suggested that the disease was highly contagious. During the eleventh and fifteenth centuries, for example, leprosy was widespread in Europe. Then a sharp decline in incidence followed in the sixteenth century. The reason for this decline and for the comparative decrease in virulence and communicability of this disease today are not known.

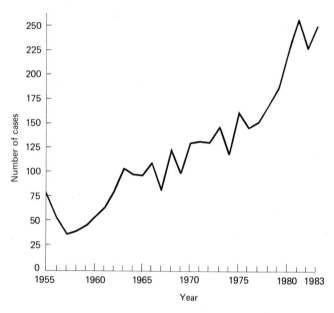

Figure 22-8 Reported cases of leprosy in the United States per year, 1955–1983. The increases in the 1970s and 1980s were due primarily to imported cases among Indochinese refugees (modified from CDC annual summaries).

Diagnosis

Bacterial diagnosis is made by direct microscopic demonstration of the presence of acid-fast bacilli in scrapings of fluids from the lesions (Figure 22-9). A skin test using an antigen called *Lepromin*, obtained from heat-inactivated extracts of infected tissues, is of some value. Clinical findings are often characteristic enough for a tentative diagnosis.

Treatment

Antimicrobial agents called sulfones, which are related to the sulfonamides, are fairly effective in arresting progression of the lesions and in allowing them to heal (Figure 22-10). These agents render patients noninfectious and allow them to return to normal daily activities as outpatients. Treatment is prolonged, for months to years, and it is not certain when or if a complete cure is ever obtained. The antibiotic rifampin has been shown to render patients noninfectious in just a few weeks, but the full effect of this promising agent is still under investigation. The other antituberculosis drugs are not effective against leprosy.

Control and Prevention

Only persons who have prolonged contact with leprosy patients under poor sanitary conditions seem to stand an increased risk of being infected. Young children are more susceptible than adults. Using good sanitary procedures when dealing with patients is

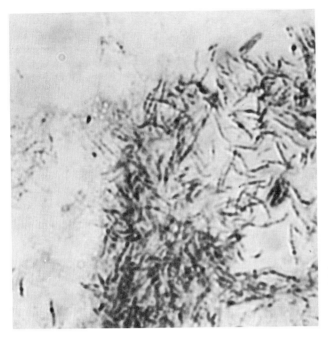

Figure 22-9 Micrograph of *M. leprae* taken from a lesion and stained by the acid-fast method. (Courtesy American Leprosy Missions, Bloomfield, N.J. 07003)

thus recommended. It may also be advisable, in some situations, to remove young children from infectious parents and place them on a course of preventative chemotherapy. Tattooing parlors in endemic areas should be avoided, for contaminated tattooing needles have been shown to transmit leprosy. New cases of leprosy were prevented on a Pacific island by subjecting the entire population of 1500 people to a course of sulfone treatment. Possibly such prophylactic chemotherapy could be used in other endemic areas to block the spread of leprosy.

CLINICAL NOTE

Hansen's Disease in Vietnamese Refugees

Beginning in July 1975 Vietnamese refugees 15 years of age and older living in Camp Pendleton, California, Fort Indiantown Gap, Pennsylvania, and Fort Chaffee, Arkansas, were examined for evidence of Hansen's disease. Among 27,057 adults examined, 39 definite cases were found (1.4 cases per 1000). Only 4 cases (10%) were of the infectious (lepromatous) form. Of the others, 5 were borderline, 3 indeterminate, and 27 tuberculoid. Males numbered 23. The estimated age-specific rates per 1000 (and the numbers of cases) were as follows: 15–19 years, 1.1 (6 cases); 20–29 years, 1.8 (15 cases); 30–39 years, 0.7 (4 cases); 40–49 years, 2.2 (7 cases); 50–59 years, 2.5 (5 cases); and 60+ years, 1.2 (2 cases). Five cases had been recognized in Vietnam, and treatment begun there; 34 cases were newly diagnosed. In addition, 6

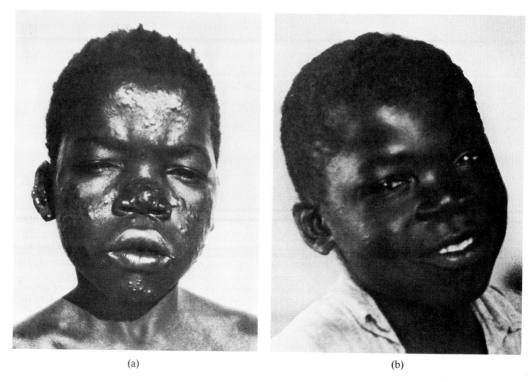

(a)   (b)

Figure 22-10   (a) A child with leprosy before treatment. (b) The same child after treatment with a sulfone. (Courtesy American Leprosy Missions, Bloomfield, N.J. 07003)

suspected but unproved cases were identified. All proved cases were either under therapy or had already completed adequate courses of therapy. Followup in each case was coordinated by respective state health departments and public health service hospitals at Carville, San Francisco, and New York.

Several additional cases of Hansen's disease have already been recognized and reported among the refugees who were not screened because they were placed with family or sponsors before July.

Because the prevalence of Hansen's disease in Vietnam has been estimated at 3 to 5 per 1000, it was expected that a number of cases would be found among the 140,000 refugees who entered the country in 1975. In addition, more cases could be expected to develop over the next decade. The risk to U.S. residents, however, is small. The only important risk of untreated lepromatous Hansen's disease patients is to their family contacts. A study in the Philippines showed that the risk of secondary cases of Hansen's disease in such contacts was 6.2 cases per 1000 persons per year. In the years 1949 to 1972 an average of 30 cases of lepromatous Hansen's disease per year were recognized in immigrants to this country. Nevertheless, cases of Hansen's disease in U.S. citizens who have never lived in a leprosy-endemic area are rare. And the few lepromatous cases among the Vietnamese refugees are not thought to be an important additional risk. Early diagnosis and treatment are important, however, to prevent progression of the disease and disability (*MMWR 24*:455, 1976).

ACTINOMYCETES AND RELATED MICROBES

Actinomycetes and related microbes are gram-positive bacteria; some species are acid fast and related to the mycobacteria. These organisms grow in long filaments with extensive branching and thus resemble the morphology of fungi (Chapter 29). They are procaryotes, however, and possess bacterial-type cellular morphology. Widespread in nature, they are found in soil and are noted for the production of antibiotics and decomposition of organic matter. Some of these organisms are associated with diseases in humans and animals. The more prominent human pathogens are briefly discussed here.

Nocardia

The most frequently encountered *Nocardia* species is *Nocardia asteroides*. It is acid fast and is a common inhabitant of soil. Generally it is an opportunistic pathogen-causing disease in patients with other medical problems that have compromised their basic resistance to infections. Lung infection is the most common disease caused by *N. asteroides* and may be misdiagnosed as tuberculosis. The infection may spread from the lungs to the blood and involve various other parts of the body, especially the brain. *Nocardia* species may also cause penetrating lesions of the skin, subcutaneous, or deeper tissues that are localized and have connecting passages (sinuses) to the surface through which pus drains. Characteristic clumps (granules) made of compact colonies of nocardia are present in the pus. Infections are usually best treated with sulfa drugs.

Actinomyces

Actinomyces are anaerobic gram-positive, non-acid-fast, filamentous organisms with or without branching. The species *Actinomyces isrealii* is the major human pathogen. *A. bovis* is a common pathogen of cattle only and causes a disease called lumpy jaw. *A. isrealii* is normally found in the mouth of humans and usually acts as an opportunist by causing infections in damaged tissues. The following types of infection are produced:

1. Head and neck infections following injury to the mouth or jaw, such as tooth extractions or other dental procedures
2. Pulmonary infections resulting from aspiration of infectious material from the mouth

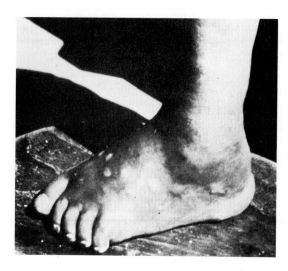

Figure 22-11 Actinomyces infection of the foot. (Centers for Disease Control, Atlanta)

3. Abdominal infections, probably resulting from swallowing organisms after abdominal surgery or injury

4. Human bites that directly introduce the organisms into the tissues or any injury that breaks the skin; foot infections are common in some areas (Figure 22-11).

Infections are often characterized by draining abscesses with the actinomyces filaments embedded in yellowish granules in the pus. Diagnosis is based on clinical appearance and the presence of typical organisms in the granules. Actinomyces are susceptible to various antibiotics, including penicillin, the antibiotic of choice. Surgical removal of the abscess is often necessary before successful treatment is possible.

Streptomyces

Streptomyces form long branching filaments that segment into beadlike structures called *conida*. Each conidium can develop into a new colony. Most streptomyces are nonpathogens and are found in the soil. Many of the commonly used antibiotics are produced from these organisms. The species *Streptomyces somaliensis*, and perhaps a few other species, causes localized swollen lesions that are indistinguishable clinically from lesions caused by *Nocardia* species.

SUMMARY

1. Members of the genus *Mycobacterium* are causative agents of two chronic diseases of great historical interest and significance, tuberculosis and leprosy. The mycobacteria are unique in that their cellular composition includes a high con-

centration of lipid and wax. Because of their staining characteristics, they are known as acid-fast bacteria. They are strict aerobes.

2. Tuberculosis is caused by a number of mycobacteria other than *M. tuberculosis* (MOTT). These MOTT are not transferred from person to person but produce a disease that is similar to that caused by *M. tuberculosis*.

3. Tuberculosis therapy has been difficult, requires long periods of antimicrobial use, and has been quite effective. Relatively large numbers of compounds are commonly used in therapy. A vaccine called BCG is available and has produced reliable results in areas where tuberculosis is a major health concern.

4. Leprosy is an age-old human disease. There are millions of cases of this disease throughout the world, but it is infrequently found in the United States. New approaches to therapy have enabled many leprosy patients to have normal lives.

5. The actinomycetes are very similar in structure and composition to the *Mycobacteria*. They are much less often involved in human infections but the infections are serious and often life threatening.

Haemophilus, Bordetella, and Brucella

23

The bacterial species of the three genera *Haemophilus*, *Bordetella*, and *Brucella* are all small gram-negative coccobacilli. Based on current classification methods, however, these three genera are not closely related and so each is discussed separately in this chapter.

HAEMOPHILUS INFECTIONS

Bacterial species of the genus *Haemophilus* (sometimes called *Hemophilus*) require special growth factors that are found only in blood and other body fluids. The name *haemophilus* means blood loving (Greek, *Haemo* = blood, *philus* = loving). Some species are nonpathogens whereas others are primary pathogens.

Bacteria

Haemophilus influenzae is the major disease-producing species of this genus. Several other species, such as *H. aegyptius* and *H. ducreyi*, are virulent but are less common agents of serious human infections. *H. influenzae* is a small (1 × 0.3 μm), coccobacillary, gram-negative bacterium. It requires blood products—specifically hemin and a coenzyme called NAD—in the artificial media for growth. Most isolates possess a capsule and can be divided into six different types, based on differences in capsular antigens. The types are designated *a* through *f* with type *b* most commonly associated with diseases in humans. The capsule helps retard phagocytosis and an enzyme produced by pathogenic strains specifically splits IgA molecules. These traits may contribute significantly to the virulence of this bacterium. The bacterium does not survive well outside the body and is found only in humans.

Pathogenesis and Clinical Disease

H. influenzae colonizes in the respiratory tract and as many as 50% of young children may be carriers. Only a small number of persons who carry this bacterium develop a clinical disease, which usually appears in young children. Thus *H. influenzae* generally functions as an opportunist. Clinical diseases may begin as a nose and throat infection (nasopharyngitis). The infection may spread to the sinus and middle ear or develop into pneumonia. In a small percentage of cases, the bacteria spread to the blood and then to the meninges. *H. influenzae* is the most common cause of bacterial meningitis in children between 3 months and 3 years of age. *Haemophilus* meningitis is a serious disease and often fatal without vigorous treatment. Infections of the epiglottis and larynx occur less frequently but are serious due to possible obstruction of the respiratory tract, which constitutes a true medical emergency.

Other infections associated with *H. influenzae* are less serious but fairly common. Included are otitis media or inner ear infection, contagious conjunctivitis, sometimes referred to as pink eye, cellulitis and osteomyelitis in children, and pneumonia in adults. Pneumonia caused by nontype b haemophili is currently being found in increasing numbers in elderly persons.

Transmission and Epidemiology

The *Haemophilus* bacteria are widespread in humans; most persons develop active antibody immunity against them before reaching adulthood. Newborns receive passive immunity from their mothers and hence valuable protection during the early months of life. Most cases are sporadic, except for conjunctivitis, which is highly contagious, and many result when the host's resistance becomes lowered. In this regard, larger numbers of infection may occur in conjunction with an epidemic viral respiratory disease, such as influenza. The name *H. influenzae* was applied to this bacterium because early studies mistakenly thought it was the primary cause of influenza. Approximately 10,000 cases of *Haemophilus* meningitis occur in the United States each year. The death rate is 5% and a significant number who recover have permanent, residual damage of the central nervous system.

Diagnosis

Often diagnosis of *H. influenza* meningitis can be made by direct microscopic observation of the bacteria in the spinal fluid. The quellung test (p. 226) on bacteria in spinal fluid, using specific antiserum, will confirm if the observed bacteria are *H. influenzae*. Bacteria can be cultured on chocolate agar and then specifically identified. Some cases are diagnosed through serological procedures that can detect free bacterial capsular antigens in body fluid like blood or spinal fluid.

Treatment

The proper treatment given early prevents death in most cases, while delay in treatment greatly reduces the chance for therapeutic success. Ampicillin and chloramphenicol, tetracyclines, and sulfa drugs may be effective. Sensitivity tests to determine the most effective chemotherapeutic agent are generally completed on all strains isolated from serious disease conditions.

Prevention and Control

Because of the widespread nature of this bacterium, little can be done to prevent exposure. The most effective means of preventing deaths and minimizing neurologic damage are early diagnosis and treatment of meningitis. Most children develop natural immunity during the first six years. Currently a vaccine made of capsular antigens of type b *H. influenzae* is being tested; if successful, it may be recommended as a routine vaccine for infants. Unfortunately, infants do not respond as well as older children and adults to this antigen.

Other Haemophilus Species

Several other species of *Haemophilus*, such as *H. aphrophilus*, *H. haemolyticus*, and *H. parainfluenzae*, are sometimes involved in human infections. In certain geographical areas *H. ducreyi* is commonly isolated from patients suffering from a sexually transmitted disease known as *chancroid*. This infection is characterized by the development of a small papule or pustule at the point of infection, usually the genitalia. The pustule ruptures and forms an ulcer similar to the chancre observed with syphilis. The ulcer is often accompanied by swollen and suppurative (draining pus) regional lymph nodes. Specific diagnosis is made by isolating *H. ducreyi* from the lesion or lymph nodes. Treatment with sulfonamide or tetracycline is generally effective.

CLINICAL NOTE

Outbreak of Haemophilus influenzae Type b Disease in a Day-Care Center: Kansas

Four episodes of serious *Haemophilus influenzae* type b infection occurred in three children attending a day-care center in Lawrence, Kansas, during 8 days of October 1976. This outbreak accounted for a third of all *H. influenzae* type b disease reported in Lawrence from January 1, 1974, through October 31, 1976.

The patients were among 13 infants, ages 5 to 14 months, cared for in the same room at the day-care center. There were 59 older children at the center, none of whom became ill. Two children became ill on the same day, one with meningitis and the other with cellulitis of the cheek and bacteremia. Eight days later another child developed meningitis and cellulitis of the cheek. After the child who initially had bacteremia and cellulitis was treated for 6 days with intramuscular ampicillin (100 mg/kg/day), a repeat blood culture was taken; it was negative. However, 7 days after completing this initial therapy, the child developed meningitis. The three children were not related and had no contact with each other except at the day-care center. All *H. influenzae* type b isolates were sensitive to ampicillin.

Children, staff members, and family contacts of patients received ampicillin or rifampin as antibiotic prophylaxis in an attempt to eradicate carriage and prevent transmission of organisms, particularly to young children. Rifampin was prescribed according to recent recommendations for prophylaxis of meningococcal disease and ampicillin was given orally for 5 days. No further cases developed. Although *H. influenzae* is the most common cause of bacterial meningitis in the United States, outbreaks of clusters of the disease are considered unusual (*MMWR 26*:201, 1977).

WHOOPING COUGH

The clinical term for whooping cough is *pertussis*. Historically it has been one of the prominent childhood diseases and before the advent of an effective vaccine was a frequent cause of death in young children. Today vaccination has greatly reduced the number of cases of pertussis in developed countries.

Bacterium

Bordetella pertussis is the causative agent of whooping cough. Morphologically it is similar to *H. influenzae*. It differs from *Haemophilus*, however, in that it does not require specific blood components for growth and will grow on various types of culture media. Agar containing blood, potato starch, charcoal, and cefalexin is the culture medium of choice. This bacterium survives for only a short time when expelled from the body in respiratory secretions.

Pathogenesis and Clinical Disease

B. pertussis is aerosolized from the throat of a person with whooping cough and is transmitted to others by the airborne route. This bacterium selectively attaches to the epithelial cells of the respiratory tract and growth is limited to the superficial tissues. After an incubation period of 10 days, generalized symptoms of an upper respiratory infection occur, such as sneezing, runny nose, and coughing (the term catarrhal refers to such symptoms). This first, or prodromal, stage lasts a week or two. The second stage progresses into episodes (paroxysm) of uncontrollable coughs. Each paroxysm may consist of 5 to 20 rapid coughs, with the patient unable to breathe between coughs. At the end of the paroxysm a forced inspiratory breath causes the "whooping" sound. This coughing and whooping form the basis for the common name for this disease. Such prolonged coughing may lead to anoxia (decreased oxygen in the blood), expelling of mucus, and vomiting. The second stage may continue for 1 to 6 weeks. The third stage may include some coughing during convalescence and may last for several more weeks. Various toxins produced by *B. pertussis* are thought to induce the accumulation of mucoid materials and the extensive coughing. The central nervous system is affected and contributes to the morbidity and mortality associated with whooping cough. Respiratory distress and secondary bacterial pneumonia also contribute to the seriousness of many cases of whooping cough, particularly in young children. About 25% of the cases are mild or subclinical and are passed off as a nonspecific respiratory infection.

Transmission and Epidemiology

B. pertussis is found only in humans and is transmitted, in most cases, only by persons with an active infection. Up to 90% of the unimmunized household contacts of a clinical case may develop whooping cough. Pertussis is found worldwide and has no seasonal distribution. Widespread immunization in the United States has caused a steady decline in the number of cases. In 1950, for instance, 120,000 cases with 1100 deaths occurred compared to 1032 cases in 1982 with just a few deaths. Similar decreases are seen in other countries where wide-scale immunization is used. Reported cases in the United States are shown in Figure 23-1.

Diagnosis

Fluorescent-tagged antibodies can be used for a rapid and specific identification of *B. pertussis* obtained directly from nasopharyngeal swabs (swabs passed through one nostril into the nasopharynx). Culture can be obtained by having the patient cough directly onto the open plate or by streaking the plate with the nasopharyngeal swab.

Treatment

Although no antibiotic is always successful, the antibiotic erythromycin is the most effective chemotherapeutic agent. Tetracyclines and chloramphenicol have also been used but are somewhat less effective. Removal of respiratory secretions, oxygen therapy to aid breathing, and general supportive measures are of value in treating patients with severe symptoms.

Prevention and Control

A killed pertussis vaccine has been widely used for many years and is associated with a steady decline in the number of cases of whooping cough. The vaccine is usually

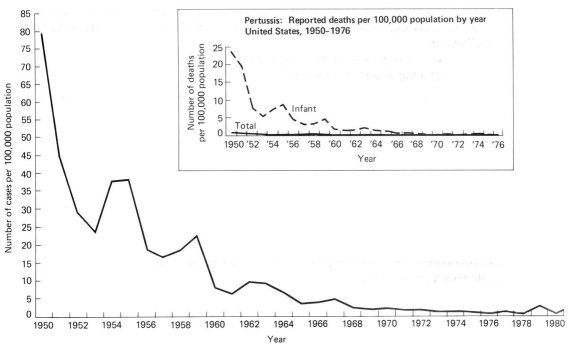

Figure 23-1   Reported yearly cases and deaths (insert) from pertussis (whooping cough) in the United States, 1950–1980 (*CDC Annual Summary*, 1980).

given in combination with tetanus and diphtheria toxoids as the DPT vaccine. Little passive immunity to this disease is transferred to newborn infants; therefore vaccination should be initiated as soon as possible. The first immunization of a series of three should be given at about 6 weeks of age and the other two at monthly intervals. Booster immunizations should be given at about 1 year of age and again just before starting school. When a person under 4 years of age who has been immunized is exposed to someone with whooping cough, a booster injection should be given. When exposed, unimmunized children should be given prophylactic treatments with erythromycin for about 10 days.

Brain damage has been reported in about 1:100,000 vaccinated infants; consequently, some countries with low rates of whooping cough have begun limiting the use of the vaccine in young infants. Still, young infants are the ones who need the protection most; the balance between benefits and hazards in the use of this vaccine is sometimes difficult to determine. When use of this vaccine was discontinued in England for a period of time, a dramatic rise in the number both of cases and fatalities due to whooping cough occurred. There is current interest in developing an improved whooping cough vaccine.

CLINICAL NOTE

Pertussis: Maine and Georgia

Two outbreaks of pertussis, one in Maine, the other in Georgia, have been reported to the Centers for Disease Control in Atlanta. Details of these outbreaks are as follows.

Maine. Pertussis was diagnosed in a 2-year-old girl from Bridgeton, Maine, in April 1977 after a 6-week history of cough. The child had been seen several times both as an outpatient and in the hospital, where diagnoses of asthma, bronchitis, and cystic fibrosis were considered before the diagnosis of pertussis. Direct fluorescent antibody (FA) stain of a nasopharyngeal smear from the patient and from an ill sibling confirmed pertussis in both. Two other siblings, the parents, and a neighbor's child also had had a clinical illness compatible with pertussis. All the children had received the recommended number of immunizations for diphtheria and tetanus toxoids and pertussis vaccine (DPT) for their age. The cases were treated with erythromycin and an immunization clinic was set up in the community.

Georgia. An outbreak of pertussis occurred among students of a Decatur, Georgia, elementary school over a 5-week period in May and June 1977. Of the school's 580 students, 26 had a clinical syndrome of fever and catarrhal symptoms, followed by prolonged cough, as did 4 preschool siblings of sick children. None developed clinical pneumonia or required hospitalization and most had a relatively mild cough. Of the 30 cases, 26 were students in the third grade or their contacts.

Nasopharyngeal swabs were obtained for culture and FA staining from 28 ill schoolchildren and their siblings. *Bordetella pertussis* was isolated from 6 children; it was identified by FA staining in 1 culture-positive child and 3 other children.

Immunization histories of the ill children were compared with those of the well children. Of 75 children who gave a history of complete DPT immunization for their age, 18 were ill. Of 19 children who had a history of incomplete immunization, 12 became ill. No child had a certain history of no prior pertussis immunization. The majority of children with incomplete immunization lacked a preschool booster of DPT. Thus complete immunization provided 62% more protection than partial immunization.

Editorial Note: Pertussis occurs more frequently than is generally recognized. It is often not considered in the differential diagnosis of cough (as with the index case in the first outbreak) or in older children because the disease may be mild and manifested simply as a persistent cough (as in the second outbreak). Diagnosis is further complicated by the various capabilities of laboratories in identifying the organism by culture or FA staining (*MMWR* 26:250, 1977).

BRUCELLOSIS

The disease brucellosis is caused by species of the genus *Brucella*. The natural infections occur in various animals; humans become infected by contact with contaminated animal products.

TABLE 23-1 SPECIES OF *BRUCELLA*, COMMON RESERVOIR HOST AND HUMAN INFECTIONS

Brucella species	Reservoir host	Human disease
B. abortus	cattle	Brucellosis (undulant fever)
B. canis	dogs	Brucellosis
B. melitensis	goats	Brucellosis (Malta fever)
B. neotomae	rodents	none
B. ovis	sheep	none
B. suis	swine	Brucellosis (Bang's disease)

Bacteria

Of the three most common *Brucella* species, *B. abortus* normally causes infections of cattle, *B. melitensis* is usually found in sheep and goats, and *B. suis* commonly infects swine (Table 23-1). Humans are susceptible to all three species. Brucellae are small, gram-negative, pleomorphic, coccobacillary-shaped bacteria. Because they grow slowly on artificial culture media, incubation for several days to several weeks is sometimes necessary before colonies develop. These microorganisms may survive from several days to several weeks when shed in the body fluids of an animal.

Pathogenesis and Clinical Disease

The *Brucella* organisms enter the body via lesions or cuts, ingestion, or inhalation. The bacteria are readily phagocytized by white blood cells; however, they are able to survive inside both PMNs and macrophages and much of the pathogenesis of brucellosis is associated with this intracellular survival.

Bacteria are carried with the phagocytic cells through the lymphatic system to the blood and into such organs of the RES as the liver and spleen, which may, in turn, become enlarged. Circulating antibodies are produced but are unable to neutralize the bacteria sequestered inside the white blood cells.

The onset of clinical symptoms of brucellosis is usually gradual and often occurs weeks or months after exposure. Clinical symptoms are quite generalized and include fever, weakness, malaise, body ache, headache, and sweating. The fever may occur in cycles with febrile periods alternating with afebrile periods. The fever pattern has prompted the use of the name *undulant fever* for this disease. When cell-mediated immunity develops, the body is better able to contain or eliminate *Brucella* infections. Recovery from the disease is gradual and partial disability frequently prolonged. Some infections are not apparent or go unrecognized. Brucellosis induces abortions in animals, an important factor in the economics of the cattle and swine industries. It is not, however, a feature of the human disease.

Transmission and Epidemiology

Large numbers of *Brucella* organisms are shed in urine, placental fluids, milk, and other secretions of infected animals. Transmission among animals occurs by direct

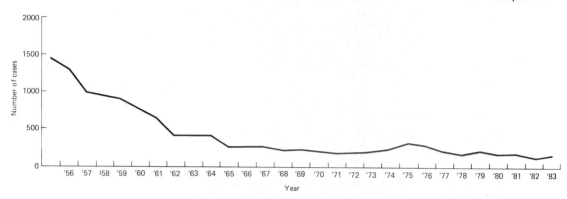

Figure 23-2   The reported occurrence of brucellosis in the United States, 1955–1983 (modified from CDC annual summaries).

contact with contaminated materials. Similarly, transmission to humans is by contact with contaminated animal products. Thus infections are most often seen in persons who work with animals or in meat-processing plants. Between 1965 and 1975, 2302 cases of brucellosis were reported in the United States. More than half were in persons working in meat-processing jobs. But the number of cases of brucellosis has decreased significantly in the past three decades (Figure 23-2) due to intensive control programs with domestic animals. Currently many states are certified as being free of brucellosis. Still, a slight increase in the number of cases has occurred in the past few years among persons working with cattle. Drinking of unpasteurized milk is a major transmission route of brucellosis in some parts of the world.

Diagnosis

Various clinical findings in persons most likely to be exposed are suggestive of the disease in humans. Diagnosis is confirmed by cultivation of the *Brucella* organism from the blood or tissues of the patient. A significant increase or high levels of serum antibodies also help to confirm a diagnosis. Skin tests are available to detect those who have had brucellosis.

Treatment

Tetracyclines are the most effective antibiotics and generally cure the clinical disease within a few days. Prolonged therapy for 3 to 4 weeks is recommended, however, to ensure killing of the bacteria sequestered in the white blood cells and to prevent relapses. Streptomycin is sometimes used in conjunction with tetracyclines to help prevent recurrences of this disease.

Prevention and Control

Pasteurization of milk is effective in preventing transmission of brucellosis. Most control efforts are directed against the animal reservoir and extensive serologic and skin testing of domestic animals is required by law in most states. Infected animals are destroyed. An effective living vaccine is available for animals. Serologic tests or certification of vaccination is required to transport cattle into brucellosis-free areas or across state lines. These measures have resulted in a general decline in the number of brucellosis infections in both humans and animals.

SUMMARY

1. *Haemophilus influenzae* is responsible for a number of serious infections ranging from meningitis to pneumonia and cellulitis. It is an organism that evokes fear among medical personnel because of its ability to produce rapidly fatal infections in children. Other members of the genus are rarely involved in disease and include one species that is sexually transmitted.

2. Whooping cough, a common killer of children prior to development of a vaccine, has remained a not infrequent cause of disease even today. *Bordatella pertussis* is difficult to culture in the laboratory, is a gram-negative bacillus. Infection with this organism is not easily treated and may require several weeks of patient convalescence.

3. A classic zoonotic disease, brucellosis is usually transmitted to humans through contact with contaminated animals or animal products. Individuals in the animal industry, particularly males, have an increased risk of getting the disease. Meat, milk, and meat products have been implicated in the spread of infection. Several species exist. In the United States the most common cause of human disease is due to *Brucella abortus*.

Yersinia
and
Francisella

$$24$$

The bacterial species now classified under the genera *Yersinia* and *Francisella* were previously included in the genus *Pasteurella*. More refined studies, however, have shown that these microorganisms are quite distinct from each other as well as from other species of *Pasteurella* and so these two genera were created. Some bacteria are still classed under the original *Pasteurella* genus and several species of *Yersinia* are known. Most of the *Pasteurella* are associated with animal diseases. The most prominent species is *P. multocida*, which causes fowl cholera and is frequently found colonized in the mouth and respiratory tract of various animals, including dogs and cats. *P. multocida* may be transmitted to humans by animal scratches or bites and may result in serious wound infections or pneumonia.

The most commonly known human pathogens of the genera *Yersinia* and *Francisella* are similar in that their primary hosts are various wild and domestic animals. They cause plague and tularemia, respectively, in humans.

PLAGUE

The bacteria species *Yersinia pestis*[1] is the cause of epidemic plague or the "black death" of the Middle Ages. Due to improved living conditions, and perhaps changes in other factors influencing host-parasite relationships, plague is no longer the devastating disease it once was. Yet sporadic cases still occur in the western United States

[1]It has been proposed that this name be changed to *Yersinia pseudotuberculosis* subsp. *pestis*. We find this change confusing and awkward and have chosen to continue use of the name *Y. pestis*.

and continual monitoring of this disease is required to avoid conditions that might cause epidemics.

Bacterium

Y. pestis (Figure 24-1), a gram-negative coccobacillus, shows bipolar staining that produces a "safety-pin" appearance when viewed with an optical microscope. It can easily be grown on common laboratory media.

Pathogenesis and Clinical Disease

Y. pestis is able to multiply in a variety of different mammalian and insect hosts and exists in three cycles. The first is apparently the natural cycle; here the disease is found in wild rodents and is called *sylvatic plague*. Sylvatic plague is transmitted among the rodents by fleas. The most frequent carriers of plague are squirrels, mice, prairie dogs, and chipmunks; over 200 different animals have been shown to be susceptible, however. The susceptibility of wild rodents to plague varies. Some animal species die of the disease whereas others experience subclinical infections.

The second cycle occurs when plague is spread to urban rodents, mainly rats, that live in close proximity to humans. This cycle is called *urban* or *domestic plague*. Urban rats frequently die of plague, which causes their fleas to seek new hosts and

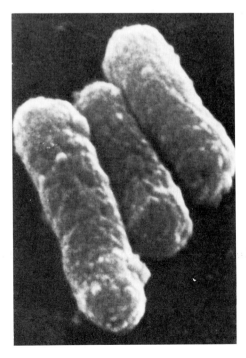

Figure 24-1 Scanning electron micrograph of *Y. pestis* magnified 40,000×. (T. H. Chen and S. S. Elberg, *Inf. Imm. 15*:972–977, Figure 4, with permission from ASM).

results in the increased spread of the disease among the rats and an increased chance of spread to other animals as well as humans.

   The third cycle, called *human plague*, starts when humans are bitten by an infected flea from either the sylvatic or urban cycles. Generally the flea bite occurs on the legs and the bacteria spread to regional lymph nodes in the groin, where extensive multiplication and swelling occur. The swollen lymph nodes are called *buboes*, especially in older medical writings, and this form of the disease is called *bubonic plague* (Figure 24-2). The buboes usually appear less than a week after the flea bite. Fever, chills, nausea, malaise, and pains may precede and accompany the buboes. The spread of the bacteria is not stopped by the lymph nodes and so bacteremia results. The presence of the *Y. pestis* in the blood is called *septicemic plague*. Massive involvement of blood vessels occurs, resulting in purpuric (purple) lesions in the skin. This manifestation was responsible for the "black death" title earlier applied to this disease. Clumps (emboli) of bacteria may become trapped in the lungs, where the lesions erode into the air sacs and cause *pneumonic plague*. Pneumonic plague gives an added dimension to this disease, for the bacteria can be readily transmitted from the patient to other persons by the airborne route. Those contracting pneumonic plague in this way rapidly develop severe signs of the disease and die within 2 or 3 days. The epidemiology and pathogenesis of plague are shown in Figure 24-3.

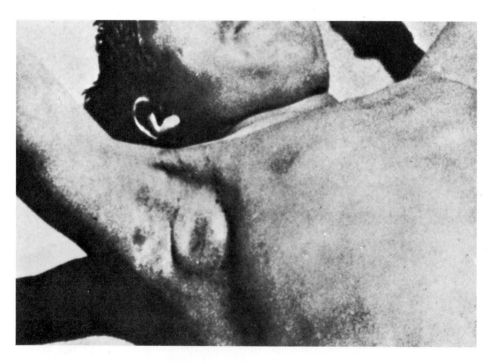

Figure 24-2   Swollen axillary lymph nodes (bubo) in a patient with plague. (Armed Forces Institute of Pathology, AFIP MIS #219900(7-B))

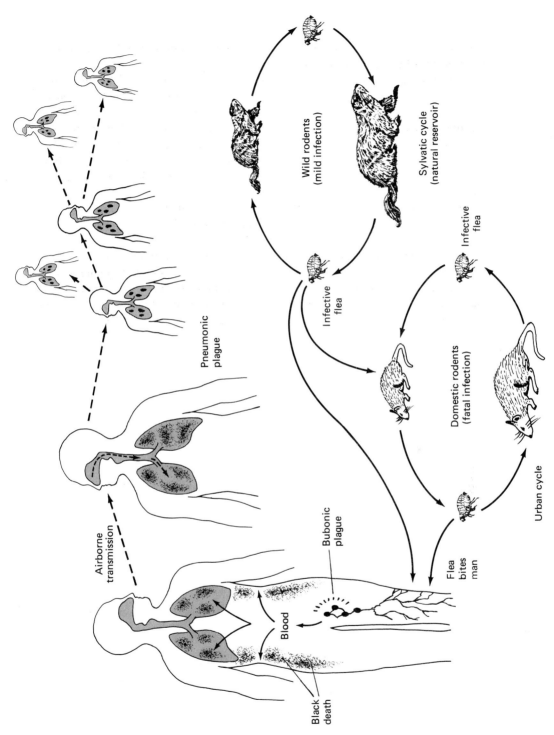

Figure 24-3 The epidemiology and pathogenesis of plague.

The death rate from untreated bubonic and septicemic plague is 50 to 75% whereas pneumonic plague is close to 100%. Some persons do develop mild nonfatal cases of plague.

Transmission and Epidemiology

Plague has occurred in pandemics in earlier periods and throughout history was one of the most devastating diseases of mankind. The first well-documented pandemic occurred in A.D. 550 and resulted in an estimated 100 million deaths over a 60-year period. The next major pandemic took place in the fourteenth century when 25% of the population of Europe died. Smaller epidemics continued until about 1800; then a general decline set in. The last major epidemic happened in China at the end of the 1800s. During the nineteenth century plague was carried to most parts of the world by rat-infested ships, including to the West Coast of the United States. Today most cases of plague are reported in southeast Asia. Virtually all plague seen today results from flea bites and not from airborne transmission from person to person. Sylvatic plague, however, still exists in the western United States in over 50 species of rodents and their fleas. Most cases seen in the United States occur among persons who live in rural areas or who camp in the West. At present, 10 to 20 cases of plague per year have been diagnosed in humans in the United States (Figure 24-4). Urban plague from domestic rats in seaport cities is a possible threat; however, no such outbreaks have occurred for many years.

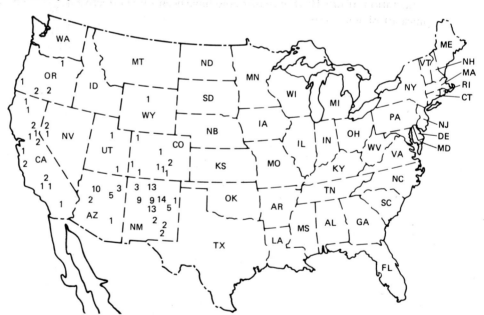

Figure 24-4 Geographic distribution of the 136 human plague cases, by county, occurring in the United States, 1970–1981 (*MMWR 31:*74, 1982).

Diagnosis

Preliminary laboratory diagnosis may be made by direct microscopic examination of smears of fluids from lymph nodes or lesions. The appearance of gram-negative, bipolar-staining coccobacilli is suggestive of *Y. pestis*. A confirmed diagnosis can be made by culturing the bacteria and by serologic tests. Extreme care is needed to prevent laboratory-acquired infections when working with plague.

Treatment

Y. pestis is highly susceptible to streptomycin, tetracyclines, and chloramphenicol. Early treatment is extremely important, especially for pneumonic plague because treatment after the first day may not be successful. Proper early treatment of bubonic plague reduces the mortality to less than 5%.

Prevention and Control

Both living and killed vaccines are available. Three doses of the killed vaccine are used in the United States and this dosage is recommended for persons going to southeast Asia. Plague vaccinations were effective in protecting U.S. military personnel during the Vietnam War. In general, plague can be controlled by improved living conditions that reduce close contact between humans and rodents. Efforts to prevent the importation of rats by ship or airplane have been quite effective and are a necessary phase of plague control.

CLINICAL NOTE

Plague: South Carolina

On August 5, 1983, plague was diagnosed in a 13-year-old girl in South Carolina. She became ill while en route to Maryland from her previous residence in Santa Fe, New Mexico, and subsequently died. The area in which she had lived had been recognized as a locality where sylvatic plague was enzootic.

On July 25, the girl, a horsewoman who spent considerable time outdoors, handled and then released a wild chipmunk. On July 27, she flew to Atlanta, Georgia, and spent the night with friends; the following day she was driven to Seneca, South Carolina. That evening, she complained of a sore throat and tenderness in her right groin and reportedly had a temperature of 40.0°C (104°F). On July 29, she saw a physician, who noted an oral temperature of 38.3°C (101°F), pharyngeal erythema, tender cervical lymph nodes, and a 1-x-2-centimeter tender right inguinal lymph node. Laboratory tests, including complete blood count, urinalysis, and throat culture, and tests for mononucleosis, were done, and oral penicillin was prescribed. Three days later she was seen again, still febrile and with expanding right inguinal nodes. Her white blood cell count was 20,500, and a chest x ray was normal. Because of her history of residence in a plague-enzootic state, a diagnosis of plague was considered. She was hospitalized and given parenteral therapy, including streptomycin. By the following morning, she was tachypneic (rapid, shallow respiration), with productive bloody sputum, and appeared moribund. She was transferred to a large, regional medical center where, despite intensive supportive care and therapy with intravenous chloramphenicol, she developed overwhelming sepsis and died on August 2. A chest radiograph taken before death revealed extensive pulmonary infiltrates.

Antemortem aspiration of the right inguinal lymph node demonstrated gram-negative bipolar staining bacilli on Giemsa stain. Both this aspirate and multiple cultures of blood yielded *Yersinia pestis.* In addition, fluorescent antibody (FA) stains for *Y. pestis* were positive for specimens consisting of blood smears, culture material, and pulmonary secretions.

Editorial note: This is the fifth documented case of plague east of the hundredth meridian (south-central Texas to north-central North Dakota), excluding laboratory accidents, since 1920. All five patients were exposed in enzootic areas (four in the western United States, one in Vietnam). Considering this patient's outdoor activities and area of residence, exposure possibilities are numerous; her exact exposure will probably never be known, since the chipmunk was not captured. That she was able to handle the animal suggests that it was not healthy.

Because the patient had no evidence of pneumonia before hospitalization, no chemoprophylaxis was recommended for the friends with whom she stayed in Georgia; there were no secondary cases. Based on the clinical picture and the positive FA results from sputum, it appears that pneumonic plague and the potential for human-to-human transmission existed terminally. Local health-care providers had placed her in complete isolation before this development. Hospital staff directly in contact with her at this point were placed on prophylactic tetracycline and followed up for evidence of illness. No secondary cases appeared during the expected incubation period (*MMWR 32*:417, 1983).

YERSINIA ENTEROCOLITICA INFECTION

By far the major disease in humans caused by *Yersinia* is that caused by *Y. enterocolitica*. This bacterium is primarily associated with domestic animals but may be transmitted to humans through contaminated foodstuffs or directly from such animals as poultry and swine.

The infection is characterized by acute abdominal pain, profuse (sometimes bloody) diarrhea, and headache. Vomiting may occur in some patients. These symptoms are characteristic of many cases of appendicitis and so have led to the removal of normal appendixes in patients with this infection. Patients may also have an inflammation of the abdominal lymphatic structures, a condition referred to as mesynteric adenitis. Recovery is usually uneventful and complete.

Y. enterocolitica can be isolated by plating a stool specimen on a selective medium. When present in low numbers, it can be cultured by a cold-enrichment procedure in which the culture specimen is held in saline at 4°C for up to 3 weeks. Periodic cultures are made from the cold enrichment to regular media and incubated at 35°C to recover the organism.

TULAREMIA

Bacterium

Francisella tularensis is the cause of the disease tularemia. It is a small (0.5 × 0.3 μm), gram-negative coccobacillus. Cysteine and blood or serum must be present in culture media before this bacterium will grow and even then growth is slow.

Pathogenesis and Clinical Disease

Tularemia is a widespread disease in many species of animal and insects. Humans become infected by being bitten by an infected insect, by handling blood or tissues from infected animals, or by drinking contaminated water. An ulcer-type lesion usually develops at the site of inoculation or bite (Figure 24-5) and regional lymph nodes become swollen and painful. Systemic signs, such as dizziness, headache, chills and

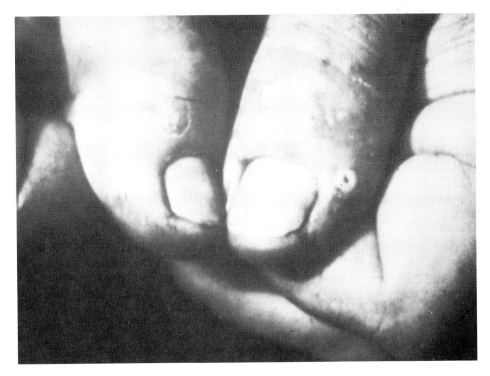

Figure 24-5 Lesions at the site of exposure to *Francisella tularensis*. (Centers for Disease Control, Atlanta)

fever, sweating, and prostration, develop. Gastrointestinal symptoms may result from ingesting contaminated water or meats. Pneumonia may also be part of the clinical picture, either as a result of airborne exposure or as an extension of the systemic disease. The lesion heals in 4 to 7 weeks without treatment and complete recovery may require 3 to 6 months. Some relapses may occur, for *F. tularensis* is able to remain sequestered inside certain host cells and not be removed by normal host defense mechanisms. Unless treated, a death rate of 10% is possible, but death rates are less than 1% with antibiotic therapy.

Transmission and Epidemiology

Most cases occur in rural areas and among persons who came in contact with wild animals or who are routinely exposed to ticks, deerflies, or other biting arthropods. Rabbits and rodents are the most common animal sources of human infection and transmission occurs during handling or dressing of an infected animal. Tularemia is sometimes referred to as "rabbit fever" or "deerfly fever." Open streams of water may become contaminated from infected beavers or muskrats. Infections can be maintained in ticks by the passage of *F. tularensis* from the female to her offspring (transovarian passage). No human-to-human transmission happens under natural conditions and the occurrence of diseases in humans is sporadic. From 100 to 200 cases are reported each year in the United States (Figure 24-6).

Diagnosis

Growth of *F. tularensis* occurs slowly even on some specialized culture media and isolation of the microbe from clinical specimens is difficult. Diagnosis is usually made on the basis of clinical symptoms and a history of possible exposure. Serologic agglutination tests are available; a sharp rise in antibodies against *F. tularensis* is needed to confirm the diagnosis.

Treatment

Streptomycin, the treatment of choice, is highly effective against *F. tularensis*. It is more effective than some other broad-spectrum antibiotics in preventing recurrent diseases. Penicillin is ineffective.

Prevention and Control

The best methods of preventing tularemia are to avoid possible infected animals, especially sick rabbits, and to take precautions to reduce the chance of being bitten by arthropods. When working with *F. tularensis*, care should be taken to prevent laboratory-acquired infections. Because of the widespread nature of this disease in wild animals and arthropods, it cannot be controlled by the eradication of these natural hosts.

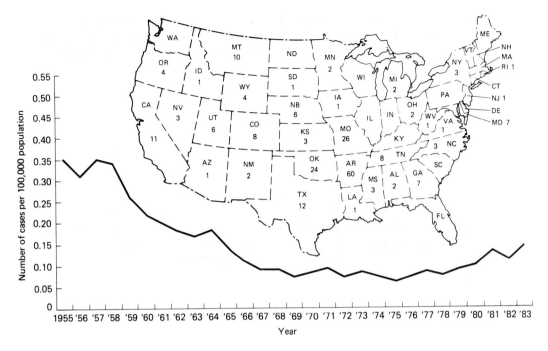

Figure 24-6 Reported cases of tularemia in the United States, 1955–1983. Map shows distribution of the total number of cases occurring in 1980 (modified from CDC annual summaries).

A live attenuated vaccine is available to persons who have a high risk of exposure, including laboratory personnel working with this microorganism, sheep herders, and those who work with wild animals or process hides or other products from these animals.

CLINICAL NOTE

Tularemia: Colorado, Alaska, and Georgia

Through October 13 of 1979, CDC received reports of 166 cases of tularemia. Three reports exemplify several clinical and epidemiologic characteristics commonly observed with this disease.

Colorado. A sheep-shearing crew was working west of Rangely during the week of April 23 when 4 of 9 members became ill with fever and headache. Three persons developed left axillary lymphadenopathy (enlarged lymph nodes) with lesions on the dorsum of the left hand. The other patient, who did not have adenopathy or a skin lesion, suffered a more severe illness associated with a pulmonary infiltrate. All patients consulted a physician approximately 10 days after the onset of illness and recovered with tetracycline therapy. One patient had a fourfold rise in antibody to *F. tularensis* whereas the other 3 had single titers of >1:160. Before becoming ill, these men had sheared sheep that seemed ill and that were covered with wood ticks (*D. andersoni*). The presence of lesions on only the left hand is explained by the procedure that the workers use in shearing sheep. The men part fleece with their bare left hand while shearing with the right hand—often rupturing ticks in the process and spilling blood onto the left hand.

In late June a 31-year-old laboratory technician was hospitalized in Grand Junction, with an illness of 2 weeks, a duration that began several days after working with an isolate of *F. tularensis*. Symptoms included fever to 105.8°F (41°C), headache, and pleuritic chest pain; pneumonitis and pleural effusion were confirmed by x ray. A diagnosis of tularemia was made, based on a sixteenfold rise in titer. The patient recovered with streptomycin therapy.

Alaska. On August 31 a 49-year-old man in Fairbanks became ill 3 days after dressing a rabbit killed by his dog. Initial symptoms were a fever of 105°F (40.5°C) and vomiting; within 2 days he developed bilateral axillary adenopathy, with two ulcerations just proximal to a cut on his left hand. Culture of a lymph node aspirate grew *F. tularensis* and the patient made an uneventful recovery with tetracycline therapy. A number of dead rabbits were recently observed in the area.

Georgia. In mid September two boys aged 10 and 11 from Calhoun became ill after handling a dead rabbit they had found. Both boys developed fever, swollen axillary lymph nodes, and ulcerative lesions on their hands. When seen on October 1, both patients were still ill and cultures of both hand lesions and one lymph node aspirate grew *F. tularensis*. Both patients recovered following streptomycin therapy (*MMWR 28*:529, 1979).

SUMMARY

1. The *Yersinia* and *Francisella* are very small gram-negative bacilli. These organisms are often the cause of disease in lower animals and are characteristically transmitted to humans through the bite of an insect vector. *Yersinia* has been responsible for the great, distinctive plagues of the past and lives endemically in the rodents of western deserts of the United States.

2. Tularemia, resulting from infection by *F. tularensis*, is a not uncommon infection of humans, particularly in some areas of the world. Because of its normal habitat—rodents—it is most often a disease found or contracted in a rural setting. Antibiotics have been successful in treating the infection.

Enteric and Related Gram-Negative Bacilli

25

Many bacteria discussed in this chapter and the following one are members of the family Enterobacteriaceae. This family consists of related bacteria that primarily inhabit the large intestines of humans and animals. Some are also found in soil, water, and decaying matter. Because of the close relationship of many of these microbes, it is sometimes difficult to determine the exact classification categories. Over the years various classification arrangements were used and the names of some species were periodically changed. For example, as of 1972 there were only 12 genera and 26 species in this family. Table 25-1 lists the accepted 21 genera of Enterobacteriaceae in 1984, and the number of species exceeds 81 with additions being made regularly. In the following discussion references are chiefly to the genus or species names and less emphasis is given to larger taxonomic categories. In the clinical setting these microorganisms are referred to as the gram-negative or the enteric bacilli. Also included in this broad category of gram-negative bacilli are some members of the genera *Vibrio* and *Pseudomonas* that are taxonomically distinct from the Enterobacteriaceae but cause similar diseases and have similar epidemiologic patterns.

Some of these bacteria are of moderate-to-high virulence and are able to cause disease when they infect susceptible hosts. They are referred to as the frank pathogens and include species of the genera *Salmonella*, *Shigella*, and *Vibrio*, the causative agents of typhoid fever, dysentery, and cholera, respectively. Most other enteric bacilli are of lower virulence and function as opportunistic pathogens; these organisms are regular inhabitants of the intestinal tract of humans or are routinely found in the general environment. The opportunistic species only cause disease when they gain access to other body compartments or tissues or when the host defenses become com-

TABLE 25-1 GENERA OF THE FAMILY ENTEROBACTERIACEAE

Buttiauxella	*Ewingella*	*Providencia*
Cedecea	*Hafnia*	*Rahnella*
Citrobacter	*Klebsiella*	*Salmonella*
Edwardsiella	*Kluyvera*	*Serratia*
Enterobacter	*Morganella*	*Tatumella*
Erwinia	*Obesumbacterium*	*Yersinia*
Escherichia-Shigella	*Proteus*	*Xenorhabdus*

promised. The frank pathogens are discussed in this chapter and the opportunistic pathogens in the subsequent one.

GENERAL CHARACTERISTICS OF THE ENTERIC BACILLI

The members of the family Enterobacteriaceae are relatively small, $0.5 \times 2\mu m$, non-spore-forming bacilli. Some are motile; others are not. Some have capsules, but others do not. They ferment a variety of different carbohydrates and the patterns of carbohydrate fermentation are used to help differentiate and classify these bacteria. The bacterial colonies appear similar on nondifferential media. Various differential and selective media, however, are used to help in the preliminary classification of the Enterobacteriaceae. Once these microorganisms have been classified by biochemical tests to the genus or species level, further differentiation is made by serologic tests.

People in a clinical bacteriology laboratory spend much time identifying and differentiating the species of these gram-negative bacilli. Being widespread, normal inhabitants of the body, they are often found in clinical specimens and it is a rather laborious task to determine if pathogenic strains are present among the nonpathogens. When dealing with an infected patient, particularly a compromised host, it is also necessary to determine if the disease is caused by a low-virulent strain. Trying to find the involvement, if any, of these bacteria in a given clinical disease is a challenge to physicians and laboratory workers.

Because these bacteria are found in large numbers in the intestinal tract, they are often transmitted by the anal-oral route and are frequent contaminants of food and water. The enteric bacilli are able to survive for extended periods when adequate moisture is present. They can be carried in water supplies over long distances and may be found on foods or in other environmental niches where moisture is present. Freezing does not destroy these bacteria and frozen foods or ice can remain contaminated for extended periods. They are responsive to relatively low concentrations of common disinfectants and are effectively reduced in water supplies treated with small amounts of chlorine. The species *Escherichia coli* is a predominant facultative anaerobic bacterium of the intestinal tract and is used in the United States as an indicator organism to determine fecal or sewage contamination of water supplies.

The endotoxins contained in the cell walls of these enteric bacteria may play an important role in the pathogenesis of the diseases they cause. Some pathogenic strains also produce exotoxins, called enterotoxins, that specifically affect the intestinal tract, causing diarrhea and fluid loss from the body. Various species of the Enterobacteriaceae are able to cause pneumonia and are also the most common cause of urinary tract infections. These microorganisms are now recognized as a major cause of wound infections and other infections acquired in hospital patients. They may also cause systemic infections and occasionally meningitis, especially in infants. It has been estimated that infections by these enteric bacilli may be contributing factors in about 100,000 deaths per year in the United States. Infections caused by these bacteria are often difficult to treat with routinely used chemotherapeutic agents.

SALMONELLOSIS

The genus *Salmonella* consists of three species, *S. choleraesuis*, *S. typhi*, and *S. enteritidis*, and these three species contain some 1500 different serotypes of biochemically related enteric bacilli. The major diseases caused by the salmonellae are typhoid fever and gastroenteritis.

TYPHOID FEVER

Pathogenesis and Clinical Disease

Typhoid fever is caused by *S. typhi* which attaches to and penetrates the epithelial lining of the small intestines. Following penetration, the bacteria are phagocytized by macrophages; unfortunately, they are not destroyed but are actually able to multiply within the macrophages. The macrophages carry the *S. typhi* into the blood and throughout the RES. The bacteria are released from the macrophages, into the bloodstream. These events occur during the first week of infection and may be accompanied by fever, malaise, lethargy, and aches and pains. During the second week extended bacteremia is present and the foci of infection may occur in various tissues; in particular, the gallbladder becomes infected. Bacteria may be shed from the gallbladder back into the intestinal lumen. During this time ulcerative lesions of Peyer's patches may develop and the patient is often severely ill with a constant fever as high as 40°C (104°F), abdominal tenderness, diarrhea or constipation, and vomiting. By the third week, in uncomplicated cases, the patient is exhausted, may still be febrile, but shows improvement. Death may result in up to 10% of the untreated patients. After people recover from the clinical disease, *S. typhi* may continue to multiply in the gallbladder of about 3% of the patients. These persons may become chronic carriers and serve as a source of future outbreaks. The pathogenesis of typhoid fever is shown in Figure 25-1.

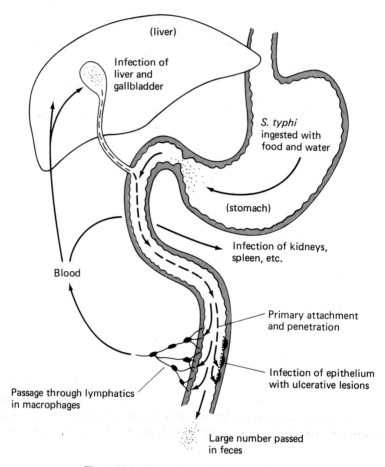

Figure 25-1   The pathogenesis of typhoid fever.

Transmission and Epidemiology

The primary mode of transmission of the typhoid bacillus is through contaminated food or water. Typhoid fever cases have declined significantly because of adequate water and sewage systems in developed countries. Most outbreaks of typhoid fever in the United States today are associated either with failures in water or sewage systems or with persons living in undeveloped areas. The threat of typhoid is always present when normal water and sewage systems are disrupted by disasters like floods and earthquakes. Carriers who work in food-handling jobs may also be a source of limited outbreaks. The typhoid fever rate in the United States is seen in Figure 25-2.

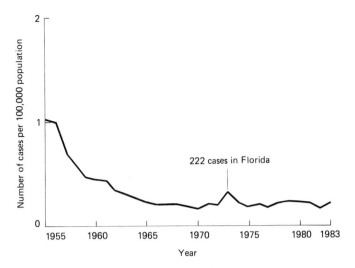

Figure 25-2 Reported case rates for typhoid fever by year in the United States, 1955–1983. The number of cases has remained relatively constant since 1970. About one-half of the cases reported in the United States are acquired during foreign travel. The source of domestically acquired typhoid is usually a chronic carrier of *S. typhi* (modified from CDC annual summaries).

Diagnosis

Typhoid fever, particularly in early stages, is easily confused with other diseases. A positive diagnosis depends on the isolation of *S. typhi* from the blood and feces or other parts of the body. Agglutination tests showing a rise in specific antibodies are also used.

Treatment

Treatment is with ampicillin or cholamphenicol. It must be continued for several weeks to ensure killing bacteria that became sequestered in the phagocytic cells. Carriers are best cured by daily treatment with ampicillin for three months. If this treatment fails, surgical removal of the gallbladder may be necessary.

Prevention and Control

Proper water treatment and sewage disposal are the most important factors in controlling typhoid fever. Pasteurization of milk and exclusion of chronic carriers as food handlers are also helpful. Killed vaccines have been used for many years and may be of some value.

CLINICAL NOTE

Typhoid Fever: Michigan

During October and November 1981, 18 cases of typhoid fever were diagnosed in Jackson, Michigan, among 310 United Way volunteers who consumed a luncheon served at a community banquet hall on October 8, 1981. Although no specific food could be incriminated, a probably chronic carrier of *Salmonella typhi* was identified among the food handlers who prepared the luncheon.

Dates of onset ranged from October 12 to November 11, 1981, for an incubation period of 4 to 33 days (mean = 13.5). Older individuals tended to have shorter incubation periods. The attack rate was 5.8%. Sixteen of the 18 cases were confirmed by blood and/or stool culture. All isolates of *S. typhi* were phage type E_1 and were sensitive to chloramphenicol, ampicillin, and trimethoprim-sulfamethoxazole.

All patients experienced fever [mean temperature 103.3°F (39.6°C)], fatigue, and headache, and most had chills, sweats, and anorexia; 39% reported diarrhea, and 33% had constipation. No instances of gastrointestinal hemorrhage or perforation were reported. There were no deaths and no evidence of secondary transmission.

Self-administered questionnaires asking about foods eaten at the luncheon and subsequent illness were distributed to all attendees; 289 (93%) returned completed questionnaires. Food histories of the 16 culture-confirmed cases were compared with those of asymptomatic controls and failed to incriminate any food item.

A probably chronic carrier of *S. typhi* was identified among the food handlers. This individual, an asymptomatic 68-year-old female with previously undiagnosed cholelithiasis (gallstones), had participated in the preparation of all or most of the foods served. *S. typhi* of the same phage type and antimicrobial-sensitivity pattern as that obtained from cases was isolated from her rectal swab and all her stool specimens; her serum antibody titer was 20. She subsequently underwent cholecystectomy (removal of gall bladder) in combination with high-dose amoxicilin therapy. Culture of the gallstone after antimicrobial therapy and all follow-up stool cultures have been negative (*MMWR 31*:544, 1982).

GASTROENTERITIS

Pathogenesis and Clinical Diseases

Many serotypes of *Salmonella* are found in the intestinal tract of various animals and birds. When ingested by humans, the salmonella proliferate in the intestines and symptoms of gastroenteritis begin within 18 to 36 hours. Such symptoms as fever, abdominal pain, and diarrhea are common. This disease is usually self-limiting and complete recovery occurs within several days. Extensive dehydration may occur in very young and old persons and the resulting fluid imbalance may be life threatening. Human infection by these organisms is usually limited to the lumen of the intestine. Such infections constitute a form of infectious food poisoning.

Transmission and Epidemiology

Salmonellosis is one of the most common infectious diseases in the United States. An estimated 2 million cases are reported annually. Infection results from ingesting salmonella-contaminated foods. Poultry products, including eggs, are the most common source of salmonella infections, but meat products, in general, are frequently contaminated. As salmonellae are normal intestinal bacterial flora of domestic animals, foods may become contaminated with intestinal contents during slaughter; if not thoroughly cooked, the salmonellae may survive to proliferate during storage when refrigeration is not used. Any food that comes in contact with rodents or animal products may become contaminated. Pets or other animals may harbor salmonellae and transmit the infection directly to humans. Pet turtles are often infected; consequently, their sale is regulated in many states. Outbreaks of *Salmonella* gastroenteritis often occur after such holidays as Thanksgiving and Christmas. The increased use of widely distributed mass-produced foods may result in an increase in the rate of salmonellosis in the United States. The numbers of reported cases of salmonellosis occurring in this country are shown in Figure 25-3.

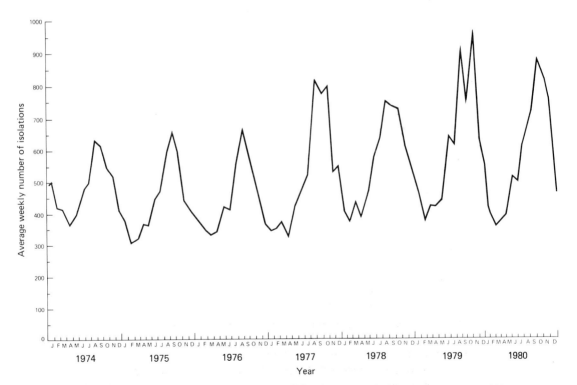

Figure 25-3 Reported isolations of salmonella from humans in the United States, 1974–1980. Each point represents the weekly average number of isolates for the month (*CDC Annual Summary,* 1980).

Diagnosis

Isolation of salmonella from the intestinal tract is required for a positive diagnosis.

Treatment

Supportive therapy is the recommended treatment. Antibiotics are not recommended except in extreme cases of disseminated disease or cases involving infants or elderly persons.

Prevention and Control

Proper cooking and refrigeration of meats eliminate or prevent the growth of salmonella. Sanitary procedures in slaughterhouses help reduce the level of contamination. Some foods are routinely monitored for the presence of salmonella.

CLINICAL NOTE

Multistate Outbreak of Salmonellosis Caused by Precooked Roast Beef

In the first week of August 1981, three outbreaks of salmonellosis that affected more than 100 people in three northeastern states were reported to CDC. The first two outbreaks were traced to precooked roast beef from a Philadelphia meat-processing plant, and the third to delicatessen-style sliced sandwich meat served at a hospital cafeteria. Some of these meat slices were of the precooked roast beef processed in the Pennsylvania plant.

The first outbreak followed a wedding reception held on July 25 at Claymont, Delaware, attended by approximately 150 people, mostly residents of Delaware County, Pennsylvania. Of the 58 persons contacted for interview, 37 had had diarrhea. *Salmonella* group B was isolated from the stools of 13 patients (11 *S. chester*, 2 *S. typhimurium*). Illness was significantly associated with eating precooked roast beef at the reception. None of the meat served at the reception was available for culture.

The second outbreak followed a wedding reception held on July 25 in southern New Jersey; 47 of 92 persons who attended became ill, and illness was again associated with eating precooked roast beef. *Salmonella* was isolated from 18 of 20 stool cultures (17 *S. typhimurium*, 1 *S. newport*). *S. typhimurium* and *S. johannesburg* were isolated from an opened package of precooked roast beef provided by the caterer of the reception. Another unopened package of the same brand from the same caterer contained *S. typhimurium*, *S. newport*, and *S. anatum*.

The third outbreak, which occurred in a hospital in Philadelphia, Pennsylvania, was first recognized on July 24 after two patients had severe diarrhea. Subsequent investigation revealed 42 cases of diarrheal illness between July 20 and August 11. Six of the persons involved were inpatients, and 36 were hospital employees. *Salmonella* group B was isolated from stools from 18 persons (including 4 patients);

Salmonella group C₂ was isolated from 1 employee. *Salmonella* group B was isolated from 5 of 71 asymptomatic dietary and nursing staff in a stool-culture survey. Preliminary analysis of a case-control study demonstrated an association between illness and eating sandwich-meat slices served at the hospital cafeteria. The meat slices included the same brand of precooked roast beef involved in the other outbreaks. Some of the infected persons had not eaten the beef; the other meats may have been contaminated by it. The suspected beef samples were not available for culture, but *Salmonella* group B was recovered from meat drippings in a tray containing remnants of meat from the cafeteria delicatessen.

On August 5, the U.S. Department of Agriculture (USDA) asked the Philadelphia producer to temporarily halt further distribution of the implicated beef. *S. typhimurium* was isolated from 1 of 64 specimens tested by the USDA. Assessment of the internal temperature of these products by the protein coagulase test showed that the core temperature ranged from 130°F to 152°F, ± 5° (54.4°C to 66.7°C ± 2.8°). On August 10, the USDA issued a recall order of all precooked roast beef that had been processed by the Philadelphia company before August 6, 1981.

Editorial note: This is the first reported multistate outbreak of salmonellosis attributable to commercially produced precooked roast beef in 4 years. Until 1977, when multiple outbreaks of the disease involving several meat-processing companies were reported from Connecticut, Georgia, New York, New Jersey, Pennsylvania, and Virginia, the USDA instituted regulations requiring that raw beef be cooked until heated throughout to at least 145°F (62.8°C).

The outbreaks reported here may have resulted from failure to achieve the required minimum temperature, as indicated by the USDA study. Also, recent evidence shows that under certain conditions even heating raw meat to 145°F (62.8°C) may not produce a completely *Salmonella*-free product. Further studies on the survival of *Salmonella* in raw beef may be indicated (*MMWR 30*:391, 1981).

BACILLARY DYSENTERY

Bacteria

The *Shigella* are primarily pathogens of humans. The four species of the genus *Shigella*—*S. dysenteriae*, *S. flexneri*, *S. boydii*, and *S. sonnei*—can all cause dysentery in humans. *S. dysenteriae* causes the most severe type.

Pathogenesis and Clinical Disease

Usually the shigellae are not able to penetrate into the deeper body tissues or into the blood. After ingestion, the shigellae pass to the small intestines, where multiplication begins. The bacteria are carried to the large intestines; here they specifically attach to and penetrate into the epithelial cells, where further multiplication occurs. Generally penetration is not deeper than the submucosal cells. Inflammation, together with sloughing of the epithelial cells, results in ulcerative lesions. After 1 to 3 days of incubation the patient experiences a sudden onset of symptoms—abdominal cramps, fever, and diarrhea. The diarrheal stool frequently contains mucus and blood. Significant loss of water and salts may occur and in young and/or debilitated patients this dehydration and electrolyte imbalance may cause death. In otherwise healthy persons the disease is usually self-limiting and recovery occurs in 3 to 7 days. The death rate from dysentery in young children is significant in countries with poor sanitation and nutrition. Most residents in areas where dysentery is endemic, develop immunity to the disease either through clinical or subclinical cases. Many such persons, however, remain carriers of the organism and serve as a source of infection for new susceptibles, such as visitors or newborns entering the population.

Transmission and Epidemiology

Transmission is from human to human via the fecal-oral route by "fingers, food, feces, and flies." The disease is endemic in underdeveloped countries. In other countries outbreaks may occur in closed groups living in such areas as summer camps and mental hospitals. Historically dysentery has been a problem in military populations and entire armies have become temporarily disabled when living under unsanitary conditions existing during combat. Often people from countries like the United States contract bacillary dysentery within a short period after entering a country where dysentery is endemic. Still, about 20,000 cases of dysentery are reported each year within the United States itself (Figure 25-4).

Diagnosis

Diagnosis is made by isolating shigellae from the feces or intestinal tract.

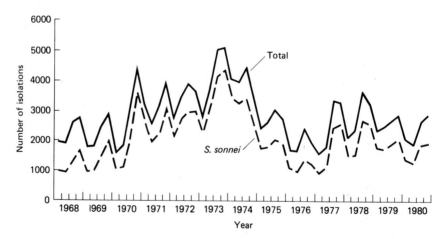

Figure 25-4 Reported isolations of shigella from humans in the United States, 1968–1980. *S. sonnei* accounted for 70% of the isolates in 1980, while most of the other isolates were *S. flexneri* (*CDC Annual Summary*, 1980).

Treatment

Most cases should be treated. Ampicillin and other broad-spectrum antibiotics are used, together with supportive therapy, to maintain fluid balance.

Prevention and Control

Prevention of person-to-person transmission by following good sanitary practices is the most effective means of avoiding this disease. Patients with the disease should be isolated.

CLINICAL NOTE

Outbreak of Shigellosis: Fort Bliss, Texas

An outbreak of food-borne shigellosis occurred on November 5, 1976, in a tactical unit conducting field-training exercises at Fort Bliss, Texas. Of 850 soldiers at risk, 176 became ill with diarrheal disease; 53 were hospitalized.

The onset of the majority of the cases (92) was between 1 A.M. and noon on November 5; an additional 34 cases occurred during the second half of the day. Excluding the suspected index case, the range of onset was from November 4 to 9.

The disease was characterized by rapid onset with fever up to 41°C (105°F), abdominal cramps, profuse diarrhea (bloody in several cases), and frequent vomiting. Many of the more serious cases with high fevers complained of severe myalgia with backache. The mean duration of the disease was 4 days, with a range from 1 to 8 days. The longest period of hospitalization was 5 days; however, most hospitalized cases were discharged within 48 hours. All cases recovered without sequelae. Stool cultures were positive for *Shigella boydii*, serotype 2, in 29 individuals.

The distribution of times of onset and the nature of the illness typified a food-borne infection originating from a common source. Although the unit was operating under field conditions, most of the personnel ate their meals in a common mess hall. A limited number of meals were prepared separately and delivered to troops at various outlying areas; most of these meals were distributed at noon.

Interviews with a large sampling of soldiers concerning food ingestion on November 3 and 4 revealed a statistically significant association between eating spaghetti at the evening meal on November 3 and subsequent diarrheal disease.

The mean incubation period calculated from the time of ingestion of the spaghetti at the evening meal of November 3 was 50.5 hours. The spaghetti was not available for culturing. However, water, milk, and several other foods that were available failed to demonstrate any contamination with enteric pathogens.

Of the 26 food handlers working in the mess hall at the time of the outbreak, 12 were symptomatic with diarrheal disease. Positive stool cultures for *S. boydii*, serotype 2, were reported for 9 of the symptomatic and 1 of the asymptomatic food handlers. One food handler responsible for preparing the spaghetti reported having had diarrheal disease at the time he did so. This food handler had spent the preceding weekend (October 30–31) in Juarez, Mexico; 2 days later he had onset of illness.

The meat sauce was prepared on the morning of the outbreak whereas the spaghetti was prepared in the afternoon, several hours before being served. The spaghetti and sauce were reportedly reheated before serving. Field mess facilities, including those for hand washing, were limited, however, and there is some question whether the reheating was performed as prescribed.

The following control measures were taken:

1. All food handlers associated with the outbreak were removed from the mess line and rectal swabs were taken. The food handlers were not allowed to work at that job until they had consecutive negative cultures taken at least 24 hours apart. Cultures were not taken until at least 48 hours after discontinuance of antimicrobials. (Symptomatic food handlers were placed on 2 g ampicillin daily for 7 days.)

2. Meticulous attention to food preparation procedures, especially hand washing for mess personnel, which included brushing of fingers and nails, was instituted. All food service personnel were continuously monitored for signs or symptoms of disease and proper food handling techniques were emphasized.

3. All persons who were ill or had a positive culture were instructed in proper sanitary practices by a community health nurse. Special attention was given to soldiers with families to ensure that secondary cases did not occur in family units. All family contacts were instructed to report any occurrence of diarrheal disease (MMWR 26:107, 1977).

CHOLERA

Bacterium

Vibrio cholerae, the causative agent of human cholera, is similar to the enteric bacilli in many respects and so is discussed in this chapter. In current classification schemes, however, it is placed in a family called *Vibrionaceae*. This bacterium can be grown on simple media and differentiated from the enteric bacilli by using selective and differential media. The bacilli are slightly curved on initial isolation, giving comma-shaped cells (the first name given to this bacterium was "Kommabacillus"). *V. cholerae* has been subclassified into various biotypes. The biotypes *classical* and *El Tor* are responsible for the more serious epidemics.

Pathogenesis and Clinical Disease

The disease of human cholera, often referred to as *Asiatic cholera*, can be devastating, especially in crowded populations with poor sanitary and medical facilities. The term *cholera* itself means any conditions characterized by violent diarrhea. The bacterium is transmitted via contaminated food or water. The organisms attach to and proliferate in the small intestines but do not invade the tissues. It has now been discovered that the pathogenesis of cholera results from the production of an enterotoxin. This enterotoxin stimulates enzymatic reactions within epithelial cells lining the intestinal tract, which, in turn, causes the loss of fluids and electrolytes into the lumen of the intestines. The incubation time averages 2 to 3 days and the onset is abrupt. The initial signs are vomiting and diarrhea. The solids in the intestinal tract are purged early in the disease and the subsequently voided fluid is watery, without odor, and contains such electrolytes as sodium chloride, potassium, and bicarbonate. As much as 15 to 29 liters of fluids may be lost in one day. Death results from rapid dehydration and resulting electrolyte imbalance.

The patient develops sunken eyes and cheeks and the skin becomes wrinkled. Without treatment, death rates are known to exceed 60%. With treatment, death rates may be reduced to less than 1%.

No direct tissue damage occurs. *V. cholerae* remains in the intestinal tract after recovery and the patient may act as a carrier and continue to shed the bacteria up to a year. Persons over 50 years of age may become chronic carriers and intermittently shed the organism for many years. The pathogenesis of cholera is outlined in Figure 25-5.

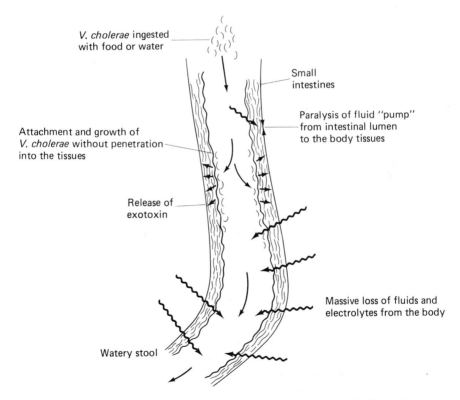

Figure 25-5   The pathogenesis of cholera showing the toxin-mediated effects of the *V. cholerae* on the intestinal mucosa.

Transmission and Epidemiology

Transmission follows the typical fecal-oral routes with carriers and clinical cases serving as sources of infection. The role of animals as carriers is not clear. Shellfish have been incriminated in the latest outbreaks of cholera in the United States.

Cholera is endemic in regions of India and Bangladesh and periodic epidemics erupt throughout Asia and Africa. Occasional outbreaks occur in other parts of the world. Because of today's rapid international travel, cholera could break out in any part of the world.

During the mid-1800s major outbreaks of cholera occurred along the Mississippi and Missouri river valleys. No cases were reported between 1911 and 1973. In 1973 a single case occurred in Texas. Then in 1977 a case developed in Alabama and in 1978 eleven cases were reported in Louisiana. Subsequently cases have continued to occur along the Gulf Coast. (See clinical note.) Their sources were shown to be due to improperly cooked shellfish. The source of infection of these shellfish is not known, but evidence now indicates that *V. cholerae* is widespread along the Gulf Coast. This situation offers a challenge to epidemiologists.

Diagnosis

Isolation of *V. cholerae* from the patient is needed to confirm diagnosis. A serologic test of acute and convalescent serum may be helpful in confirming the diagnosis. Direct fluorescent antibody tests on stools from patients have been successful in making a rapid diagnosis.

Treatment

Effective treatment of cholera, if initiated soon enough, is amazingly simple. Inasmuch as death results from loss of fluids and not tissue damage, the patient can be maintained by replacing the lost fluids and electrolytes. For severe cases, intravenous isotonic electrolyte solutions are given until the patient recovers, often within hours. The fluid balance can then be maintained by oral administration of electrolyte solutions containing glucose. Fluid therapy is continued until antibodies are produced to neutralize the enterotoxin. Oral therapy alone can be highly effective, especially if the initial fluid loss is not excessive. Such a procedure is appropriate for clinics in rural areas that are staffed with paramedical personnel. Under proper treatment death rates may be reduced to less than 1%. Tetracyclines are effective and help eliminate the organism from the intestinal tract.

Control and Prevention

Proper sewage treatment and water purification systems are the most important preventative measures. Countries with adequate systems have few, if any, outbreaks of cholera. Rapid detection, isolation, and treatment of patients and carriers are also important.

Persons traveling in countries where cholera exists should avoid consuming uncooked fruits or vegetables, raw seafood, and nonsterilized beverages. Considering the outbreaks along the Gulf Coast in the United States, care should be taken to properly cook shellfish taken from these waters.

A killed vaccine has been used for many years and numerous countries require an international certificate of vaccination against cholera from travelers arriving from cholera-infected areas. The killed vaccine is not highly effective and work is currently underway to develop more effective vaccines.

Other Vibrios

The bacterium *Vibro parahaemolyticus* and the newly discovered species *V. mimicus*, *V. fluvialis*, and *V. hollisae* are found in marine estuaries throughout the world. These organisms cause a self-limiting gastroenteritis of several days' duration. It is now recognized that about half the cases of diarrhea during the summer in Japan are caused by these bacteria. Outbreaks also occur in the United States and other countries. The source of infection is almost always raw or inadequately cooked or improperly refrigerated seafood.

CLINICAL NOTE

Followup on *Vibrio cholerae* Infection: Louisiana, 1978

According to the record, 4 more cases of cholera and 2 asymptomatic infections were identified in Louisiana, bringing the total number of persons known to be infected in August and September 1978 to 11. The 6 most recent infections were discovered after a 58-year-old woman from Lafayette had onset of a diarrheal illness on September 24, was hospitalized, and had *Vibrio cholerae* isolated from her stool. On September 22 she ate crabs that were caught in White Lake, boiled, and then held without refrigeration for approximately 6 hours. Investigation found that 5 of 9 other persons who ate the crabs at the same time also developed diarrheal illnesses; *V. cholerae* organisms were isolated from the stools of 3 of these ill persons. Some of the boiled crabs left over after the meal had been refrigerated and *V. cholerae* organisms were isolated from one of them. Other crabs, caught in White Lake at the same time by the same man, were boiled separately on September 22 and eaten at once by 6 persons; none became ill, but *V. cholerae* organisms were isolated from the stools of 2 of the 6 persons. All previously reported isolates of *V. cholerae* from Louisiana in August and September were also of the same serotype.

The 8 infected persons with symptoms had eaten boiled or steamed crab within 5 days before onset of illness. A case-control study of foods eaten by the first five symptomatic patients and 10 age- and sex-matched neighbor controls found that none of the controls had eaten crabs during comparable periods. The 3 asymptomatic infected persons had eaten crabs within 9 days before culture. As noted, *V. cholerae* was isolated from a boiled crab. The organism was also isolated from raw shrimp caught south of Pecan Island. These epidemiologic and laboratory data indicate that crabs collected in Louisiana in the area between Mud Lake, west of Cameron, and Vermilion Bay, south of Abbeville, have been the vehicles of infection for the cases of cholera. Crabs prepared in large lots by commercial establishments have not been implicated.

Preliminary results of studies on the effect that boiling has on crabs artificially infected with *V. cholerae* from one of the Louisiana cases showed that the organism can be isolated from iced crabs individually boiled after 2, 4, 6, and 8 minutes of boiling but not after 10 minutes. At 8 minutes the crab shell was red and the meat was firm; so these criteria are not adequate to determine when crabs are safe to eat. In practice, crabs are cooked in varying numbers and via a variety of methods and containers. The crabs eaten by the persons with cholera were reportedly steamed for up to 35 minutes or boiled for 10 to 20 minutes (*MMWR 27*:388, 1978).

CAMPYLOBACTER INFECTIONS

Bacterial species now belonging to the genus *Campylobacter* were classified as vibrios for many years. Campylobacter means curved rod (Greek) and describes the shape of these bacteria. They are gram-negative, motile, microaerophilic microorganisms and are best isolated on a selective agar medium in an atmosphere of 5% oxygen. Long recognized as part of the intestinal microbial flora of many mammals and birds, these bacteria have been incriminated as a cause of abortions in domestic animals. Today it is recognized that campylobacter, primarily the species *C. jejuni*, cause enteritis in humans.

The most common infection is acute gastroenteritis, which is generally characterized by fever, diarrhea, and abdominal pains. The pains may be severe and mimic acute appendicitis. Nausea and vomiting are sometimes experienced. Recovery usually occurs without treatment in less than a week. Although intestinal infection occurs in patients of all ages, it is most common in young children and may account for up to 30% of all acute diarrhea in children under 8 months of age living in underdeveloped countries. Campylobacter infections may spread to the blood and other tissues in compromised patients of all ages. A less frequent campylobacter infection involves the developing fetus and usually results in the death of the fetus.

Diagnosis is made by isolating *C. jejuni* from the feces, using selective media. Supportive treatment is given for diarrhea and erythromycin, gentamicin, or chloramphenicol, depending on the susceptibility of the isolated organism, is used to treat systemic infections. Control is best achieved by good hygiene, with special emphasis on avoiding transmission of microorganisms from animals to food and water consumed by humans.

CLINICAL NOTE

Outbreak of *Campylobacter* Enteritis Associated with Raw Milk: Kansas

During the week of March 23, 1981, the Wichita–Sedgwick County Department of Community Health was notified that a patient admitted to a local hospital with gastrointestinal illness had *Campylobacter jejuni* isolated from his stool. The hospital's clinical laboratory, which routinely reports isolations from communicable agents, noted that the patient regularly drank raw milk from a commercial dairy. *C. jejuni* was isolated from rectal swabs from two of three other members of the patient's family, all of whom also drank raw milk from the same dairy. The dairy voluntarily stopped selling raw milk on April 1 and cooperated in an investigation of the problem.

News coverage of the preliminary investigation prompted telephone calls from persons in 104 families (representing 264 individuals), who reported that members of their families had recently had a gastrointestinal illness and that the families purchased raw milk from the same dairy. *C. jejuni* was isolated from the stools of 60 of 116 (52%) persons in households that had one or more ill family members.

A cohort study was conducted of families who belonged to a local food cooperative that purchased raw milk from the dairy in question the week of April 6. Then 17 of 24 member families completed a questionnaire about exposure to pets, live poultry or cattle, and persons outside the household who had diarrhea. Questions also concerned recent travel and food-intake patterns, including consumption of chicken, rare meat, uncooked eggs, cheese, raw milk, and water.

No significant association was found between illness and any risk factor except raw milk. Gastrointestinal illness had affected members in all 11 families that purchased raw milk from the dairy but did not affect 6 families that did not purchase the milk. Of those who drank raw milk, 39 out of 55 (71%) were ill, as were 4 of 36 (11%) persons who did not drink raw milk ($p < .01$, t test). These 43 persons all became ill in the period March 1–April 4. Predominant symptoms included diarrhea, abdominal cramps, and headache. Duration of illness ranged from 1 to 9 days; few people sought medical advice. *C. jejuni* was isolated from 17 of 29 (59%) ill and 4 of 8 (50%) well persons; all 21 isolates were from persons who drank raw milk.

Rectal swabs collected on April 8 from well cows and those with mastitis at the implicated dairy and from well cows (none with mastitis was seen) from two other local dairies that also sell raw milk were positive for *C. jejuni*. Cultures of milk samples obtained at all three dairies were negative for *C. jejuni*. In the period March 31 to April 7 bulk-tank milk samples from the implicated dairy, but not samples from the other two dairies, exceeded the generally recommended standard plate count level of 100,000 organisms/ml. The count fell below this level on April 8 and 9.

The dairy implemented hygienic measures during the investigation, such as not using milk from cows suspected of having mastitis, using a disinfectant solution to wash teats, and immersing milking claws in a disinfectant solution before putting them on each cow. The dairy began selling milk again on April 10. No new cases of raw-milk-associated gastrointestinal illness had been reported as of May 6 (*MMWR 30*:565,1981).

SUMMARY

1. The enteric bacilli consist of a large group of gram-negative bacilli that are normally found in the intestinal tract of humans and animals. They are transmitted by the fecal-oral route and usually are commensals with only a few primary pathogens, such as *Salmonella* and *Shigella.*

2. Typhoid fever, a disease caused by *Salmonella typhi,* is of considerable significance worldwide. Most frequently transmitted in contaminated water, this organism causes a serious life-threatening illness. Proper sewage and water treatment, as well as adequate food-handling laws, are necessary to prevent the spread of this organism. Other salmonellae cause disease in humans but are nearly always transmitted through contamination of our environment by animal feces.

3. Shigellosis or bacillary dysentery is a human disease and is transmitted through human fecal contamination of food, water, or inanimate objects. The disease is severe but usually self-limiting.

4. Asiatic cholera is a disease known for its great human plagues. This fecally transmitted disease can cause death in its victims within hours of infection. Infections have resulted from eating improperly cooked shellfish and drinking contaminated water.

5. *Campylobacter* produces a painful, sometimes serious gastrointestinal disease. Probably transmitted from domestic animals, the disease is generally self-limiting.

6. Each of these serious intestinal infections—shigellosis, cholera, and campylobacteriosis—results from the production of a potent enterotoxin that causes a profuse outpouring of water into the lumen of the intestine because of its action on cyclic AMP.

Opportunistic Pathogens

26

ENTERIC BACILLI AND RELATED BACTERIA

The bacteria discussed in this section are generally of low virulence and are often present as normal or transient inhabitants of the intestinal tract and other tissues of humans and animals. Some are also found in water, sewage, and soil. All except *Pseudomonas* are members of the family Enterobacteriaceae. Members of the genera *Escherichia*, *Klebsiella*, *Enterobacter*, *Serratia*, and *Citrobacter* ferment the sugar lactose and share a number of other properties; they are sometimes called *coliforms*.

All these opportunistic bacilli are capable of producing similar infections. When they gain access to such tissues as the urethra, bladder, lungs, wounds, or internal organs, they may be capable of causing disease, particularly in a compromised host. The most frequent problems are urinary tract and wound infections. Pneumonia, gastroenteritis, septicemia, and meningitis may also result from these microbes.

The more commonly encountered genera or species are discussed briefly in this section, with emphasis on some unique characteristics of each. Because these microorganisms are in a continual state of reclassification and renaming, in some cases, reference is primarily to the generic name.

Klebsiella

The major species of this genus is *K. pneumoniae*. It is a cause of primary pneumonia in older persons with such predisposing medical problems as chronic bronchitis, diabetes, or alcoholism. It is also a common cause of septicemia as well as urinary tract and wound infections. Many antibiotic-resistant strains are found in hospitals; treatment is often difficult.

Enterobacter

The *Enterobacter* are closely related to the *Klebsiella* and cause similar infections. The most commonly encountered species is *Enterobacter cloacae*. These bacteria are frequently resistant to antimicrobial therapy and therefore cause serious infections.

Serratia

Serratia marcescens is the most frequently encountered species of this genus. This bacterium may produce red-pigmented colonies when grown at room temperatures. For many years it was considered a nonpathogen and, because of the pigmented colonies, it was used in various experiments to follow the movement of airborne particles in hospitals and other environments. It is now recognized that *S. marcescens* may cause pneumonia, cystitis (inflammation of the urinary bladder), and other infections in compromised hosts. Treatment is difficult because of its resistance to many commonly used antimicrobials.

Proteus, Providencia, and Morganella

Bacteria of these closely related genera are found in water, soil, sewage, and the intestinal tracts of humans and animals. Most clinical infections are of the urinary tract and burns. These bacteria are responsible for 10% of hospital-acquired (nosocomial) infections. Treatment with antibiotics is often difficult.

Citrobacter

This genus is closely related to the *Salmonella*. *Citrobacter* have occasionally been incriminated as the cause of infections in humans, particularly urinary tract infections.

Escherichia

Escherichia coli is the most commonly occurring species of this genus. Like many other enteric bacilli, *E. coli* was considered a nonpathogen for many years. It is one of the predominant facultative anaerobic bacteria of the intestinal tract and so is used as an indicator organism in determining the amount of fecal contamination in water and food. Many strains are used in experimental work in cell research. Much of the current work in molecular biology and recombinant DNA uses *E. coli* and more is probably known about this organism than any other bacterium.

It became increasingly apparent over the past several decades that *E. coli* of varying degrees of pathogenicity exist and that these bacteria are responsible for numerous human infections. They are the primary cause of urinary tract infections and bacteremia; among the enteric bacilli, they are the most common cause of wound and systemic infections. Certain strains produce enterotoxins that function like the enterotoxins produced by *Shigella* and *V. cholerae*. These strains are a major cause of acute diarrhea in children under 2 years of age and much of the "traveler's" diarrhea often experienced by adults is due to them. The extent of such intestinal diseases is not known because most cases are self-limiting and a specific laboratory diagnosis is difficult. Epidemics in hospital nurseries have been reported and infections are probably widespread in infants living under impoverished conditions. Where infants are malnourished and supportive therapy is not given, a significant number of deaths result from dehydration and electrolyte imbalance due to *E. coli* enteritis.

Pseudomonas

Species of the genus *Pseudomonas* are widespread and are commonly found in soil, water, and intestinal tracts of humans and animals. The major species associated with human disease is *P. aeruginosa*. It is an opportunist that causes troublesome infections in compromised patients. These infections are similar to those caused by the preceding enteric bacilli. Infections by *P. aeruginosa* may occur in any tissue but are frequently seen in burns and wounds. Pneumonia and systemic infections with very high mortality rates are also caused by this microbe. *P. aeruginosa* produces a soluble bluish-green pigment with a sweet odor described as smelling somewhat like grape jelly. This pigment often gives a characteristic color to pus, along with the distinct odor. A firm diagnosis is made by isolating the bacterium from the infected tissue.

P. aeruginosa infections are among the most difficult to treat, for they are resistant to all but a few chemotherapeutic agents. Often combinations of antimicrobial agents are used in attempts to treat them.

Control and prevention rely on proper aseptic techniques when dealing with burns and open wounds. *Pseudomonas* species are able to grow in water with minimal nutrients and are found in such places as water baths used for heating baby bottles, vases for fresh-cut flowers, and water sumps in humidifiers. Certain precautions, such as not allowing fresh-cut flowers in critical areas of a hospital and routine monitoring of water held in baths and air systems, help reduce the hazard of these infections. *Pseudomonas* species are among the most resistant vegetative bacterial cells to chemical disinfectants.

CLINICAL NOTE

Otitis Due to *Pseudomonas aeruginosa* Serotype 0:10
Associated with a Mobile Redwood Hot Tub System: North Carolina

From March 19 to April 2, 1982, six cases of *Pseudomonas aeruginosa*, serotype 0:10, infection occurred following common exposure to a hot tub in Orange County, North Carolina. Clinical illness included severe hemorrhagic external otitis (inflammation of the external ear), which, although commonly associated with swimming pools, has not been previously reported in the literature for whirlpool/spa settings.

Among 24 members of a university coeducational fraternity who used the implicated tub from March 26 to 29, two had simple dermatitis, and four developed severe external otitis, one of whom, a 19-year-old male, had concurrent cellulitis of the chest wall and thigh. He was hospitalized and treated with intravenous tobramycin for 4 days. His infection began as an area of erythema approximately 1½ inches in diameter below the left nipple, accompanied by tender, swollen left axillary lymph nodes and a pustule below the right nipple. The patient also noted severe pain and drainage from his left ear. Cultures from the chest pustule and the draining left ear were positive for *P. aeruginosa* serotype 0:10 (resistant to cephalothin, ampicillin, tetracycline, and trimethoprim-sulfamethoxazole and sensitive to gentamicin and carbenicillin). His symptoms began 48 hours after last exposure to the tub. The three other persons with severe external otitis that began within 48 hours of last exposure to the tub visited the student health service for treatment. In two of those, disease was bilateral and was associated with profound erythema or bloody discharge. The first had onset on March 27; the other, with onset on March 29, had a positive culture of ear drainage for *P. aeruginosa* of the same resistance pattern as the 19-year-old male. Neither responded to topical antibiotics, but both were treated successfully with intramuscular gentamicin.

A survey of fraternity members showed an association of illness with exposure to the tub, which was rented and used from March 26 to March 29. Of 15 students who responded to a questionnaire, five (described above) met the case definition of ear infection or skin rash developing within 7 days after exposure to this tub. Total duration of exposure to the tub over the 4-day period was significantly associated with illness. Patients had a mean duration of 10.2 hours exposure; nonpatients had a mean duration of 5.1 hours exposure.

Inspection and culturing of the tub on April 15, after a previous night's usage at another fraternity, showed a pH 7.6 and free bromine level of <0.5 parts per million (ppm). Of 12 environmental swabs of the tub, four were positive for *P. aeruginosa* serotype 0:10. No other serotypes were identified in the specimens. The positive sites included a recirculation port, two areas of the dual filter, and filter intake line.

Procedures involved in maintaining and using the tub were reviewed. Usage peaked during the four evenings, when 15 or more persons at a time were in the tub. Despite written instructions to check the free-bromine level every 4 hours, water sampling was performed only once before use each day. The tub was emptied and rinsed with water from a garden hose daily, and filters were sprayed with water on March 27 and 28. No hyperbromination or scrubbing of internal surfaces was performed (*MMWR 31*:541, 1982).

NON-SPORE-FORMING ANAEROBES

This is a category of diverse and incompletely characterized microorganisms that share the characteristics of being both non-spore formers and anaerobic. They form a significant proportion of the normal flora of the human body. Bacteria from this category include from 80 to 90% of the bacteria present on the skin, in the mouth, or in the upper respiratory tract, and about 99.9% present in the intestinal tract. The anaerobic bacteria include both gram-negative and gram-positive cocci and bacilli as well as spirochetes. These bacteria are more difficult to grow and isolate in pure culture in artificial media than the nonanaerobes. Consequently, they have often been ignored or missed in the past during routine bacteriological examinations of clinical specimens. These bacteria, however, are recognized today as important opportunistic pathogens that produce a significant number of infections. Currently their classification is not complete. But because of the increased interest and research activity involving these microbes, names and classification schemes will undoubtedly undergo frequent revisions. Therefore only a listing of the genus names of some of these bacteria will be made at this time.

Because these bacteria are part of the normal flora of many body tissues, their incrimination as the cause of a given infection can be made only when they are isolated from a tissue that is normally free of these organisms. The source of these infections is usually endogenous and disease results when the integrity of the tissue is altered to allow passage of these bacteria from their normal site of growth to other tissues. Often the anaerobic environment is created by facultative anaerobes that use up the free oxygen and thus act in a synergistic manner to allow the growth of the anaerobe.

Some general clinical problems attributed to these anaerobic bacteria are briefly discussed next.

A. Infections of the abdominal cavity
Such infections result from passage of fecal material into the abdominal cavity as a result of conditions like injury, surgery, appendicitis, and cancer. Over 90% of the abdominal abscesses and infections are now thought to be caused by anaerobic bacteria. Members of the genus *Bacteroides* (*B. fragilis* in particular) are most frequently involved in these infections.

B. Infections of the female reproductive organs
About 75% of the infections and abscesses of female reproductive organs are caused by anaerobes. Such conditions as abortion, surgery, cancer, extensive manipulations, prolonged labor, intrauterine contraceptive devices, and gonorrhea may predispose the tissue to these anaerobic infections.

C. Liver abscesses
Anaerobic bacteria may reach the liver by direct spread from adjacent tissues or from the blood. One-half or more of the liver abscesses are now thought to be caused by anaerobic bacteria.

D. Respiratory tract infections
A variety of infections of the respiratory tract are caused by these anaerobes. Between 75 and 90% of such diseases as pneumonitis and lung abscesses are induced by these microbes.

E. Infection of skin and muscles
Anaerobic infections may develop in skin, muscle, and connective tissue following injury, surgery, or lack of blood supply. Human bites are a common reason for such infections.

TABLE 26-1   MAJOR ANAEROBIC BACTERIA COMMONLY ASSOCIATED WITH INFECTIONS

Bacteria	Morphology	Associated with the following types of infections
Bacteroides	Gram − bacilli	Peritonitis, liver abscesses, gynecologic, pulmonary, upper respiratory, wounds, bacteremia.
Fusobacterium	Gram − bacilli	Liver abscesses, gynecologic, pulmonary, upper respiratory, wounds, bacteremia.
Peptostreptococcus	Gram + cocci	Peritonitis, liver abscesses, gynecologic, pulmonary, upper respiratory, wounds, bacteremia.
Peptococcus	Gram + cocci	Peritonitis, liver abscesses, gynecologic, pulmonary, upper respiratory, wounds, bacteremia.
Propionibacterium	Gram + bacilli	Upper respiratory (pathogenicity uncertain)
Eubacterium	Gram + bacilli	May be isolated from infected tissues, but pathogenic role, if any, is not known
Veillonella	Gram − cocci	May be isolated from infected tissues, but pathogenic role, if any, is not known

F. Septicemia

Invasion of the blood system may result from any of the preceding anaerobic infections. About 10% of all blood infections detected in hospital patients are caused by these anaerobes. Death rates from such infections are 10%.

G. Brain abscesses

Bacteroides and anaerobic cocci are the most frequent etiologic agents of brain abscesses. Without proper surgical and antimicrobial intervention, these abscesses give the patient an extremely poor prognosis.

Treatment of these anaerobic infections is often difficult. Drainage and surgical removal of dead tissue, when possible, are most helpful. No easy, routine method for testing antibiotic sensitivity is available. The broad-spectrum antibiotics, especially tetracyclines, are moderately effective; many resistant strains are found, however. Penicillins, both natural and semisynthetic, are effective against most anaerobes. An antibiotic called clindamycin seems very active against *Bacteroides fragilis*, which is the anaerobe most frequently involved in human infections.

The genus names and characteristics of the most frequently encountered non-spore-forming anaerobes are listed in Table 26-1.

SUMMARY

The majority of the enteric bacilli are opportunistic commensals. Disease results when these organisms are displaced from their normal intestinal habitat into the body tissues or spaces of a compromised patient. Control of such disease constitutes a major problem for hospital personnel.

Mycoplasma and Legionella

MYCOPLASMA INFECTIONS

The mycoplasmas are a group of free-living and parasitic microorganisms that are unique in that they possess no cell wall. They are widespread and are found as natural flora in the mouth, throat, and genitourinary tract of mammals and birds. There are three genera of mycoplasma, the genus *Acholeplasma*, which includes the free-living forms, and the genus *Ureaplasma* and genus *Mycoplasma*, which contain only parasitic agents.

Mycoplasma cells, except for the lack of a cell wall, have the same intracellular components and metabolic activities as other bacteria. The cell membrane differs from that of other bacteria and their shapes are variable due to the flexibility of this membrane (Figure 27-1). Smallest cell sizes are about 300 nm in diameter for the spherical-shaped cells. Other forms may be filament or branch shaped. Multiplication is by binary fission, which sometimes takes the form of fragmentation into groups of daughter cells. Mycoplasma can be grown in enriched agar media and produce small colonies about 0.5 mm in diameter that have the appearance of a fried egg (Figure 27-2).

Pathogenesis and Clinical Disease

Various diseases caused by the mycoplasmas have been diagnosed in mammals and birds. The first mycoplasma to be discovered was isolated from cattle suffering from a disease called pleuropneumonia; consequently, other mycoplasmas have often been referred to as pleuropneumonialike organisms or PPLOs. The best-known disease of

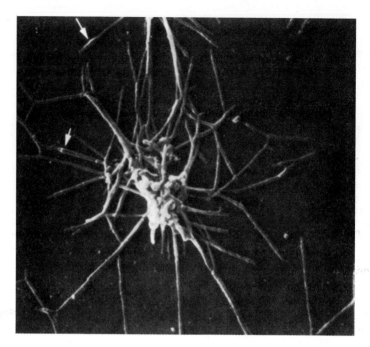

Figure 27-1 Scanning electron micrograph of a small colony of *Mycoplasma pneumoniae* showing a filamentous shape around the periphery and pleomorphic shapes in the center. Bulbous swellings (arrows) are seen in some individual cells. (K. E. Muse, D. A. Powell, and A. M. Collier, *Inf. Imm. 13*:229–237, Figure 1b, with permission from ASM)

humans caused by mycoplasma is called primary atypical pneumonia; the causative microbe is *Mycoplasma pneumoniae*. This form of pneumonia is called atypical because it does not have the characteristics of the typical bacterial pneumonias but resembles pneumonias caused by viruses. The species *Ureaplasma urealyticun* appears to be the cause of a form of nonspecific (nongonococcal) urethritis that is transmitted by sexual contact. Mycoplasmas are also incriminated as the possible agents of such diseases of humans as lupus erythematous and rheumatoid arthritis, for which other specific microorganisms have not yet been shown to be responsible. Nevertheless, there is not yet enough evidence to prove that mycoplasmas cause these diseases.

Transmission and Epidemiology

Primary atypical pneumonia is widespread and may account for 20% of pneumonia in urban populations. It is chiefly responsible for pneumonia in persons between 5 and 30 years of age. Outbreaks are often associated with schools, families, summer camps, or military barracks. The organisms seem to be transmitted efficiently by aerosol from person to person during the acute stages of the disease, which lasts for 1 to 2 weeks.

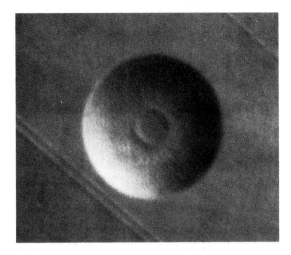

Figure 27-2   Figure of *Mycoplasma hominis* colony showing the "fried egg" colony appearance. This unusual colony form is produced by the colony growing down into the medium as well as across the surface of the agar.

Diagnosis

Pneumonia caused by mycoplasma can be differentiated from viral or rickettsial pneumonias by clinical and laboratory tests. Both specific and nonspecific serologic tests can be used. The most common test is for cold agglutinins—substances that agglutinate red blood cells when held at about 4°C and occur in about 80% of the patients with mycoplasma pneumonia. *M. pneumoniae* can be cultured from the respiratory tract by using enriched media.

Treatment

Antibiotics of the tetracycline and erythromycin groups are effective in reducing the severity and duration of the disease. Such antibiotics as penicillin that affect only bacterial cell walls are obviously of no value against microorganisms that have none.

Prevention and Control

The best prevention is to avoid contact with persons suspected of having the disease. Antibiotics can be taken prophylactically to prevent the spread of infection to members of a group or family where a known index case has been diagnosed. Research is being conducted to develop a vaccine, but as yet no effective vaccine is available.

LEGIONELLOSIS

The disease now called the *Legionnaires' disease* or legionellosis is a pneumonialike illness that went unrecognized as a specific disease until the late 1970s. Attention was dramatically focused on it in the summer of 1976 when some 5000 members of the American Legion attended a convention in Philadelphia. Within 2 weeks of the convention's close, many of these Legionnaires complained of chills, fever, and muscle aches. Over the next week 12 of the Legionnaires died of a pneumonialike illness. During the ensuing weeks 170 of those attending the convention were hospitalized with pneumonia; 29 deaths occurred.

An extensive investigation was immediately launched to find the cause of this newly recognized disease. Tests were run with all known pathogenic microorganisms or toxins that might be responsible and all tests were negative. After several months of continued research a previously unidentified bacterium was found to be the culprit.

Bacterium

The causative bacterium grows in guinea pigs, in the yolk sac of embryonated eggs, and on special nutrient media containing extra amounts of the amino acid cysteine and iron. The bacterium seems to have the shape of a bacillus (Figure 27-3). It does not stain well with the gram stain and special stains, such as the Gimenez silver-impregnation stain, are used to demonstrate the presence of these cells. When grown

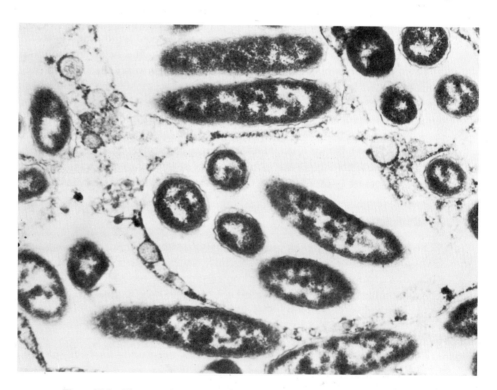

Figure 27-3 Electron micrograph of *Legionella pneumophila*. (Centers for Disease Control, Atlanta)

in yolk sacs, the cells have both coccoid and bacillary forms. The shape is pleo-morphic when grown on culture media but is predominantly bacillary. These bacteria are quite stable and may remain living for up to one year in water. Evidence indicates that they may be free living in soil or streams and possibly in water held in air-condi-tioning systems. No close relationship has been found between this bacterium and any of the previously characterized bacteria. Thus a new genus called *Legionella* has been established for it. Presently there are six species within the genus, the most prominent being *Legionella pneumophila*. It is anticipated that other species may yet be identified.

Pathogenesis and Clinical Disease

The pathogenesis of Legionnaires' disease most closely resembles lobar pneumonia and begins 2 to 10 days after exposure. Some early symptoms are diarrhea, weakness, headache, muscle aches, malaise, anorexia, and a dry cough. An increasing tempera-ture to 40°C (104°F) may be seen after several days, along with prostration and pulmonary consolidation. Some patients experience stupor and show signs of in-volvement of the kidneys and liver. The primary involvement, however, appears to be in the lungs. The duration of the disease is from 5 to 16 days. Most cases are seen in older or immunosuppressed persons, although all ages may be afflicted. Unless treated, 20% of those patients requiring hospitalization die. Evidence now indicates that many mild or subclinical cases may occur.

Transmission and Epidemiology

Person-to-person transmission does not seem involved. When clusters of cases occur, it appears that exposure was from a common environmental source (Figure 27-4). Some evidence suggests that this organism may grow in the soil, in streams, in water found in air-conditioning systems, or in domestic water supplies. Airborne dissemi-nation via dust or water sprayed in air-conditioning systems or from showers has been suggested.

Once the causative bacterium was isolated, thus providing a known antigen, it was possible to study serum samples that had been collected from patients who had suffered from unknown types of pneumonia before 1976. Many of these samples con-tained specific antibodies against *L. pneumophila*, indicating that this disease has been around for many years. Since the initial recognition of this disease in 1976, nu-merous outbreaks have been recognized in all parts of the United States and in many foreign countries. Many isolated cases occur as well as some clusters of infection. Several hundred severe cases are diagnosed each year in this country (Figure 27-5). An estimated 20,000 to 30,000 additional mild or subclinical cases are thought to occur yearly here. It is presently determined that between 3 and 6% of all hospital-associated pneumonias are due to *L. pneumophila*. Legionellosis has repeatedly oc-curred in compromised patients in hospitals.

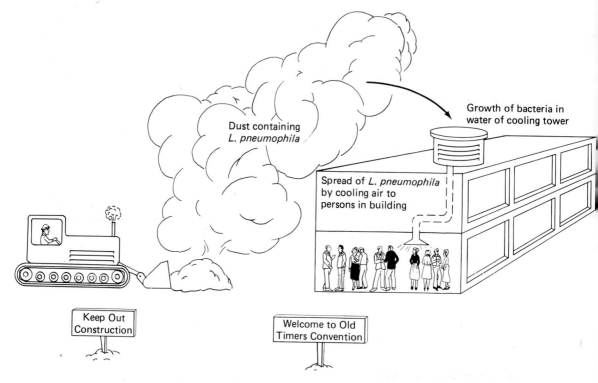

Figure 27-4 A proposed mechanism of transmission of *L. pneumophila* to humans.

Diagnosis

A tentative diagnosis is based on symptoms when no other causative agent can be demonstrated. Cultivation of *L. pneumophila* from the lung tissues or blood is possible but is often difficult. Specific laboratory tests rely mostly on serologic procedures that show specific increases in or high levels of antibodies against the *L. pneumophila*. The presence of *L. pneumophila* in sputum or lung tissues can sometimes be demonstrated by direct microscopic examination, using special stains or specific fluorescent-labeled antibodies.

Treatment

Erythromycin has been the most effective antibiotic in treating this disease. Often recovery is prompt and dramatic following the use of this agent. Therapy usually lasts for about 2 weeks. Prompt treatment greatly decreases the death rate. Rifampin may also be effective.

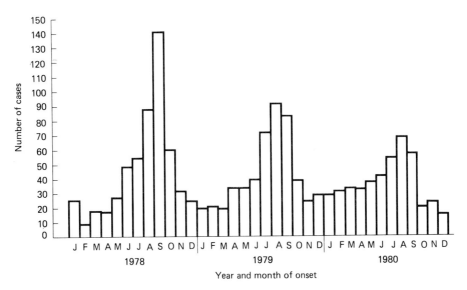

Figure 27-5 Reported sporadic cases of legionellosis by month of onset in the United States, 1978–1980. Seasonality is seen with 51% of all reported cases having onset in July to October (*CDC Annual Summary*, 1980).

Prevention and Control

No vaccines are available. Elimination of possible contamination of water used in some air-conditioning systems may reduce the number of cases. Avoiding exposure to high concentrations of dust from such activities as soil excavation could be helpful. Protecting compromised patients from excessive dust is recommended. As more is learned about the epidemiology of this disease, additional preventative measures can be developed.

CLINICAL NOTE

Isolates of Organisms Resembling Legionnaires' Disease Bacterium from Environmental Sources: Indiana, 1978

Organisms identical to *Legionella pneumophila* were isolated from two environmental specimens collected in the investigation of the outbreak of Legionnaires' disease in Bloomington, Indiana. The positive specimens included water from an air-conditioning cooling tower atop the Indiana Memorial Union, a hotel student union complex in which 19 of 21 confirmed cases had stayed overnight in the 2 weeks before onset of illness, and water from a creek approximately 50 m from the Union.

The water specimens were initially examined for *L. pneumophila* by direct fluorescent antibody (FA) methods and were positive. Aliquots were inoculated into guinea pigs. Guinea pigs were sacrificed when fever was noted or, if no fever was noted, 7 days after inoculation. Splenic tissue was negative by direct FA, but FA-positive organisms were recovered from yolk sacs of embryonated hens' eggs inoculated with suspensions of guinea pig splenic tissue. The organisms were isolated directly on charcoal yeast extract agar from the splenic tissue of a guinea pig inoculated with the creek water. The isolates from the cooling tower were strongly FA positive, but the creek water isolates gave weak FA staining. Organisms from both sources had colonies on special agar typical of pneumophila. Subcultures did not grow on trypticase soy agar or trypticase soy blood agar. Isolates from each water specimen showed a pattern of cellular fatty acids on gas-liquid chromatography typical of the *L. pneumophila*. Studies of the DNA relatedness of these isolates showed them to be the same as *L. pneumophila*.

The cooling tower is located on the roof of the Union, adjacent to and higher than the wing with guest rooms. Studies are underway to determine whether water droplets released from the cooling tower in the process of evaporative cooling could be drawn into air intakes serving hotel rooms and meeting areas. Procedures were undertaken to decontaminate the cooling tower water (*MMWR 27*:191, 1978).

SUMMARY

1. Mycoplasma are unique bacteria without cell walls. They produce a number of diseases in animals but only one in humans. This primary pneumonia is common among children and young adults. Older individuals seem somewhat refractory, probably due to antibodies from earlier infection.

2. Legionnaires' disease is due to a bacillus normally present in watery environments. Individuals with pulmonary compromise are usually the victims of this organism. Frequently nosocomial, the infection represents upward of 5 to 6% of all pneumonias in hospitalized individuals. Diagnosis is difficult because the organism is characteristically refractile to the analine stains used in early diagnosis.

Rickettsiae and Chlamydiae

28

RICKETTSIAE

Rickettsiae are a group of small bacteria that traditionally have been considered separately from the typical bacteria. In fact, the rickettsiae have many characteristics, such as methods of laboratory cultivation and modes of transmission, that suggest a close relationship to the viruses. For many years the rickettsiae were considered a separate group of microorganisms positioned between the bacteria and viruses and the study of rickettsial diseases was usually included in the general subject area of virology. It is now well established, however, that rickettsiae are small obligate parasitic bacteria.

Most rickettsiae and rickettsial diseases share some common features. These features are discussed first and are then followed by several of the more important rickettsial diseases of humans.

General Characteristics

Rickettsiae are about 0.3 μm in diameter and up to 1.0 μm in length (Figure 28-1). Their shape ranges from pleomorphic to coccobacillary to bacillary and they are procaryotic cells. Their metabolic activities are highly dependent on energy received from living host cells and all but one (*Rochalimea quintana*) are able to multiply only inside the living host cells and are thus called *obligate intracellular parasites*. They are grown in the laboratory in cell cultures, embryonated eggs, or in animals, much like viruses (see Chapter 31). Most rickettsiae are readily inactivated once they leave the

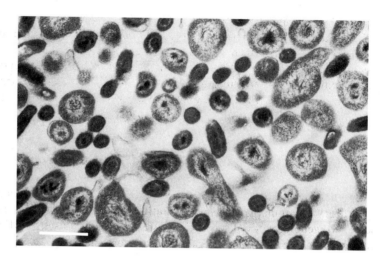

Figure 28-1 Transmission electron micrograph of the rickettsia *Coxiella burnettii* showing the pleomorphic nature of this microorganism (bar = 0.6 μm). (T. F. McCaul and J. C. Williams, *J. Bact. 147*:1063–1076, Figure 1b, with permission of ASM)

host. Therefore their transmission depends on direct contact or vector transmission and all rickettsial diseases except Q-fever require an arthropod vector for successful transmission between hosts. Three genera of rickettsiae are described: the genus *Coxiella* contains only the Q-fever agent, *Rochalimea* contains the agent of trench fever, and *Rickettsia* contains the other species (Table 28-1).

General Pathogenesis

The rickettsiae are usually introduced into the tissues by the bite of an arthropod and have a predilection for the cells that line the small blood vessels (endothelial cells). These bacteria multiply and spread along the blood vessels of the body. The signs and symptoms result from inflammation and swelling of the small blood vessels. This

TABLE 28-1 DISEASES CAUSED BY RICKETTSIAE

Disease	Reservoir	Vector	Rickettsial species
Trench fever	human	human louse	*Rochalimaea quintana*
Q-fever	lower animals	tick	*Coxiella burnetii*
Rocky Mountain spotted fever	tick	tick	*Rickettsia rickettsii*
Epidemic typhus	human	human louse	*Rickettsia prowazekii*
Endemic typhus	rodent	flea	*Rickettsia typhi*
North Asia tick typhus	rodent	tick	*Rickettsia sibirica*
Boutoneuse fever	rodent	tick	*Rickettsia conorii*
Rickettsial pox	mouse	mite	*Rickettsia akari*
Scrub typhus	rodent	mite	*Rickettsia tsutsugamashi*

condition may cause blockage or a reduced blood flow to some tissues and some leakage of blood into the surrounding tissues. The leakage of blood in the skin produces the spots and rashes seen with most rickettsial diseases (Figure 28-2). Headache, chills, and fever are due to the generalized inflammation; and stupor, delirium, and shock may occur due to alterations in blood flow to the brain and other vital organs. Symptoms may last for several weeks. Death rates may be as high as 70% with epidemic typhus or less than 1% with rickettsial pox. Lifelong immunity usually results after recovery.

Diagnosis

Most rickettsial diseases are diagnosed by patient history and clinical signs or in the laboratory by an increase in specific antibodies between the acute and convalescent sera. Two general types of serologic tests exist. The first uses specific rickettsial antigens prepared by growing the rickettsiae in embryonated eggs. Methods of measuring antigen–antibody reactions like complement fixation, agglutination, or immunofluorescence may be used. The second type, called the *Weil-Felix* test, is an agglutination test that uses certain strains of *Proteus* bacteria as the antigens. Some antigens present in these strains of *Proteus* cross-react with antibodies against certain rickettsiae. Earlier this procedure was widely used because it is relatively simple to run and is

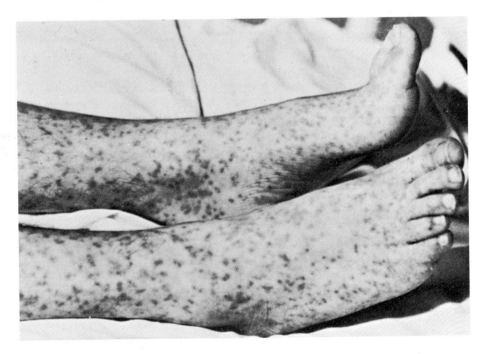

Figure 28-2 The rash of Rocky Mountain spotted fever consisting of sharply defined spots over most of the body.

less expensive than using rickettsial antigens. Unfortunately, neither the sensitivity nor the specificity of the Weil-Felix test makes it a reliable procedure and currently it is seldom used.

Treatment

Rickettsial diseases respond well to treatment with tetracyclines. Chloramphenicol is also effective, but its use is restricted due to its greater toxicity to humans. Death rates are drastically reduced when chemotherapy is applied.

Prevention and Control

Two general methods are used to prevent rickettsial diseases. First, vaccines developed to fight some rickettsial diseases may be used on persons who have a high risk of being exposed to a specific rickettsial disease. The second method is to eliminate or reduce the animal reservoir and/or the arthropod vector of a given rickettsia.

SPECIFIC RICKETTSIAL DISEASES

Epidemic Typhus

Epidemic typhus is caused by the species *Rickettsia prowazekii*, named after Ricketts and von Prowazek, two early investigators of this disease. Both scientists died following accidentally acquired laboratory infections of typhus. Without treatment, death rates from epidemic typhus may be as high as 70%.

The typhus rickettsia infects humans and the body louse of humans. The louse becomes infected when it feeds on infected humans and it leaves when the human body temperature significantly increases or decreases from normal. The louse can only move a short distance when searching for a new host. The louse will die of typhus in 1 to 3 weeks, but during this period the rickettsiae proliferate in its digestive tract and are excreted in the feces. When the infected louse infects and bites a new human host, louse feces are deposited on the skin. The louse bite causes itching, which is scratched, and the scratching forces the contaminated feces into the bite wound, thus initiating a new infection. Because of the short distance the louse can travel from human to human, epidemic typhus is associated with conditions of poor hygiene where humans are crowded together. These conditions are found in times of war, flooding, or other major disruptions of normal human activities. These conditions have existed often enough over the years to have allowed epidemic typhus to be a major killer of mankind. Armies of the past were frequently stricken with typhus fever and the outcome of many military campaigns was determined not so much by the strategies of the generals as by the epidemics of typhus fever. In 1489 during the Spanish siege of Granada, for example, 3000 Moorish troops died in battle and 17,000 died of typhus; in 1528, as the French army was on the verge of victory at Naples, typhus struck down 30,000 French troops and the tide of battle changed,

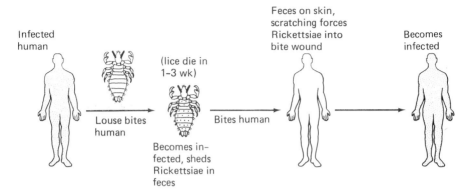

Figure 28-3 The transmission of epidemic typhus from human to human by the body louse.

resulting in a French defeat. During his campaign to conquer Moscow Napoleon's army of 500,000 troops was reduced to fewer than 200,000 by disease. About 180,000 died of typhus. The last major epidemic typhus outbreaks occurred in southeastern Europe during World War I and in Russia just afterward. In the Russian epidemic an estimated 30 million people contracted the disease and over 3 million deaths resulted. The mode of transmission of epidemic typhus is shown in Figure 28-3.

Epidemic typhus has greatly decreased over the past 60 years. A few limited outbreaks occurred during World War II, but effective use of DDT as a delousing agent and vaccination of military personnel have generally controlled this disease.

Some humans who have recovered from typhus can apparently carry the rickettsiae in their tissues for the remainder of their life. Some of these carriers may experience a mild case of clinical typhus, called *Brill-Zinsser disease*. These persons could serve as a focus of a new epidemic if part of a crowded, deprived environment where body lice are present.

Endemic or Murine Typhus

This disease, which is caused by *Rickettsia typhi*, is milder than epidemic typhus. Only sporadic cases are seen in humans; the death rate is less than 5% among untreated cases. The natural infection is found in rats, mice, and other rodents and is sporadically transmitted to humans by fleas. The disease in rodents and fleas is mild or subclinical and *R. typhi* may be carried in these hosts as a latent infection. The infection is occasionally transmitted to humans when they are bitten by an infected flea. Persons who live, work, or play around rodent-infested areas stand the greatest risk of infection. No human-to-human transfer occurs. Endemic typhus is found worldwide. In the United States it appears mostly in the southeastern states. Generally fewer than 75 cases per year are reported in this country. Deaths are rare when chemotherapy is applied. The transmission of endemic typhus is seen in Figure 28-4.

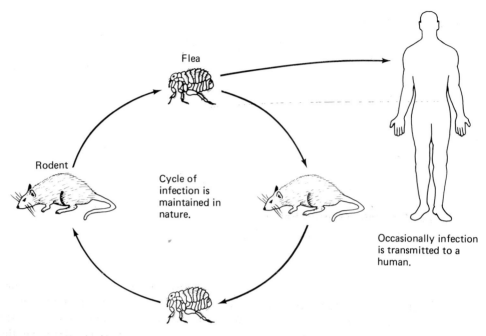

Figure 28-4   The transmission cycle of endemic typhus involves rodents and fleas.

CLINICAL NOTE

Outbreak of Murine Typhus: Texas

A cluster of cases of murine (endemic) typhus has been reported from Texas. From October 25 to November 11, 1982, five persons became ill with fever [temperature ≥ 40°C (≥ 104°F)], headache (three patients), and myalgia (two patients). On the 4th or 5th day of illness, three patients developed a macular rash that began on the trunk and spread to the extremities. Blood specimens obtained on December 16, 1982, from three patients demonstrated indirect fluorescent antibody titers of 1:512 or greater to typhus-group rickettsiae; cross-absorption studies performed at CDC using antigens to *Rickettsia typhi* (the causative organism of endemic typhus) and *R. prowazekii* (the causative organism of epidemic typhus) indicated the former as the cause of the elevated titers. No serum specimens were obtained from the other two patients. Four patients received appropriate antimicrobial therapy with tetracycline; all five recovered without sequelae.

Three patients—a 27-year-old male, a 25-year-old female, and a 6-year-old female—lived in a house that had been unoccupied for 5 years before being moved in July 1982 to its present site on a peanut farm in Comanche County in north-central Texas. The other two cases occurred in a 24-year-old female who visited this family at their home every week or 2, and a 48-year-old female, the grandmother of the 6-year-old, who lived ¼ mile away and visited the house at least once a month. Inspection of the house revealed holes in the roof, walls, and floors, and a large space beneath the house. Family members had heard rodents in the attic before the outbreak, and a mouse had recently been killed in the bathroom. Two or 3 weeks before the outbreak, rat poison had been placed inside the house. Five cats, present in the home before the outbreak, died during the outbreak period, four of unexplained causes, one in an accident. The cats slept indoors and had fleas. The family also owned three dogs, which usually slept underneath the house; they remained healthy during the outbreak period. None of the patients recalled being bitten by fleas.

An exterminator visited the house on November 19, 1982, and applied insecticide and rat poison. No further illnesses among family members or visitors to the house have been reported (*MMWR 32*:131, 1983).

Rocky Mountain Spotted Fever

This disease was first recognized around the year 1900 in the Rocky Mountains—hence the name. Yet it is found throughout North and South America and in Russia. Currently the greatest number of cases in the United States occur in the southeastern regions. The causative agent, called *Rickettsia rickettsii*, is primarily a parasite of ticks. This rickettsia infects many tissues of the tick without apparent ill effects. The eggs of the female tick may be infected and so the infection is passed directly to her progeny. This process is called *transovarian passage*. The rickettsiae are in the saliva of the tick and are transmitted to humans or animals by a tick bite. Ticks may become infected by feeding on infected animals or by transovarian passage from tick to tick without the involvement of an animal reservoir. No human-to-human transfer occurs. Death rates vary in different areas, suggesting that strains of varying degrees of virulence exist. Overall the death rates are generally from 5 to 10%. About 1000 cases are reported each year in the United States, but the number of cases seems to be increasing (Figure 28-5). The transmission of Rocky Mountain spotted fever is shown in Figure 28-6.

Q-fever

A rickettsia called *Coxiella burnetii* is the cause of Q-fever. The name *Q-fever* comes from "Query" fever, for the cause of this disease was not known for some time. *C. burnetii* is more stable than other rickettsiae and is able to survive for long periods outside the host, allowing transmission by indirect means. Current research indicates that this rickettsia forms a resistant endospore (Figure 28-7). Natural infections are found in many species of ticks and apparently can be spread by tick bites to birds and mammals in which asymptomatic infections develop. Rickettsiae are shed in saliva, urine, and milk. High concentrations are present in the placenta and amniotic fluids of infected animals. These rickettsiae remain viable on drying and may be carried on dust particles by the airborne route. Humans may be infected by the bite of ticks, ingesting contaminated milk, direct contact with infected tissues, or by the airborne route. The airborne infection results in pneumonitis whereas other routes may pro-

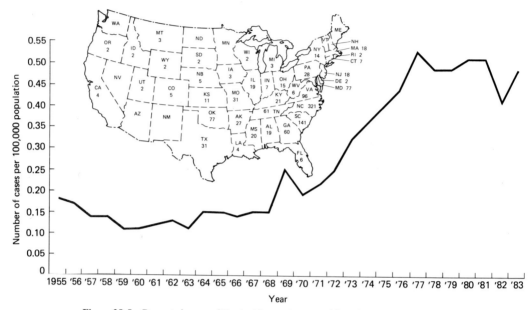

Figure 28-5 Reported cases of Rocky Mountain spotted fever in the United States, 1955–1983. Insert map shows the distribution of the 1163 cases reported in 1980 (modified from CDC annual summaries).

duce a nondescript disease with chills, malaise, and fever. A rash is not seen with Q-fever. Asymptomatic infections seem widespread in cattle and rickettsiae may be found in unpasteurized milk. No milk-borne epidemics have been reported, however. Q-fever is found throughout the world.

Other Rickettsial Diseases

In addition to the preceding varieties, other rickettsial diseases are found in different geographic areas throughout the world. Scrub typhus, which occurs over a wide area of southeast Asia, is the most important. The rickettsial diseases of humans are listed in Table 28-1.

CLINICAL NOTE

Q-Fever at a University Research Center: California

During the first three months of 1979, 11 confirmed and more than 30 presumptive cases of Q-fever occurred among researchers and employees of the University of California, San Francisco (UCSF). One person died. Most, if not all, of the infections were introduced by pregnant sheep used in research. In the preceding 15 years only 4 cases had been recognized at UCSF.

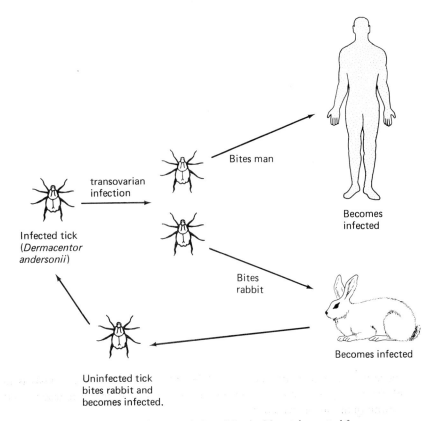

transovarian
infection

Bites man

Becomes
infected

Infected tick
(*Dermacentor
andersonii*)

Bites
rabbit

Becomes infected

Uninfected tick
bites rabbit and
becomes infected.

Figure 28-6 The transmission of Rocky Mountain spotted fever.

Preliminary results of a serologic survey of 580 employees revealed that 114 (19.6%) had complement-fixing (CF) antibodies (>1:8) to *Coxiella burnetii*. In comparison, there were only 4 positives (0.2%) among 2200 specimens submitted to the Microbiology Laboratory of the San Francisco Department of Public Health (SFDPH) since routine testing of patients with respiratory infections began 2 years ago. At USCF the highest prevalence of CF antibodies was in animal technicians and cage cleaners, plus those who worked on the floors where sheep were studied. Out of 9 employees who worked with soiled linen in the campus laundry, 5 had positive titers. Many other employees with positive titers had no direct contact with the research sheep but used corridors and elevators where sheep were transported in open carts.

Approximately 600 pregnant ewes are supplied annually to UCSF researchers. In November 1978, 47% of 122 sheep in the supplier's flock were positive for Q-fever antibodies. After the outbreak was recognized in April 1979, the sheep were removed to a separate building, which is in the process of being brought up to the National Institutes of Health's third level of containment standards through the addition of negative air pressure, air locks, and high-efficiency particulate filters on exhaust ducts.

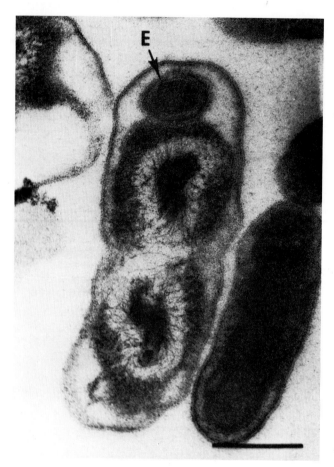

Figure 28-7 Transmission electron micrograph showing the presence of an endospore (E) in the rickettsia *Coxiella burnettii*. This cell is undergoing division (bar = 0.2 μm). (T. F. McCaul and J. C. Williams, *J. Bact. 147*:1063–1076, Figure 3c, with permission of ASM)

Editorial Note: Q-fever is a rickettsial zoonosis readily transmitted by the airborne route in areas contaminated by tissues, such as the placenta, or by excreta of infected animals. Sheep, goats, and cattle are natural reservoirs; their infections are usually inapparent. In humans the infection generally produces mild, influenzalike respiratory disease but sometimes pneumonia, hepatitis, or endocarditis, and, rarely, death (*MMWR 28*:333, 1979).

CHLAMYDIAE

The chlamydiae, like the rickettsiae, were considered more closely related to the viruses than to bacteria for many years. It is now known that chlamydiae are small procaryotic cells and so they are classed as small bacteria.

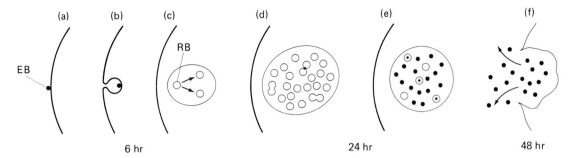

Figure 28-8 Stages in the replication of chlamydiae. (a) attachment of elementary body (EB) to cell membrane; (b) phagocytosis of EB; (c) EB changes into a reticulate body (RB) that divides by binary fission; (d) continued replication of RBs inside of vacuole; (e) RBs change into EBs, and (f) lysis of cell membrane and vacuole with release of EBs.

General Characteristics

Chlamydiae are obligate intracellular parasites that depend completely on the host cell for energy, for they have no ability to produce their own ATP molecules. They go through a unique developmental cycle inside intracytoplasmic vacuoles of the host cell (Figure 28-8). The basic structure, called an *elementary body*, is 0.2 to 0.4 μm in diameter. It is infectious and enters the host cell by phagocytosis. The replication occurs in the phagosome, which becomes enlarged and is called a vacuole. Before replication can occur, the elementary body changes into a larger structure, 0.7 to 1.0 μm in diameter, that is called a *reticulate body*. The reticulate body is not infectious but is the replicating form of chlamydiae. It divides by binary fission to fill the vacuole with new particles. The reticulate bodies next change into the smaller, infectious elementary bodies that are not able to multiply. The growth of chlamydiae may cause the death and breaking up of the host cell that result in the release of the elementary bodies.

Two species of the genus *Chlamydia—C. trachomatis* and *C. psittaci*—cause diseases in humans.

Diseases Caused by C. trachomatis

Three categories of diseases of humans caused by *C. trachomatis* are listed in Table 28-2 and include (a) trachoma, (b) a complex of diseases transmitted by direct (primarily sexual) and indirect routes, and (c) lymphogranuloma venereum. The ability of a single species to cause such varied clinical diseases probably stems from slightly different variations in virulence or host tissue affinity for different serotypes of this microbe. Specific serotypes of the chlamydiae are characteristically associated with the different disease manifestations. This diversity is also a function of the different routes of transmission and the degree of natural resistance of the persons being infected. In many cases, the chlamydiae are apparently able to persist in the cells of the host for prolonged periods without causing disease.

TABLE 28-2   DISEASES FOR WHICH CHLAMYDIAE HAVE BEEN IMPLICATED
AS ETIOLOGIC AGENTS

Chlamydia	Normal host	Disease in humans
C. psittaci	birds	Psittacosis, ornithosis
C. trachomatis sero groups A, B, C	humans	Trachoma
Sero groups D–K	humans	Nongonococcal urethritis (NGU), inclusion conjunctivitis, infant pneumonia
Sero groups L_1–L_3	humans	Lymphogranuloma venereum

Trachoma

Trachoma (Figure 28-9) is an infection of the eyelid (conjunctivitis) and, in some
cases, of the cornea (keratitis). Cases of varying degrees of severity appear and range
from asymptomatic infections to those showing extensive scarring of the cornea with
resultant blinding. This disease is widespread in areas where poverty, overcrowding,
and unsanitary conditions exist. Humans are the only hosts; infection is spread by
direct and indirect contact. Trachoma is most prevalent in Asia and Africa. An estimated 400 million people worldwide suffer from this disease and of them about 6
million are blind. The number of persons with severely impaired vision or blindness
in countries where trachoma is prevalent definitely impairs socioeconomic progress.
Trachoma ranks among the major infectious disease problems of mankind. Most trachoma seen in the United States appears on Indian reservations in the Southwest or in
Appalachia. This disease is rarely seen in persons living under modern sanitary
conditions.

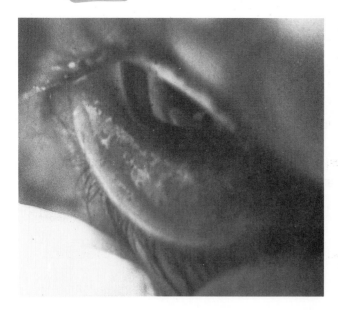

Figure 28-9   Trachoma with infection of
the eye lid (conjunctivitis). (Centers for
Disease Control, Atlanta)

Inclusion conjunctivitis, urethritis, and associated diseases

These clinical conditions are caused by serotypes of *C. trachomatis* that are passed by sexual contact. In many cases, these infections are asymptomatic or involve only mild symptoms that go undiagnosed. This form of urethritis is commonly called *nongonococcal* (NGU) or *nonspecific urethritis* (NSU) and is now recognized as a common sexually transmitted disease. *C. trachomatis* can be isolated from approximately 60% of males suffering from NGU. This infection seems to be widespread but is often without symptoms in females. As many as 10% of cervical specimens taken from females without symptoms who were undergoing routine medical examinations contained chlamydiae. Some females, however, will experience clinical diseases, such as inflammation of the cervix (cervicitis) or uterine tubes (salpingitis). This infection is readily transmitted to infants during birth from an infected mother. The infected infant may then develop conjunctivitis or a serious form of pneumonia. This form of conjunctivitis may be seen in as many as 25% of the infants born in some areas of the United States. Still, this disease is less severe than trachoma, is often self-limiting, and does not infect the cornea. Generally blindness does not result. Sporadic cases may occur in adults whose eyes become infected through contact with contaminated towels, fingers, and similar items. Transmission can also occur in unchlorinated swimming pools.

Lymphogranuloma venerium (LGV)

This disease is transmitted by sexual contact and is caused by distinct chlamydial serotypes. A variety of nonspecific symptoms may be experienced in the early stages of illness, with lesions on the skin and mucous tissues of the genital organs. This condition is followed by the characteristic signs of enlarged and painful lymph nodes in the inguinal area (buboes).

Diagnosis

C. trachomatis infections are diagnosed by observing inclusion bodies (the vacuoles filled with the chlamydiae) in cells scraped from infected tissues, by culturing the chlamydiae in cell cultures or embryonated eggs, and by showing a rise in specific antibodies.

Treatment

Sulfonamides, tetracyclines, and rifampin are effective agents in treating these chlamydial infections.

Prevention and Control

Vaccines have been tried but generally do not induce a high enough level of protection to warrant their use. Proper hygiene and sanitation are the most effective means of preventing eye infections. Some persons may remain chronic carriers and serve as a reservoir of infections, a factor that makes control difficult.

Diseases Caused by *C. psittaci*

C. psittaci is able to infect a wide range of birds and animals. This microbe was first recognized as an infection of psittacine birds, such as parrots and parakeets; hence the name psittacosis. Today the disease is also known as *ornithosis* because it infects many species of birds besides those of the Psittacine family.

Many tissues of the bird are infected and a wide variety of clinical signs may be seen. Diarrhea is a common finding in infected birds and chlamydiae are shed in the feces. Many birds have latent infections that may develop into acute diseases when such stresses as crowding and shipping occur. Ornithosis can be a major problem in the shipping and holding of pet birds and in the poultry industry.

Persons who work or live closely with birds stand the greatest risk of being infected. Exposure is usually by the airborne route via contaminated dust. Symptoms in humans are varied and may be subclinical or mild and simply passed off as a common minor respiratory disease. Occasionally (about 50 to 100 cases per year in the United States) severe respiratory infections develop. Some deaths result, but early treatment with antibiotics usually reduces the mortality rate.

CLINICAL NOTE

Psittacosis Associated with Turkey Processing: Ohio

An outbreak of psittacosis occurred among employees of an Ohio turkey-processing plant in July 1981. Approximately 27 of the plant's some 80 employees were ill; 3 were hospitalized. Turkeys being slaughtered at the plant were the probable source of infection, but no specific group of birds could be implicated.

Most patients had an illness characterized by weakness, headache, fever, chills, and cough. To a lesser extent, patients had photophobia, conjunctivitis, generalized joint pains, stomach cramps, and diarrhea. Eight patients who had chest x rays showed evidence of pneumonia consistent with psittacosis.

Paired serum specimens from 27 workers were tested for complement-fixing antibodies to chlamydial group antigen. Of 15 workers who had recently had an illness compatible with psittacosis, 7 had a ≥ four-fold titer rise, and 5 had a titer of ≥ 16 in at least 1 specimen. Of 12 workers who had not recently had a compatible illness, none had a significant titer change. Single serum specimens were obtained from 29 other workers 1 to 3 days after onset of the last-recognized case in the employee group. Eight of 11 workers in this group who had recently had illness compatible with psittacosis had a titer of ≥ 16; 2 of 18 who had not had such an illness had a titer ≥ 16.

The plant, which operates approximately 40 hours/week, 10 months a year, processes turkeys only, which are delivered by truck from various locations, and slaughtered and defeathered on the day of arrival in the "kill-pick" area. Then they are conveyed on a continuously moving line into the evisceration area, where deep tissues are exposed, the birds are inspected and trimmed, edible organs are removed, and the remaining inedible internal and external parts are discarded.

Because most employees worked in various job stations in several departments on a given day, it was difficult to assess the relative importance of respiratory, skin, and conjunctival exposure. However, the attack rate by work department was significantly higher for workers in the kill-pick and evisceration areas than in other departments of the plant. Furthermore, there was no apparent correlation between degree of skin exposure and clinical psittacosis, suggesting that infections were the result of aerosol transmission or that multiple routes of exposure may have been involved (*MMWR 30*:638, 1981).

SUMMARY

1. The rickettsiae are obligate energy parasites of animal cells, are not found as free-living forms, and are accidental parasites of humans. They are transmitted to humans by vectors and produce serious generalized infections characterized by high fever and a rash. Members of the genus *Coxiella* may be found in domestic animals and can be transmitted to humans by the airborne route. These infections respond well to antibiotic therapy and vaccines are available for some diseases.

2. The chlamydiae are also obligate intracellular parasites and are parasites of humans or animals. Numerous diseases occur from these organisms, including trachoma, a sexually transmitted disease, and a serious but usually not fatal form of pneumonia. These diseases respond well to therapy.

Fungi

29

Fungi are eucaryotic organisms existing both as single cells, as in the case of yeast, or as multicellular filaments, as seen in the molds and mushrooms. The multicellular fungi are plantlike in their structure, but they carry out no photosynthetic activities and depend on preformed organic matter for their nourishment.

The term *mycology* refers to the study of fungi and is derived from the Greek term *mykes*, which means mushroom. Fungi are widespread, with approximately 100,000 species having been identified. Fungi are actively involved in the decomposition of organic matter and play an important role in the recycling of organic compounds in nature. Many plant diseases are caused by fungi; however, these diseases will not be covered in this book. Only about 100 species of fungi are associated with diseases in humans or animals. Most fungal diseases of humans are caused by only 10 to 15 different fungi. This chapter summarizes the major fungal (mycotic) infections of humans.

MORPHOLOGY AND REPRODUCTION

Yeast

Yeast are single oval or spherical cells ranging from 3 to 20 μm in diameter. As a rule, they reproduce by budding, which first entails dividing the nucleus, followed by passage of one nucleus to a bud that forms from the wall of the mother cell. A wall forms between the bud and the mother cell. The bud separates from the mother cell and becomes a daughter cell. Many daughter cells form from a single mother cell. Initially

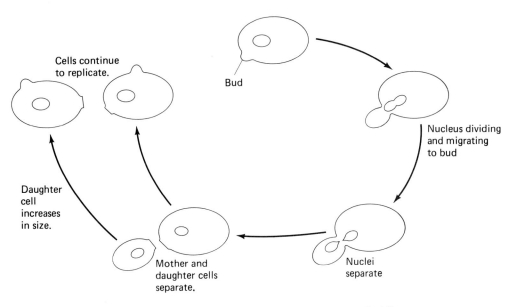

Figure 29-1 Replication of yeast cells by budding.

the daughter cell is smaller than the mother cell, but it gradually increases in size and, in turn, produces its own buds (Figure 29-1).

Molds

The growth of a mold usually starts with the germination of a spore (also called conidium), which sends out a filament that grows by elongation at its tip. This filament is the basic structure of growing molds and is called a *hypha*. Many branches of hyphae are formed and masses of hyphae are called *mycelium*. Some hyphae grow above the surface of the substrate, resembling branches of a plant, and are called aerial hyphae or aerial mycelium. Other hyphae grow into the surface to absorb nutrients, similar to roots of plants, and are called the vegetative hyphae. The hyphae vary from about 2 to 10 μm in diameter, depending on the species of mold. Many nuclei are contained within the hyphae; in many species crosswalls called *septa* are located at frequent intervals along the hyphae.

Molds reproduce by developing spores (conidia) on the aerial hyphae. Spores act as "seeds" for new colonies of molds. A reproductive cycle of one type of mold is shown in Figure 29-2. Many variations are seen in the morphology of the mycelium, spores, and reproductive structures of molds. These features are useful in identifying the different species. Some general structural variations of common molds are shown in Figure 29-3.

A typical mold colony is able to produce many reproductive structures and each structure may produce hundreds of spores. These spores are easily disseminated through the air and so mold spores are carried to virtually every unprotected environ-

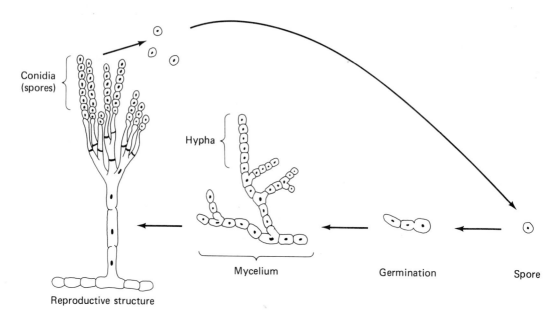

Figure 29-2 An asexual reproduction cycle of a conidial-type fungus.

mental habitat on the earth. The preceding type of reproduction is called asexual. Some fungi carry out a form of sexual reproduction in which two different reproductive bodies connect and haploid cells from each body fuse to form diploid cells.

Certain species of fungi are able to grow as either the yeast or the filamentous form—a trait called *dimorphism* (Figure 29-4). Under certain growth conditions the yeast form will develop whereas the filamentous form is produced under other conditions. This phenomenon is important in the diagnosis of some fungal infections be-

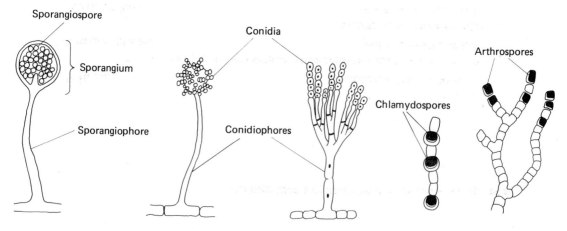

Figure 29-3 Some of the different types and arrangements of fungal spores.

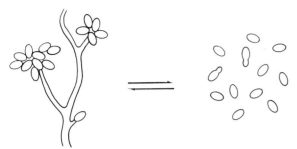

Filamentous form with
conidia when grown on
Sabouraud's agar at room
temperature

Yeast form when grown
on blood agar or in
animal tissues at 37°

Figure 29-4   Dimorphism of the fungus
Sporothrix schenckii.

cause certain pathogenic fungi exist in the yeast phase when growing in body tissues but change to the filamentous form when growing on an artificial laboratory medium. Most fungi can be cultivated on artificial media in the laboratory, through variations of the same basic methods used to cultivate bacteria.

FUNGAL DISEASES

Fungal diseases are called *mycoses.* When found in humans, these diseases can be divided into four groups, based on the level of penetration of the infection into the body tissues, as follows:

1. *Superficial mycoses.* Diseases caused by fungi that grow only on the surface of skin and hair.
2. *Cutaneous mycoses or dermatomycoses.* Included are such infections as athlete's foot and ringworm in which fungal growth occurs only in outer layers of skin, in nails, or in hair shafts.
3. *Subcutaneous mycoses.* Fungal infections that are able to penetrate below the skin and involve the subcutaneous, connective, and bone tissues.
4. *Systemic or deep mycoses.* Fungal infections that are able to infect internal organs and become widely disseminated throughout the body.

Superficial Mycoses

The superficial mycoses are of minor importance because the infections are limited to hair surface or to the surface of the skin. The resulting tissue damage is minimal. These diseases are seen most often in warm climates. The lesions appear as scaley or pigmented areas on the skin or as nodules on the shafts of hair. Treatment involves removing the skin scales with a cleansing agent and removing the infected hair. Good hygiene generally prevents these infections.

Dermatomycoses

The fungi that cause these infections are only able to infect the epidermis, hair, or nails. About 30 different species of the genera *Epidermophyton*, *Microsporum*, and *Trichophyton*, collectively referred to as dermatophytes, cause these infections. Dermatomycoses are known by such lay terms as "athlete's foot," "jock itch," and "ringworm." The term *tinea*, along with the area of the body involved, is also used when referring to these infections. For example, *tinea capitis* is an infection of the scalp (Figure 29-5), *tinea corporis* is an infection on the body (Figure 29-6), *tinea cruris* is in the groin area, or "jock itch," and *tinea pedis* is "athlete's foot."

Many dermatophytes may cause similar types of infections; so specific diagnosis can only be made by laboratory tests. Although these diseases do not cause death and are rarely serious, they may produce uncomfortable symptoms and sometimes unsightly lesions. The hyphae of the dermatophytes grow into the tissues of the epidermis, into the hair shaft, or into finger- or toenails. In young children growth of these fungi in the epidermis of the scalp moves outward in concentric circles. The term *ringworm* was applied to this type of lesion years ago when it was thought that the lesion was caused by worms coiled under the skin. *Athlete's foot* refers to lesions on the feet, often starting between the toes as small fluid-filled vesicles. The vesicles rupture, leaving shallow lesions that itch and may become secondarily infected with bacteria. Infections of the nails cause puffy-chalky lesions (Figure 29-7). Infections may persist for years in some persons if not treated whereas in others the cure is spontaneous. Reinfection may occur because typical antibody-type immunity does not seem to develop.

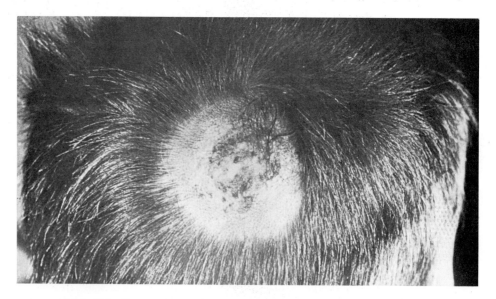

Figure 29-5 *Tinea capitis*, or ringworm infection, on the scalp of a child. (Centers for Disease Control, Atlanta)

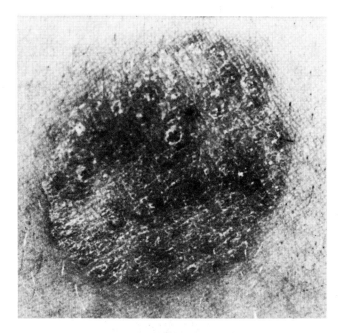

Figure 29-6 Dermatomycoses on the arm. (Centers for Disease Control, Atlanta)

Epidemiology

Dermatophytes are usually parasites of humans and animals. Transmission is apparently from person to person by direct or indirect contact with bits of sloughed-off tissues that contain the fungus. *Tinea capitis* is seen mostly in children, *tinea pedis* in adolescents and adults. Some dermatomycoses are transmitted from pets and other domestic animals to humans. Infections are found worldwide and a significant number of people have been or are currently infected. Clusters of "ringworm" infection may occur in elementary-school-age children.

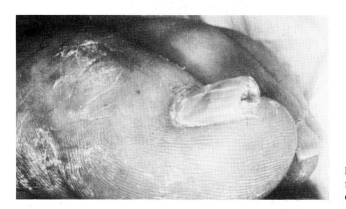

Figure 29-7 *Tinea unguium*; fungal infection of toe nails. (Centers for Disease Control, Atlanta)

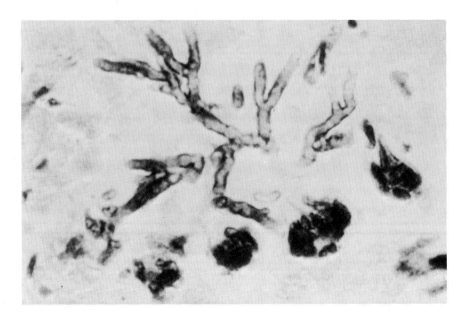

Figure 29-8 Microscopic appearance of fungal hyphae in infected tissue. (S. S. Schneierson, *Atlas of Diagnostic Microbiology*, p. 45. Courtesy Abbott Laboratories, Abbott Park, IL.)

Diagnosis

Dermatomycoses are usually diagnosed by clinical signs and symptoms. Microscopic examination of tissue scrapings shows the presence of hyphae (Figure 29-8). Tissue scrapings can be inoculated onto an agar medium and after incubation at room temperature for a week or two, fungal colonies develop. Specific species can be identified by the gross appearance of the colony and by microscopic examination of the structure of the fungus. This procedure uses Sabouraud's agar medium, which contains antibiotics and a low pH to inhibit bacterial growth.

Treatment

Numerous ointments, powders, and solutions are available as nonprescription treatments. Many are effective in providing symptomatic relief; when combined with good hygiene, they may help to produce a cure in some persons. The most effective systemic treatment is the antibiotic griseofulvin. When taken orally, it accumulates in the keratin tissues and exhibits a fungistatic effect. Treatment must be continued long enough to allow the infected tissues to be sloughed off. For infections of the scalp and skin, treatment for 2 to 3 weeks is required. Longer periods are needed for infections of nails. Infected nails may be removed surgically if prolonged treatment with griseofulvin is not practical.

Subcutaneous Mycoses

Some fungi that are normal inhabitants of the soil or organic matter are able to cause infections when introduced into the skin. These infections tend to remain in the adjacent subcutaneous tissues but on occasion may spread to deeper tissues. The most common type of subcutaneous mycoses is caused by the fungus *Sporothrix schenckii* and the disease is called sporotrichosis (Figure 29-9). This infection is seen in all parts of the world and occurs most often in gardeners, farmers, or other workers who come in contact with soil. An ulcerative lesion develops at the site of inoculation; then infection may spread to regional lymph nodes, where swelling occurs. Diagnosis is made by culturing the fungus from lesion exudate. This fungus is dimorphic with a yeast phase at 36°C and a mycelial phase at room temperature (Figure 29-4). Treatment is often difficult, but doses of potassium iodide over a 4- to 6-week period are fairly effective.

Other forms of subcutaneous mycoses occur primarily in the tropics and subtropics. The two major forms, *chromomycosis* and *maduromycosis*, are caused by several different fungal species. Lesions are usually on the feet or lower extremities where the fungi have the most likely chance of entering traumatized tissues. The lesions of chromomycosis appear as ulcerative, warty, cauliflowerlike growths. The lesions of maduromycosis are deeper and purulent, with openings draining to the outside. Treatment is often difficult but usually includes surgical removal of diseased tissues in the case of maduromycosis, with chemotherapy being used to control secondary bacterial infections. The lesions of maduromycosis appear similar to the subcutaneous lesions caused by *Nocardia*, *Actinomyces*, or *Streptomyces* (Chapter 22);

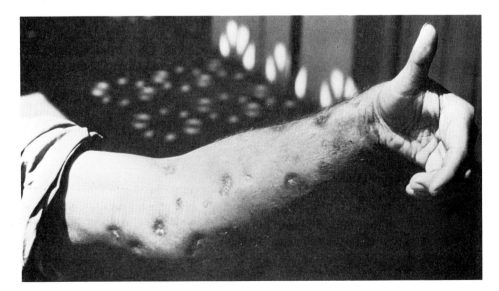

Figure 29-9 Sporotrichosis on the arm. (Centers for Disease Control, Atlanta)

it is important to determine which agents are causing the disease, for it can be treated with antibiotics if bacterial agents are responsible.

Systemic Mycoses

General pathogenesis

The systemic mycoses occur in two basic forms. The most prevalent is a subclinical or mild respiratory infection whereas the other is a severe disseminated infection involving many tissues. Unless treated, the disseminated form is usually fatal. The fungi that cause systemic mycoses live in the soil as saprophytes. The spores are inhaled into the respiratory tract, where an acute, self-limiting pneumonitis may result. This initial infection is generally mild and passed off as a common bacterial or viral respiratory disease. In a great majority of cases, the infection terminates after this mild pulmonary phase. In a relatively small number of persons, often those with compromised defense mechanisms, a chronic form of the disease develops. Slowly progressing, purulent, or granulomatous pulmonary lesions develop and resemble the lesions of tuberculosis in many ways. Often systemic mycoses of the lungs are misdiagnosed as tuberculosis. These lesions may extend directly into the tissues around the lungs or the fungi may be carried via the blood to any organ of the body, where secondary lesions will develop.

Transmission

No human-to-human transmission is known to occur. The fungi growing in soil or animal droppings produce spores that are carried by the airborne route to humans. The major systemic mycoses are discussed below; some have worldwide distribution whereas others are limited to specific geographic areas.

Diagnosis

Most fungi that induce systemic mycoses are dimorphic and diagnosis is aided by observing the yeast form of the fungus in tissue specimens. The fungi may be cultivated on various nutrient agars, in which either the yeast or filamentous forms may be produced; serologic tests are available for some infections. Delayed hypersensitivity is induced and antigens prepared from the fungi can be used in skin tests for some.

Treatment

The chemotherapeutic agents amphotericin B and 5-flurocytosine are the treatments of choice for most systemic mycoses. Surgical removal of large pulmonary lesions may be useful in some cases.

Control and Prevention

No vaccines are routinely available. Avoiding areas like bird roosts and caves where spores are most likely to be found may be wise.

Selected Systemic Mycoses

Coccidioidomycosis

This disease is caused by the fungus *Coccidioides immitis*. The fungus is found in some desert areas and is prevalent in the southwestern United States and in some areas of Central and South America. *C. immitis* grows as a mold on the soil and produces arthrospores that are carried with air currents into the pulmonary spaces, where they cause infection. As many as 50 to 80% of the people living in some areas of the central valleys of California have a positive skin test to this agent, which indicates that they have at least had the mild respiratory form of this disease. Coccidioidomycosis is called "valley fever" by residents of California's San Joaquin Valley. A small percentage of those persons infected develop the disseminated disease. *C. immitis* grows in spherical forms in tissues.

CLINICAL NOTE

Coccidioidomycosis: California

A violent windstorm in the San Joaquin Valley on December 20 and 21, 1977, created extensive dust clouds that spread to many areas of California. State and local health officials became concerned that dust bearing the arthrospores of *Coccidioides immitis* would expose people outside the regions endemic for coccidioidomycosis to the disease. During the first 24 days of January (1978) 11% of 656 sera obtained from persons with suspected coccidioidomycosis and submitted to the Kern County (California) Health Department for tube precipitin tests were positive for *C. immitis*; in comparison, 2% of 300 sera submitted in January 1977, 9% of 400 sera submitted in January 1976, and 6% of 250 sera submitted in January 1975 were positive. During the same period (January 1978) the University of California at Davis reported that 18% of 356 sera submitted were positive compared with 4% of 206 sera tested in January 1977. Several of these patients lived outside endemic regions of the state.

Editorial note: Persons who traveled through the San Joaquin Valley during the storm and those who were subsequently exposed to dust clouds from the area may have been exposed to *C. immitis*. Because the incubation period is 1 to 3 weeks, physicians should suspect the diagnosis in exposed persons who developed flulike symptoms in January. The diagnosis can be confirmed by the early appearance of *C. immitis* precipitins or by the later appearance of antibodies detected by complement-fixation or immunodiffusion tests or skin-test conversion (*MMWR 27*:55, 1978).

Histoplasmosis

The fungus *Histoplasma capsulatum* causes the disease of histoplasmosis. This fungus grows well in soil enriched by bird or bat droppings and produces infectious spores. It is most prevalent in the Ohio and Mississippi river valleys. Skin testing shows that upward to 80% of the population in some areas give evidence of having been infected. Infection results from inhaling the spores. Mild lung infections usually result and go unnoticed, but on healing they leave small, thin-walled calcified nodules that are easily mistaken for tuberculosis lesions on chest x rays. This fungus is dimorphic and grows in the form of yeast in tissues. Disseminated infections are rare.

CLINICAL NOTE

Histoplasmosis Outbreak: Tennessee

During the first weekend in May 1977 several families gathered at a friend's home in a suburb of Nashville, Tennessee, to cut and remove a large oak tree that had fallen during a thunderstorm the previous day. The tree was not noted as a prominent bird roost. There were 42 people (ages 2½ to 52 years) who either observed or helped clear debris with chain saws, hand saws, rakes, or their bare hands. Then 12 to 25 days later, 18 persons (average age, 23) developed symptoms of fever, malaise, chest pain, cough, myalgia, weight loss, and difficult breathing. Pulmonary infiltrates and/ or enlarged lymph nodes were observed on chest x rays of 13 of the 14 patients examined. Three patients were hospitalized; all recovered.

Although *Histoplasma capsulatum* could not be isolated from cultures inoculated with induced sputum from 14 patients, a majority of these patients had a titer rise in yeast phase or mycelial-phase complement-fixation (CF) antibodies in the month following illness. Two dogs present at the activities also became ill and showed a titer rise in *Histoplasma* CF tests.

Numerous soil and tree samples have been cultured; so far all have been negative. The tree was burned at the suggestion of the county health department and topsoil 2 in. deep was laid over the area.

Editorial note: This outbreak demonstrates the continued endemicity of histoplasmosis in an area that has been known since the mid-1940s to have a high prevalence of this infection. The high attack rate (43%) in this outbreak could be partially explained by the young age of the patients or by the dosage of spores to which these patients were exposed, which was sufficiently high to overcome any residual immunity they might have had.

H. capsulatum is difficult to isolate from sputum cultures; the diagnosis is often established only by serologic changes in CF antibodies or histoplasmosis immunodiffusion tests. Although spraying a 3% formalin solution on soil contaminated with *Histoplasma* spores has often been the preventive measure of choice in large outbreaks of histoplasmosis, covering the area with topsoil and burning the tree in this instance were probably adequate measures, for the soil area was small and only one tree, not notable as a bird site, was involved (*MMWR 26:*322, 1977).

Blastomycosis

This disease is caused by the fungus *Blastomycoses dermatitidis*. It probably grows in the soil as a mold and produces conidia that infect humans by the airborne route. This fungus is found worldwide, but most reported diseases occur in the central river valleys of the United States. Along with the common mild respiratory infection and the less common disseminated infection, skin lesions may also be produced. *B. dermatitidis* grows as a budding yeast in human tissues.

Cryptococcosis

This disease occurs throughout the world and is caused by the yeast *Cryptococcus neoformans*. This yeast has been isolated from soil and habitats of pigeons and exists only in the yeast form. Most infections are associated with mild respiratory tract involement. In compromised persons, however, the infection may spread through the body with a characteristic involvement of the central nervous system.

Opportunistic Fungi

Various species of fungi that are widespread in nature and generally considered of low virulence are able to cause infections in some compromised hosts. Several more frequently encountered opportunistic mycotic infections are discussed next.

Candidiasis (moniliasis)

The yeastlike fungus *Candida albicans* is often part of the normal microbial flora of the mucous membranes of the mouth, vaginal canal, and intestinal tract. Inflammation of the mouth, called *thrush*, may occur in newborn infants, who become infected during birth, or in persons with advanced cancer (Figure 29-10). Vaginal tissues may show signs of candidiasis during pregnancy or in diabetics. Candidiasis of the skin may occur where the skin is damp or irritated, such as between the upper legs or under the arms. Candidiasis seems to be more prevalent in persons on broad-spectrum antibiotic therapy, for many normal indigenous bacteria are destroyed, leaving niches into which *C. albicans* can grow. An increasing incidence of systemic candidiasis (canidia in the blood) is being recognized in various compromised patients. Candidiasis can be treated with imidazoles, various ointments, or with antifungal antibiotics, such as nystatin and amphotericin B.

Aspergillosis

Species of the genus *Aspergillus* are widespread in nature and several species are known to cause infections in humans. When persons with compromised immune defense mechanisms encounter large concentrations of aspergillus spores, infections may result. Respiratory infections are the most common and lesions containing

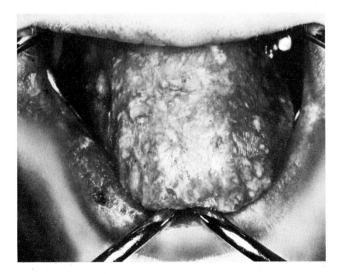

Figure 29-10 Candidiasis on the tongue and lips. (From: Council on Dental Therapeutics, American Dental Association)

masses of mycelia may develop in the lungs or bronchi. Lesions may also develop in the ear canal, sinuses, and subcutaneous tissues. Systemic aspergillosis may occur in severely immunosuppressed patients, such as those with leukemia or Hodgkin's disease. Treatment is not always successful, but amphotericin B seems to be the most effective chemotherapeutic agent.

Mucormycosis

Mucormycosis refers to fairly rare diseases produced by a variety of common fungi of the order *Mucorales*. These infections are seen in severely immunocompromised patients. The fungi may penetrate the respiratory or intestinal mucosa or enter through breaks in the skin. Localized lesions may develop, followed by spread to the blood and dissemination to all organs. Death often results from a combination of the predisposing illness and the fungal infection.

CLINICAL NOTE

**Eye Infections after Plastic Lens Implantation:
California, Florida, Montana, Ohio**

During October and November 1975 physicians in California, Florida, Montana, and Ohio noted 11 cases of unusual ocular infection in patients who had had a prosthetic plastic lens implanted in the eye after cataract extraction. The infections were suspected 2 to 6 weeks after lens implantation, when the usual short-term postoperative inflammatory changes persisted despite the topical corticosteroid therapy frequently used in these patients. Ocular cultures from 8 of the patients grew *Paecilomyces libaeinus*, a penicilliumlike organism, resistant in vitro to amphotericin B. In most cases, the plastic lens was removed after infection was suspected and local antifungal therapy was instituted. Vision was seriously impaired in all patients (*MMWR* 24:437, 1975).

SUMMARY

1. Fungi are eucaryotic, nonphotosynthetic, often multicellular organisms, some of which cause disease in humans and animals. Forms causing disease in humans include the yeasts and simple multiple-celled forms called molds. They do not have bacterial-type cell walls and infections are often difficult to treat. They are ubiquitous in the environment and cause much economic loss through their destructive growth processes.

2. Mycotic infections range from the benign athlete's foot to serious systemic disease that is frequently fatal. These diseases are far more common in compromised hosts than in normal individuals.

Protozoa

The protozoa are a group of microorganisms that are animal-like in their structure and functions.

GENERAL CHARACTERISTICS

The cell structure is eucaryotic and has many of the various intracellular components characteristic of "higher" forms of life. Most protozoa have some form of active locomotion, which is an important feature when grouping them into major subdivisions. Protozoa are quite variable in size, ranging from 5 μm to more than 100μm. They are found in soil, in most bodies of water, and in many higher forms of life, either as commensals or parasites. Of approximately 30,000 species, a relatively few are able to cause diseases in humans. Many protozoa are beneficial contributors to the various biological cycles in nature.

Protozoan diseases are generally included in the field of medical parasitology, the study of parasites found in four phyla. These phyla are the *Protozoa* of the kingdom Protista and the *Platyhelminthes* (flatworms), the *Nematodes* (roundworms), and the *Arthropoda* of the animal kingdom. The worms and arthropods are multicellular organisms, usually macroscopic in size; in fact, some, like tapeworms, may attain lengths of several meters. It is not within the scope of this book to cover the diseases caused by these multicellular types of parasites. A table listing some of these diseases, however, is included in Appendix B.

Protozoan and other parasitic diseases are common in underdeveloped, tropical, and subtropical areas. In many such areas most of the population is infected with a variety of parasites. The overall effects of these diseases on the general well-being of the inhabitants of these areas are of major importance. In industrialized nations, particularly in temperate-climate regions, parasitic diseases are of minor importance. The major concern for inhabitants of the United States is the risk of contracting protozoan diseases while visiting those areas outside the country where the infections are widespread. Yet a few protozoan diseases, such as giardiasis, amebiasis, toxoplasmosis, and trichomoniasis, are fairly widespread in the United States.

The diagnosis, treatment, and control of protozoan diseases differ in some ways from those used for other microbial diseases. The protozoa are not easily cultured on artificial media or inoculated into experimental animals or cell culture systems for isolation. Serologic tests are not as useful, for high levels of antibody do not readily form against many protozoa that infect the intestinal tract or other superficial tissues. Some infections, however, do stimulate an antibody response; and serologic tests are now available to aid in the diagnosis of these protozoan diseases. The diagnosis of most protozoan diseases depends mainly on demonstrating the presence of the parasite by microscopic methods. To determine intestinal infections, the feces are examined and the blood and/or other tissues are examined for systemic infections. Scrapings of mucosal tissues or biopsies of infected organs may also be examined. Because of their large size and distinct shapes, direct microscopic identification of the protozoa is the routine method of diagnosis. The symptoms of many protozoan diseases are quite general and often are not used as a basis for a specific diagnosis.

No vaccines are available against protozoan diseases. Chemotherapy is not as specific as it is against procaryotic microbes; however, some compounds are fairly effective against certain protozoan diseases. Toxic side effects are common with antiprotozoan drugs.

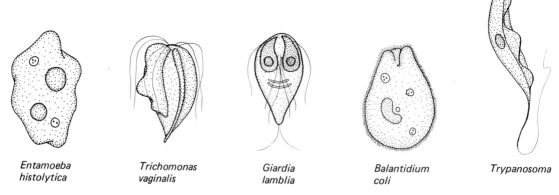

Entamoeba
histolytica

Trichomonas
vaginalis

Giardia
lamblia

Balantidium
coli

Trypanosoma

Figure 30-1 The trophozoite stages of some of the protozoal pathogens.

Some disease-producing protozoa go through a life cycle that involves more than one host and perhaps different stages of development of the parasite. Many protozoa exist in two basic forms: the active, growing form, called the *trophozoite*, and the dormant, resistant form, called the *cyst* (Figure 30-1). The trophozoite form proliferates in the tissue and causes the damage that results in the clinical disease. The cyst is able to survive in the external environment and is the form of the protozoa that is usually transmitted from host to host by indirect routes. Some protozoa go through intermediate developmental stages in blood-sucking insects and the infected insect may serve as the vector in transmitting the disease.

Protozoa that cause diseases in humans can be divided into four groups: *Sarcodina*, *Mastigophora*, *Ciliophora*, and *Sporozoa*. Several important diseases from these groups are discussed next.

PROTOZOAN DISEASES

Sarcodina

The Sarcodina (also called Rhizopodea) are protozoa that move by ameboid action—that is, by extending a section of their cytoplasm in one direction and then causing the remainder of the cytoplasm to flow into the extension. This extension is called a *pseudopodium* (false foot). The amebae are members of the Sarcodina and seven species are parasites of humans. Only one species, *Entamoeba histolytica*, however, causes widespread or major diseases in humans. The disease is called *amebiasis*; its pathogenesis is outlined in Figure 30-2. Only the cyst stage of *E. histolytica* is infectious. The trophozoite stage readily dies once out of the body; if it survives long enough to be swallowed, it will be destroyed by stomach acids. Once the cyst, which contains four nuclei, passes into the small intestine, excystment occurs; that is, the cyst changes into four small trophozoite forms of the ameba. Each continues to grow and divides by binary fission, thereby producing large numbers of offspring. These trophozoites release an enzyme that lyses tissues. This trait is the basis for the species name *histolytica*, which means tissue (histo) dissolving (lysis). The histolytic enzyme allows the amebae to penetrate into the intestinal mucosa, where subsurface lesions develop. These lesions may coalesce into extensive ulcerative areas, thus leading to severe dysentery with stools containing bloody mucus. In a small percentage of the cases, the amebae may penetrate into the mesenteric venules and lymphatics and be disseminated to various internal organs. With disseminated amebiasis, abscesses usually develop in the liver but may also develop in the brain, lungs, heart, or other tissues. Death may result from the disseminated disease.

When a person is experiencing the acute symptoms of intestinal amebiasis, called *amebic dysentery*, the contents of the intestinal tract pass rapidly through the system. Under such conditions the amebae do not have time to develop into the cyst stage and normally only the trophozoites are released. As the body begins to establish

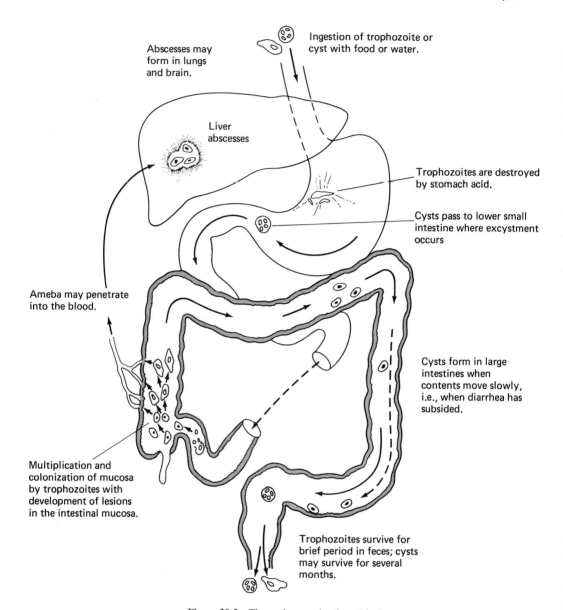

Figure 30-2   The pathogenesis of amebic dysentery.

an equilibrium with the ameba, possibly by developing neutralizing antibodies against the lytic enzymes, the lesions heal and the contents of the intestinal tract move more slowly, allowing time for the development of cysts. Thus persons showing no signs of the disease may be infectious. A large segment of the adult population in developing countries where amebiasis is prevalent lives in semibalance with this

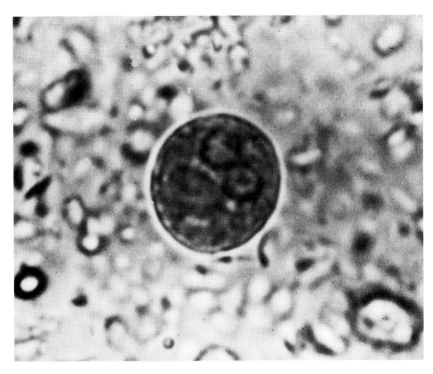

Figure 30-3 Microscopic appearance of cyst of *Entamoeba histolytica* in fecal material. (Centers for Disease Control, Atlanta)

ameba; yet they serve as a source of infection to susceptible persons. Some amebiasis is found in the United States, with most cases occurring in the South.

Specific diagnosis is made by observing the trophozoite or cyst stage of the ameba in the feces (Figure 30-3). Serologic tests are helpful in diagnosing disseminated amebiasis.

Several chemotherapeutic agents are available for the treatment of amebiasis. Tetracyclines, in combination with diloxanide furoate, is effective. A compound called metronidazole can be used with good results and chloroquine is often used in combination with the preceding drugs.

Control of amebic dysentery is best achieved by following good sanitary practices, particularly in the handling and treatment of human fecal wastes.

Ciliophora

The Ciliophora are surrounded by many fine cilia that beat in rhythmic patterns to propel the organism. Only one species, *Balantidium coli*, causes disease in humans. This organism is a large (50 to 100 μm in length), ovoid-shaped cell. Its normal habitat is the intestinal tract of hogs. Diseases in humans are rare and symptoms range from mild intestinal discomfort to severe diarrhea.

Mastigophora

The Mastigophora, also called flagellates, have whiplike flagella that serve as their organs of locomotion. Some mastigophora inhabit the superficial tissues of the intestinal or genital tract of mammalian hosts. Others require a blood-sucking arthropod for part of their life cycle with the other part of their life cycle in the blood and internal tissues of the mammalian host.

Two relatively minor diseases, *trichomoniasis* and *giardiasis*, found in the United States, and the serious diseases of *trypanosomiasis*, found in Africa and South America, are discussed next.

Trichomoniasis

This disease is caused by the protozoan *Trichomonas vaginalis*. It is a globular-shaped cell about 25 μm in length with four anterior flagella and a short undulating membrane. It exists only in the trophozoite stage and inhabits the vagina and urethra. Transmission is usually by sexual contact. A large number of cases are asymptomatic. Males having the clinical infection may experience some irritation of the urethra, with a slight discharge and pain during urination. In the female the *T. vaginalis* may cause the pH of the vagina to become slightly alkaline. This condition may be accompanied by a foul odor, a slight discharge, itching, and burning sensations. These symptoms may be caused in part by secondary bacterial infections resulting from the altered pH.

Diagnosis is made by direct microscopic examination of smears from the vaginal or urethral discharge. Treatment by oral administration of the drug metronidazole effectively cures this infection.

Giardiasis

This disease is caused by the flagellate *Giardia lamblia*. Giardia has a distinctive appearance (that resembles a human face) because of its teardrop-shaped cell, with four pairs of flagella, and two nuclei (Figure 30-1). The cell is 9 to 16 μm in length and exists in both the trophozoite and cyst stages. The cyst is able to persist for prolonged periods outside the body and transmission is by the typical fecal-oral route. Infection is in the upper small intestines; many infections are asymptomatic or go undiagnosed and are passed off as minor intestinal disturbances. Persistent gastroenteritis and diarrhea may result, along with dark, greasy, foul-smelling feces, considerable abdominal discomfort, and flatulence. The organism is the most common intestinal pathogenic protozoan of humans in the United States. Infections have occurred among campers and hikers who drank untreated water. Even water from numerous municipal sources has been implicated as a source of infection. Currently giardiasis is being diagnosed with increasing frequency among homosexual men (as are most other diseases transmitted by the fecal-oral route). Diagnosis is made by demonstrating the parasite in feces. Treatment with quinacrine or metronidazole is frequently effective. This disease may not respond to treatment, however, and may be difficult to eliminate.

CLINICAL NOTE

Giardiasis: Colorado

A multistate outbreak of giardiasis in visitors to and residents of Vail, Colorado, occurred from March 14 to April 20, 1978. At least 38 confirmed cases were reported.

On April 13 a gastroenterologist in Petoskey, Michigan, reported the occurrence of giardiasis in 6 members of the family who had vacationed in Vail, Colorado, from March 23 to 25. All had epigastric pain, nausea, and weight loss. *Giardia lamblia* was confirmed in the stool specimen of 1 of the 6 patients. Additional information obtained from the Colorado State Health Department revealed that 13 cases of confirmed giardiasis had been reported from Colorado (7 from Colorado Springs, 6 from Denver) and 12 more confirmed cases from the state of New York—all in individuals who had visited Vail during the last week in March.

An epidemiologic investigation was begun by the Colorado Department of Health and CDC. Information was obtained on 777 long-term Vail residents by means of a questionnaire and stool survey. Of those surveyed, 465 (60%) gave a history of diarrheal illness within the past 3 months. A rise in the number of acute diarrheal illnesses began March 14 to 16 and reached a peak April 1 to 12.

Preliminary analysis demonstrated no differences in attack rate by age or sex. Long-term (>7 days) and short-term (<7 days) diarrheal illness peaked at similar periods of time. The local hospital's routine examinations of stools for bacterial pathogens were negative.

Because contaminated water is a frequent cause of giardiasis outbreaks, the Environmental Protection Agency (EPA) and CDC reviewed the city's recent records of weekly sewage output. During the week of March 28 to April 3 the number of gallons of sewage produced dropped approximately 50%. This drop coincided with a sewer-line obstruction and leak into the creek supplying water to the city that was previously discovered on March 31 and corrected.

Editorial note: The fact that many cases occurred after discovery of the sewer-line obstruction is probably a reflection of the long incubation period of giardiasis (variable, but approximately 7 days) and the continued use of water from contaminated storage tanks. Illness disappeared with dilution of freshwater (*MMWR 27*:155, 1978).

Trypanosomiasis

Three species of the genus *Trypanosoma* cause serious diseases in humans. *T. gambiense* and *T. rhodesiense* cause African sleeping sickness and *T. cruzi* causes South American sleeping sickness or Chagas' disease. The morphology of these protozoa is shown in Figure 30-1.

African sleeping sickness is found only in geographic areas of Africa where the *tsetse* (glossina) fly lives. The tsetse fly is a necessary link in the life cycle of *T. gambiense* and *T. rhodesiense* and functions as the vector for transmission to humans and animals. Cattle, swine, and various wild animals are the major hosts and serve as a reservoir for the protozoa. When a person is bitten by an infected tsetse fly, the trypanosomes cause a local lesion at the site of the bite. The protozoa then spread and become lodged in the lymph nodes and produce a chronic infection. In some cases, the trypanosomes spread to the CNS and result in the well-recognized symptoms of African sleeping sickness. During this stage the patient becomes somnolent and eventually goes into a coma and dies. African sleeping sickness has a significant impact on the economy of the African continent, for large areas of otherwise productive land cannot be inhabited by humans due to the presence of infected animals and tsetse flies.

T. cruzi is found in South and Central America and is transmitted by reduviid bugs. Dogs, cats, and various wild animals serve as the reservoir of infection. The reduviid bugs bite humans at night and defecate when they feed. *T. cruzi* are in the feces, which contaminate the bite wound or other skin abrasions or are carried by fingers to the mucosa of the mouth or nose or to the conjunctiva of the eyes to cause the infection. Persons living in huts with dirt floors or walls are most likely to become infected, especially if they sleep on the floor or ground. Lesions are produced by the parasite at the site of the bite. The protozoa then spread through the body. Many infections are nondescript and may remain latent for years. Acute diseases occur in some persons, especially children, involving the heart and CNS, and result in a 10% death rate.

Diagnosis of trypanosomal diseases is generally made by demonstrating the presence of the protozoa in the blood, lymph node aspirates, or spinal fluid. There is no effective treatment for South American trypanosomiasis. Two drugs, suramin sodium and Mel B, however, are used with some success in treating the African diseases.

Sporozoa

Malaria
Of all the infectious diseases of humans malaria is probably the most important as far as total number of cases, deaths, and debilitation are concerned. Possibly hundreds of millions of people worldwide are infected with the malarial parasites. The family Sporozoa includes four species of the genus *Plasmodium* which cause most infections in humans. They are *P. vivax*, *P. malariae*, *P. falciparum*, and *P. ovale*. Most malaria is found in the subtropics or tropics. Malaria cases seen in the United States currently involve persons who were infected while visiting or residing in endemic areas outside the country. During military operations like the Vietnam War a marked increase in malaria was seen in the United States (Figure 30-4).

The female anopheles mosquito is the primary host for the malarial parasite; humans serve as an intermediate host. The life cycle of the plasmodia is quite involved, with different stages of development occurring in the human and the mosquito host. A simplified general outline of this life cycle is shown in Figure 30-5. A sexual phase of the life cycle occurs in the mosquito once it is infected by taking a

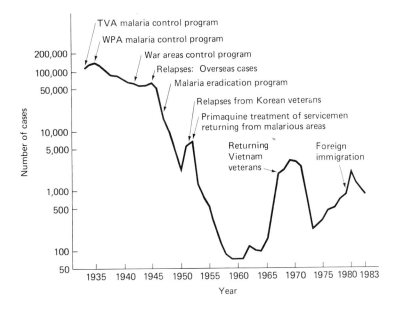

Figure 30-4 Reported cases of malaria in the United States, 1933–1983. Of all the reported cases in 1980, 81% were among foreign civilians (modified from CDC annual summaries).

blood meal from an infected person. The phases of the life cycle that occur in the mosquito result in the salivary glands accumulating large numbers of the infectious stage of the parasite, called *sporozoites*. The sporozoites are inoculated into the blood of humans bitten by the mosquito. The sporozoites are rapidly filtered from the blood and specifically infect liver cells. The parasite matures through a series of stages in the liver cells and after a week or so parasitic forms called *merozoites* are released into the blood. The merozoites infect red blood cells and go through another series of developmental stages that end with the bursting of the red blood cells, thus releasing new merozoites. These merozoites infect more red blood cells and the cycle is repeated. The cycles of infection in the red blood cells become synchronized and with each cycle more and more cells become infected and then burst. When the red blood cells burst and release cellular debris, parasites, and by-products, the onset of a malarial *paroxysm* is triggered. A paroxysm is a periodic sudden recurrence of symptoms. The paroxysms of malaria start with chills that last for 15 to 60 minutes. During this time the patient may have a headache, vomit, and generally feel nauseated. As the sensation of chilling stops, a high fever develops and lasts for several hours. It may be accompanied by a severe headache, increased nausea and vomiting, profuse sweating, and often mild delirium. The paroxysm lasts 8 to 12 hours and terminates while the patient is experiencing profuse sweating. Afterward the patient is exhausted and goes to sleep. On awakening, the patient feels relatively well. The growth of the

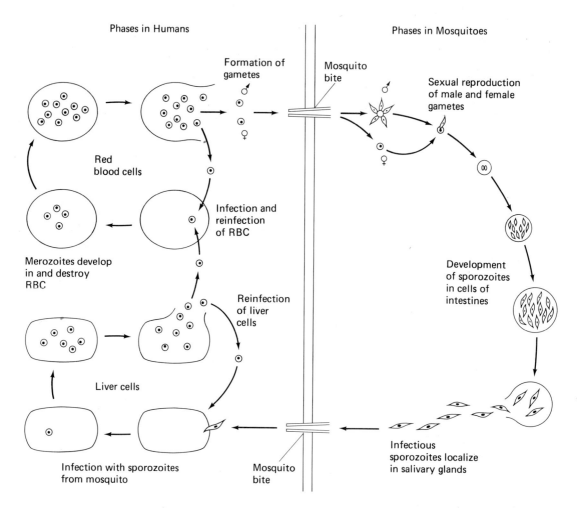

Figure 30-5 A simplified outline of the phases of the life cycle of a plasmodium parasite in humans and mosquitoes.

parasite inside the red blood cells occurs at fixed rates and this factor determines the intervals between paroxysms. The interval is 48 hours for *P. vivax* and *P. ovale*; it varies between 32 and 48 hours for *P. falciparum*; and paroxysms occur every 72 hours for *P. malariae*.

Clinical symptoms varying in severity are caused by the different species. Generally infections with *P. falciparum* are the most severe. The continued destruction of red blood cells, with concurrent damage to the capillaries, RES, and various internal organs, may lead to the death of the patient. In many patients the infection is somewhat suppressed and develops into a chronic disease. In others the infection is suppressed and remains asymptomatic for many years. Occasionally symptomatic diseases may reoccur in these chronically infected persons.

The major mode of transmission of malaria is by the bite of the anopheline mosquito. A few cases may be transmitted by other means. Occasionally a chronically infected female may congenitally transmit malaria to her offspring. Blood transfusions or unsterilized paraphernalia used in the injection of illicit narcotics may also transmit malaria. Persons who have had malaria or who have, within the past three years, visited areas where malaria is endemic, are requested not to give blood for transfusions.

Laboratory diagnosis is made by observing the malarial parasites in stained slides of blood examined with a microscope.

Perhaps more effort has been made to develop methods for the treatment and control of malaria than for any other infectious disease. And significant progress has been made, but as yet no "magic bullet" or "wonder drug" is available as an easy cure of this disease. Control of the anopheline mosquito was one of the major methods used to control or reduce the number of cases. Malaria has been significantly reduced in countries where wide-scale mosquito control programs were carried out. DDT has been a highly effective insecticide in these programs and there is concern that the reduction in the use of DDT for other environmental reasons may result in an increase in malaria in some countries. Mosquito nets and insect repellents are of some value.

Various chemotherapeutic agents have been used with some success against malaria. The two major drugs today are chloroquine and primaquine. These drugs can terminate a clinical disease, prevent recurrent attacks, and, if given long enough, result in a cure. These chemotherapeutic agents can also be used prophylactically to prevent the parasite from growing once it has infected the tissue. This type of prophylaxis is widely used when large numbers of military personnel must enter malaria-infested areas, as they did during World War II and the Vietnam War. Malaria constituted one of the major problems in these military operations. Medications taken orally on a daily or biweekly regimen can be quite effective when followed rigidly. Military personnel in the field, however, often ignored the prescribed regimen because nausea and intestinal disturbances sometimes result from the medication. Furthermore, some military personnel, particularly in an unpopular war like Vietnam, preferred to contract malaria and be sent home for a cure rather than to remain at their combat position with the possibility of an even less desirable fate. Research is currently in progress on a vaccine against malaria.

Toxoplasmosis

In contrast to many protozoal diseases found mainly in tropical regions and under unsanitary conditions, toxoplasmosis occurs in all parts of the world and can be transmitted in cosmopolitan populations. Research has shown that from 25 to 50%

of the world's population have been or are now infected with the toxoplasmosis parasite. Yet this disease in humans went virtually unrecognized until the 1940s and only a handful of cases had been specifically diagnosed during the 1950s.

The causative agent is a sporozoan called *Toxoplasma gondii*, which is a small, crescent-shaped organism (Figure 30-6), 4 to 8 μm long, with no appendages or prominent internal structures other than a nucleus. *T. gondii* is able to infect many animals and birds where it may set up an ideal parasitic relationship. Only in the past two decades has the life cycle of *T. gondii* begun to be understood. It is now apparent that the primary hosts are various felines, with domestic cats the chief transmitters to humans (Figure 30-7). Cats become infected by eating mice, birds, or raw meat; they can also be infected by the feces of other cats. The *T. gondii* goes through a sexual phase of reproduction in the intestinal tract of cats. Reproductive structures called oocysts are shed in the feces and in 3 to 4 days, if warm and damp, eight infectious sporozoites develop within each oocyst. This mature oocyst may remain viable for up to one year and infect humans and animals when ingested. No sexual reproduction of the parasite occurs in nonfeline animals and humans. However, it is able to proliferate by binary fission and circulate throughout the body. The parasite penetrates into cells and continues to proliferate until the cell bursts. As this process continues, clinical disease may result with such symptoms as fever, weakness, respiratory illness, myocarditis, or an infectious mononucleosislike illness with swollen lymph nodes. The disease is often asymptomatic or is passed off as some other disease. Only lately has a diagnosis of toxoplasmosis even been considered when dealing with such nonde-

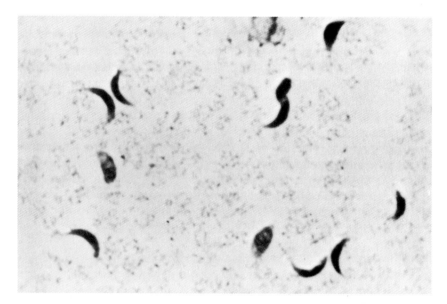

Figure 30-6 Micrograph of the crescent-shaped *Toxoplasma gondii*. (S. S. Schneierson, *Atlas of Diagnostic Microbiology*, p. 69. Courtesy of Abbott Laboratories, Abbott Park, IL.)

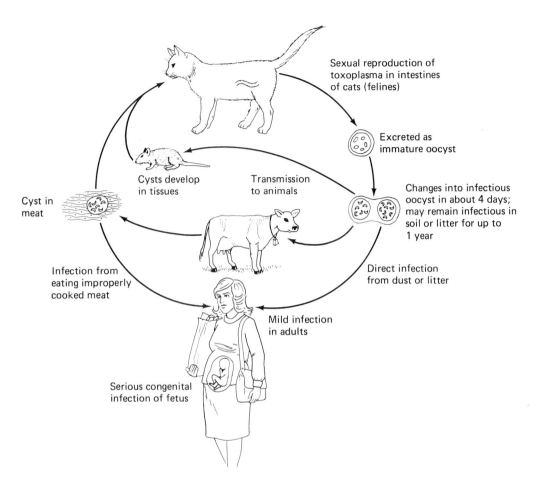

Figure 30-7   Transmission of toxoplasma in nature and to humans.

script illnesses. As the immune mechanisms of the host respond and antibodies are produced, *T. gondii* remains inside the infected cells and forms aggregates of several thousand parasitic cells that become enclosed in a fine membrane to form a cyst. The cyst evokes no further response from the host. It does not cause any tissue damage and the enclosed parasites are protected from the host's defense mechanisms. Thus a near ideal parasitic relationship is established and may persist for the lifetime of the host. These cysts, however, may serve as a source of infection to a new host that may ingest the tissues. Undoubtedly this is a major means of transmission to various carnivorous birds or animals in nature. It has also been well established that humans may become infected by eating raw or rare meat.

In a great majority of cases, toxoplasmosis is mild and self-limiting. The major concern is congenital toxoplasmosis. This condition occurs when a pregnant female develops a primary case of toxoplasmosis by being in contact with cats or by eating raw or rare meat. During the systemic phase of the infection *T. gondii* is able to pass the placental barrier and infect the developing fetus. Congenital infection is most serious if it occurs after the first trimester of pregnancy. In such cases, there is a 50% chance that serious congenital defects will develop. Generally the tissue of the brain or eyes are involved. Some infants die *in utero*; others are born with deformed brains and eyes and die shortly after birth. In some cases, infected infants show no signs of disease but carry the toxoplasma parasite as a latent infection. Later in life the parasite may begin to proliferate, causing tissue damage. Other congenitally infected infants may remain symptomless throughout life. About one of every 1000 children born in the United States has congenital toxoplasmosis, which makes this disease one of the major congenital diseases.

If a female has acquired toxoplasmosis with the resultant antibody immunity before becoming pregnant, the developing fetus is protected against congenital infection. About 30% of the women of childbearing age in the United States have antibodies against this parasite. Some health officials are recommending serologic tests for toxoplasmosis during early pregnancy and suggest that those who are negative should avoid contact with cats or their feces and also avoid rare or raw meat during their pregnancy. Such procedures should be followed by all pregnant females who have not had a serologic test for toxoplasmosis.

Diagnosis is made by examining tissues or fluids for the cysts of *T. gondii* and using serologic tests. Treatment is only effective during the systemic phase of the disease. A mixture of three different sulfa drugs in combination with the antimalaria drug pyrimethamine is used. There is no vaccine.

CLINICAL NOTE

Toxoplasmosis: Pennsylvania

On September 2, 1974, 2 male members of a wedding party became ill with low-grade fever, chills, generalized aches, fatigue, and swollen cervical lymph nodes. On September 4 another male member similarly became ill. On September 30 a female member also became ill with identical symptoms but did not have swollen cervical lymph nodes. The fever, chills, and generalized aches in these 4 persons subsided unevenly over a period of weeks: the fatigue and swollen lymph nodes persisted for months.

The patients were at first treated symptomatically and with antibiotics by their respective physicians. When the illness persisted, however, toxoplasmosis was suspected: and sera were drawn in November and December from 3 of the 4 ill persons. Results by indirect fluorescent antibody (IFA) test were positive in all 3 persons for toxoplasmosis.

These results indicated a possible common source outbreak and epidemiologic investigation revealed that on August 23, 1974, the 4 ill persons were among a group of 19 people attending a wedding rehearsal supper at a Syrian restaurant. Food histories were obtained from 15 of the 19 guests and all 15 reported having eaten Kibee Nayee, a meat dish made from raw beef. Sera obtained 2 to 5 months after the common meal were then collected from 12 more of the guests. Of the total of 15 persons from whom sera were obtained, 8 had titers of > 1:64, compatible with a recent exposure to *Toxoplasma gondii* organisms. In all cases, however, serology was performed too long after the implicated meal to demonstrate a rise in titer and to confirm the meal's possible role in transmission. Moreover, 6 of the 9 individuals with antitoxoplasma antibody titers > 1:16 had a history of habitual ingestion of rare or raw meat. Of the 8 individuals with titers > 1:64, 4 were clinically ill, but no statistically positive correlation was found between presence of symptoms and seropositivity. In cases of acquired toxoplasmosis, however, it is often impossible to obtain a history of symptomatic illness.

Editorial note: Although this investigation did not study serologic data from a control group of nonill persons, it appears likely that the illness resulted from eating raw meat at this restaurant. The high prevalence of antibodies (56%) among the 14 guests of Middle East origin may reflect their habit of eating undercooked meat. In Paris, France, where eating undercooked meat is perhaps the most important means of exposure to toxoplasma organisms, the prevalence of antibodies was 84% among 378 pregnant women studied.

Only one documented outbreak of food-borne toxoplasmosis has occurred in the United States, when 5 persons associated with the Cornell University Medical College acquired acute lymphadenopathic toxoplasmosis after eating inadequately cooked hamburger.

Because toxoplasma cysts have been found in samples of mutton, pork, and beef intended for human consumption, such meat should be heated to 56°C for 10 to 15 minutes to protect against toxoplasmosis infection. Freezing is considered a probable means of killing the tissue cysts, although viable toxoplasma organisms have been isolated from the carcass of a monkey frozen for 16 days at −20°C (*MMWR 24*:285, 1975).

SUMMARY

1. The protozoa are a diverse group that includes both free-living forms and animal parasites. A number of protozoa require a second animal host in addition to humans in order to complete their development. Such life cycles provide a variety of alternatives for exercising control measures against these organisms.

2. Protozoan diseases range in seriousness from the relatively benign giardiasis and trichomoniasis to the very common and severe diseases of malaria and amebic dysentery. Protozoan diseases are not only among the most common worldwide but are also among the most serious. Therapy of such infections remains limited and is often ineffective.

Viruses

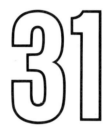

Before the germ theory of disease was established, people believed that many diseases were caused by poisons. The Latin term for poison is virus. Then as discoveries during the nineteenth century showed that microorganisms were the cause of infectious diseases, the various pathogenic microbes were identified as bacteria, fungi, or protozoa and were removed from the category of poisons or virus. Due to the inability to propagate viruses on artificial culture media or to observe them with standard optical microscopes, the virus particles went undiscovered during the so-called golden age of microbiology of the late 1800s. Yet during this time it was recognized that many diseases were caused by agents that had not been identified and such unidentified agents were still referred to as virus. Around the turn of the century it was shown that the causative agents of some diseases could pass through filters that would hold back bacterial-sized cells and by the 1930s it was possible to crystallize these agents. This latter procedure showed that they were particulate agents and not chemical poisons. By this time, however, the term virus had become permanently associated with these agents and the original meaning was, to a large extent, lost.

All forms of life seem to have specific viruses that parasitize their cells. There are viruses of animals, plants, insects, bacteria, algae, fungi, and so on. The viruses that attack bacteria are called *bacteriophage* or just *phage* and are much easier to work with in laboratory experiments than animal or plant viruses. Thus many significant discoveries on the nature of viruses were made by using phage. Fortunately, most viruses, regardless of the types of hosts they attack, function by many similar mechanisms and the information obtained through studies with phage has aided in studies of animal viruses. A great deal of information regarding the structure and functions of viruses has been obtained in the past several decades. This chapter presents a brief summarization of the major characteristics and functions of viruses that infect animals.

NATURE OF VIRUSES

The smallest viruses are 20nm and the largest 300nm in diameter. A virus possesses no independent metabolic capabilities and is thus totally dependent on a living host cell to supply all the needed energy and building blocks for its replication. A given virus contains only one molecule of one type of nucleic acid, which can be either DNA or RNA. Furthermore, the nucleic acid molecule may be either single stranded or double stranded. Some simpler viruses consist only of the single molecule of nucleic acid and a protein coat. Other viruses may possess an envelope over the protein coat; in addition, some may have internal proteins and/or small projections called *peplomers* (Figure 31-1). The complete virus particle, regardless of its structure, is called a *virion*. Five basic morphological shapes (spherical, cylindrical, brick, bullet, and tailed) are seen among the viruses and are shown in Figure 31-2.

Most animal viruses contain fairly small amounts of genetic information, which means that they are limited in the number of different types of protein molecules that can be synthesized under their direction. Many viruses that cause disease in humans contain from 5 to 15 cistrons (genes) in their nucleic acid. Many viruses must construct their protein coat, called a *capsid*, out of just one or a few different types of polypeptides. The individual protein molecules that make up the building blocks of the capsid are called *structure units*. Viral capsids are symmetrical. Many capsids are constructed as regular icosahedrons—that is, an enclosed shell of 20 triangular faces, 12 vertices, and 30 edges (Figures 31-3 and 31-4). To form the icosahedral capsid, the structure units must first form into clusters of five, called *pentamers*, and clusters of six, called *hexamers*. These clusters are called *capsomers*. The number and arrangement of the capsomers in an icosahedron are restricted geometrically. The 12 vertices

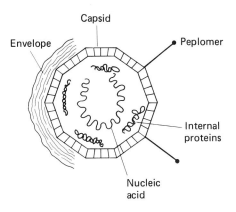

Figure 31-1 A schematic outline of a virus. The protein coat is called the capsid. An envelope is present on some viruses and not on others. Peplomers are present on some viruses. One molecule of nucleic acid is contained inside the capsid. Some viruses may have additional internal proteins. The entire virus is called a virion.

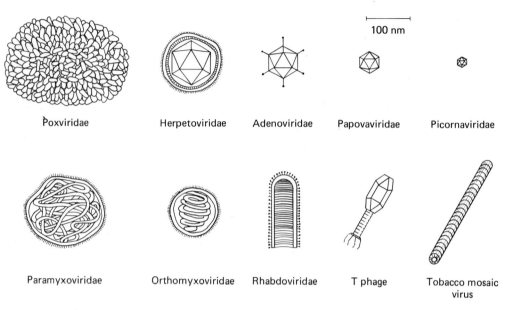

| Poxviridae | Herpetoviridae | Adenoviridae | Papovaviridae | Picornaviridae |

| Paramyxoviridae | Orthomyxoviridae | Rhabdoviridae | T phage | Tobacco mosaic virus |

Figure 31-2   The basic shapes and relative sizes of some representative groups of viruses.

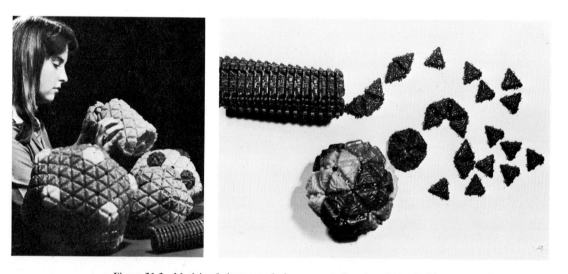

Figure 31-3   Models of viruses made from repeated copies of identical interconnecting structure units (plastic triangles) to form capsids with either cubical or helical symmetry. (Jensen Research Laboratories)

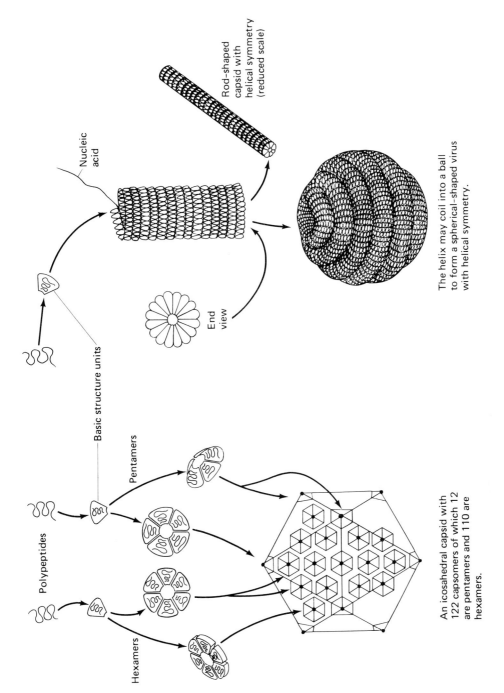

Figure 31-4 The formation of viral capsids with cubical and helical symmetry from polypeptides that form the basic structure units.

Rod-shaped capsid with helical symmetry (reduced scale)

The helix may coil into a ball to form a spherical-shaped virus with helical symmetry.

Nucleic acid

Basic structure units

End view

Pentamers

Hexamers

Polypeptides

An icosahedral capsid with 122 capsomers of which 12 are pentamers and 110 are hexamers.

must be pentamers and one of the smallest possible icosahedrons is composed of only the 12 pentamers. As the icosahedron increases in size, hexamers are added between the pentamers in regular increments. The number of pentamers remains constant at 12, however. The smallest number of hexamers that will fit is 20—that is, one for each triangular face of the icosahedron. The result is a virus with a total of 32 capsomers (12 pentamers and 20 hexamers). Other increments of capsomers that can form into icosahedrons are 42, 72, 92, 122, 162, 252, and so on. The number of capsomers for a given virus is constant and serves as a useful characteristic in classifying and identifying viruses. Icosahedral viruses are said to have *cubical symmetry*, with the nucleic acid packaged inside the icosahedral capsid.

Other viruses have *helical symmetry*, which refers to an arrangement of structure units connected side by side in a continuous ribbon that spirals into a tubular helix. The nucleic acid is connected to each structure unit much like a string that is connected along a row of beads. The tubular helix may remain extended to form a cylindrical-shaped virus or it may coil into a ball to form a spherical-shaped virus (Figures 31-3 and 31-4). A few larger viruses have more complex structures.

CULTIVATION OF VIRUSES

Viruses can only be propagated in living host cells and a major activity in a viral laboratory is to provide a suitable supply of such cells. The main sources of cells for the propagation of animal viruses are intact animals, embryonated eggs, and organ, tissue, or cell cultures. The injection of viruses in susceptible living animals gives useful information on the pathogenesis of viral diseases but is usually not a useful method of producing large amounts of viruses for vaccines or experimental studies. When dealing with human viruses, an attempt is made to find an experimental animal that will support the multiplication of the virus and produce a disease similar to that seen in humans. Such attempts are not always successful, however, for many viruses are host specific; that is, human viruses will only multiply in human cells, cat viruses in cat cells, and so forth. Yet it is possible to get some specific human viruses to multiply in such primates as monkeys or chimpanzees, an experimental procedure that is expensive and cumbersome. If there is no chance that the virus will cause death, permanent damage, or undue discomfort, human volunteers may be used in virus research. An example concerns research on the common cold; here human volunteers have been used for many years. Even though research using intact hosts has many limitations, it is often the only means available to study some diseases.

Embryonated eggs provide an inexpensive, easy-to-handle, sterile container full of a variety of living cells (Figure 31-5). Some animal viruses will multiply in embryonated eggs; others will not. Often embryonated eggs are used to produce large amounts of viruses for vaccines. A small hole can be drilled through the egg shell and virus can be injected into the appropriate embryonic tissue. Generally embryos between 7 to 10 days of age are used.

The development of methods to grow living animal cells routinely in test tubes (in vitro) greatly accelerated research work with animal viruses by making it possible

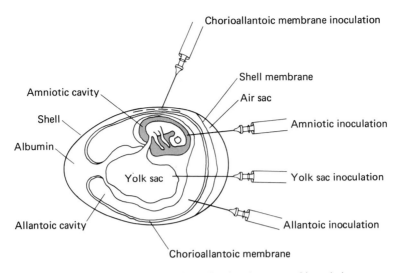

Figure 31-5 An embryonated egg showing the routes of inoculation.

to discover many new viruses, grow large amounts of viruses, and develop sensitive quantitative assays for many viruses. The impact of cell-culturing procedures is dramatized by the fact that in the late 1940s, when these procedures first came into wide use, only about 35 viruses associated with human diseases had been discovered. During the following 15 to 20 years 500 additional viruses associated with humans were identified and tremendous advances were made in our understanding of the nature of viruses. *Organ culture* is a procedure in which a section of an organ is taken from an intact host and the cells of that organ are kept alive by immersing them in a nutrient fluid in a test tube. This procedure is difficult to carry out and has limited use. The terms *tissue culture* and *cell culture* are often used interchangeably. In the technical sense, however, tissue culture means implanting tissue fragments into test tubes and allowing cells to grow out from these fragments. Cell culture is the most widely used method of growing cells in vitro. A wide variety of tissues can be used, but tissues from embryos generally work best. To produce cell cultures, the tissue is cut into small pieces and treated with an enzyme that splits proteins (proteolytic); this process causes the cells to separate into a suspension of single cells or small clumps of several cells. These cells are then washed, suspended in a nutrient medium, and placed in specially cleaned glass or plastic containers. The cells settle onto and adhere to the surface and begin to divide. Usually after several days a continuous layer, one cell deep (monolayer), will form over the surface. These cells can again be treated with a proteolytic enzyme and the cells of the monolayer will disassociate into a suspension of single cells. The cells can then be passed to new containers where they will continue to multiply. Enough cells can be obtained from one container to seed two or three new containers. Some cells can only be passed five or six times, others up to a hundred, and yet other cells adapt so well to cell cultures that they can be passed indefinitely. One particular cell culture line, called *Hela cells*, was started from human cancer tissue in 1952 and is still being passed at the present time. A procedure for setting up a cell culture is shown in Figure 31-6.

Much current work in virology uses cell cultures for the detection, propagation, and measurement of viruses. When viruses are placed on a monolayer, the cells be-

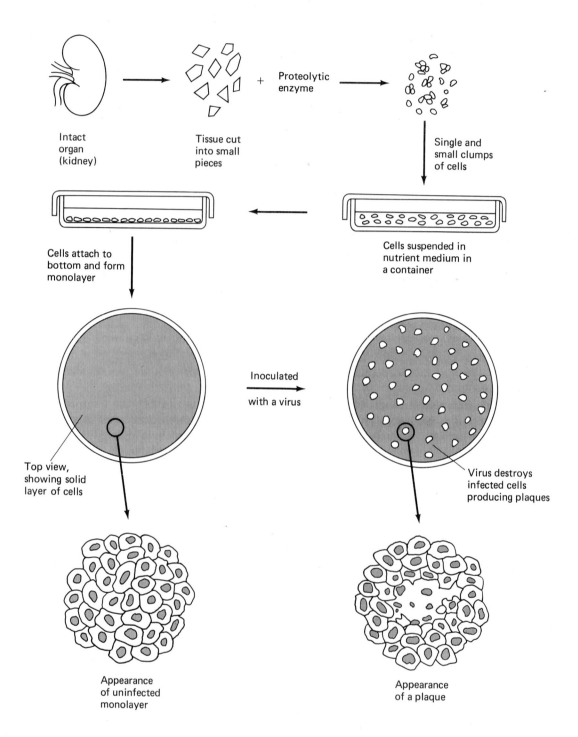

Figure 31-6 A procedure for setting up a cell culture and the production of viral plaques in the cell monolayer.

come infected and are usually destroyed. Different patterns of cell destruction, referred to as the *cytopathic effect*, are produced by different viruses and can be observed with an optical microscope (Figure 31-6). If the viruses are sufficiently dilute, an isolated area of cells in the otherwise continuous monolayer is destroyed. This area of destroyed cells is called a *plaque* and is a useful method of counting the number of viruses in a given sample.

Cell culture procedures are useful in areas of biology other than virology, for cells can be isolated from the complex interactions of an intact animal and studied under controlled conditions in a test tube. The process of isolation and subsequent growth of a single cell taken from a multicellular organism is called *cloning* and has many useful applications in various areas of biology.

MULTIPLICATION OF VIRUSES

When studying the subject of viral multiplication, the virus should be viewed as a segment of genetic information that becomes inserted into the "genetic pool" of the host cell. The only contribution of the virus is a single molecule of nucleic acid (the *viral genome*) and, in some cases, an enzyme for the transcription of this nucleic acid. All other components involved in the multiplication of the virus are supplied by the host cell. Some viruses have a profound effect on the host cell, for they redirect most of the cellular metabolic processes to the production of new viral components. Such a redirection usually results in the destruction of the infected cell. Other viruses may set up a less dramatic relationship in which they do not seriously interfere with the cell's metabolic processes and only redirect a small percentage of the cellular components into the production of new virus particles. Some viruses are able to insert their nucleic acid into the DNA of the host cell, where no influence is manifested and the viral genome replicates and rides along with the DNA of the host cell. In some cases, the viral genome that becomes inserted into the host cell DNA is partially transcribed and imparts specific traits to the host cell.

Throughout all other biological processes in nature protein synthesis is directed by the same reliable mechanism of information contained in double-stranded (ds) DNA molecules being transcribed into single-stranded (ss) *m*RNA molecules, which, in turn, direct the synthesis of polypeptides through the process of translation. These reactions are summarized as ds-DNA $\rightarrow$ *m*RNA $\rightarrow$ protein. When dealing with viruses, however, not only is the conventional ds-DNA $\rightarrow$ *m*RNA $\rightarrow$ protein pathway used but so are a variety of other modified pathways. Viruses can be divided into at least the following six classes, based on the type of nucleic acid they contain and on the pathways used to express their genetic information.

Class 1: Viruses with ds-DNA
The flow of information is ds-DNA $\rightarrow$ *m*RNA $\rightarrow$ protein. This is the classical pathway seen in all higher forms of life. An example of this class of viral multiplication is outlined in Figure 31-7.

Class 2: Viruses with ss-DNA

The flow of information is ss-DNA → ds-DNA → *m*RNA → protein. The ss-DNA must first be changed into ds-DNA, which is done by cellular enzymes after the viral nucleic acid enters the cell. Afterward the flow of information is the same as in Class 1.

Class 3: Viruses with ds-RNA

The flow of information is ds-RNA → *m*RNA → protein. This class of viruses presents a unique problem because ds-RNA is not found in normal cells. Thus no

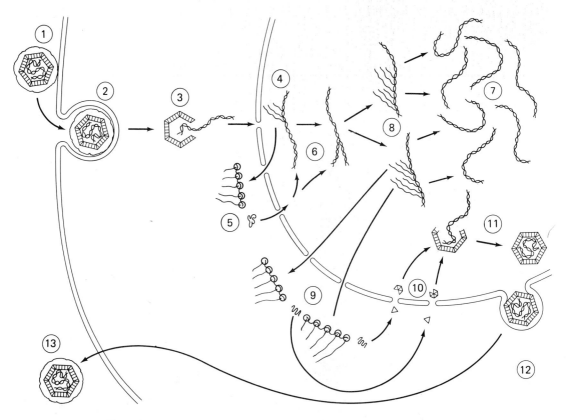

Figure 31-7 Some of the steps in the replication of a ds-DNA virus (i.e., a herpesvirus). (1) Specific attachment. (2) Penetration. (3) Release of viral nucleic acid and its migration to the cell nucleus. (4) Early transcription of viral DNA, directed by cellular enzymes. (5) Translation of viral *m*RNA and synthesis of an enzyme needed to replicate viral DNA. (6) Replication of viral DNA. (7) Synthesis of many viral DNA molecules. (8) Late transcription of viral DNA. (9) Translation of late viral *m*RNA with the synthesis of basic structure units. (10) Formation of capsomers. (11) Assembly of capsid around viral DNA. (12) Budding of virus from the nuclear membrane and picking up of an envelope. (13) Release of virus from the cell. The herpesviruses are able to produce about 500 new viruses in 10 hours from each infected cell.

enzyme is present in a cell to direct the transcription of ds-RNA molecules. To solve this problem, these viruses direct the synthesis of a special enzyme that will transcribe mRNA from the ds-RNA molecule. This enzyme is packaged inside the viral capsid along with the ds-RNA.

Class 4: Viruses with ss-RNA of the same polarity as mRNA (called ss-RNA$^+$)
The information flow is simply mRNA → protein. The viral nucleic acid acts directly as mRNA once inside the cell and completely bypasses the transcription step.

Class 5: Viruses with ss-RNA of the opposite polarity from mRNA (called ss-RNA$^-$)
The information flow is ss-RNA$^-$ → mRNA → protein. As in Class 3, this is a unique situation in which a function not found in a normal cell must be carried out—that is, the transcription of mRNA from a ss-RNA molecule. It is therefore necessary to provide a specific enzyme to accomplish this task. These viruses carry this special enzyme and also direct its formation as part of their replication process. An example of this class is outlined in Figure 31-8.

Class 6: Viruses with ss-RNA$^+$ and a special enzyme called reverse transcriptase or RNA-dependent-DNA polymerase
Viruses of this class are associated with the induction of cancer in the host cells. To do so, they must change the genetic information on their ss-RNA molecule into a ds-DNA molecule or, in other words, move backward from the normal flow of genetic information. The information flow is: ss-RNA → ss-DNA → ds-DNA → mRNA → protein. The enzyme reverse transcriptase is needed for the step from ss-RNA to ss-DNA. Normal cellular enzymes are able to direct the other functions. When the ds-DNA is formed, it may insert into the DNA of the host cell. Under certain conditions that are not well understood some of the information in this inserted DNA may be transcribed and direct changes in the cell that may cause cancer. Under other conditions the inserted DNA may be transcribed and direct the formation of new virus particles.

Steps in Viral Replication

The replication of animal viruses can be divided into the following general steps:

1. *Attachment to the cell surface.* This is a specific reaction and only cells that have the correct receptor site can be infected by a specific virus. This phenomenon accounts for the ability of a virus to infect only a certain animal species or only a given tissue within the infected animal.
2. *Penetration into the cytoplasm.* After attachment has occurred, the plasma membrane invaginates into the cytoplasm and forms a vacuole around the virus. This process is called pinocytosis.

3. *Release of viral nucleic acid.* The viral capsid is broken down by cellular enzymes and the nucleic acid is released. This procedure may occur in either the nucleus or the cytoplasm, depending on the type of virus.

4. *Transcription of viral nucleic acid.* This process occurs in the cytoplasm for some viruses and in the nucleus for others. The various modes of transcription were discussed earlier.

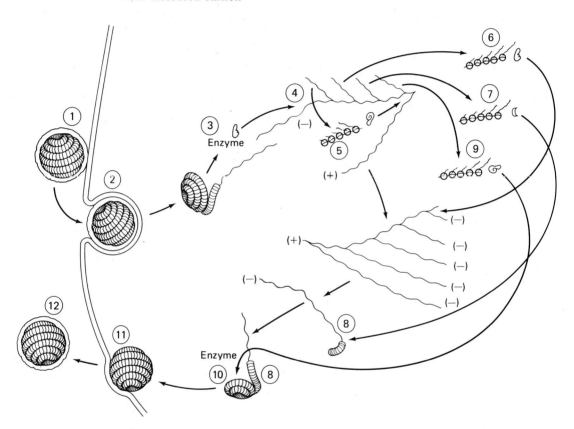

Figure 31-8 An interpretation of some of the major steps in the replication of a ss-RNA virus (i.e., a virus with a ss-RNA molecule of opposite polarity from the *m*RNA and thus it must carry its own enzyme for transcribing *m*RNA). All steps occur in the cytoplasm. (1) Attachment. (2) Penetration. (3) Uncoating with release of viral RNA and enzyme. (4) Transcription of viral RNA to *m*RNAs by the enzyme carried by the virus. (5) Translation of a viral *m*RNA with the formation of an enzyme that will direct the synthesis of complimentary copy of the viral RNA. (6) Synthesis of an enzyme that directs the synthesis of negative ss-RNA copies off the positive copies synthesized in step 5; these negative copies are identical to the original viral RNA. (7) Synthesis of structure units. (8) Formation of helical capsid around the viral RNA. (9) Synthesis of the enzyme to be packaged in the virus. (10) Packaging of enzyme in the virus. (11) Budding capsid and picking up of an envelope. (12) Release of complete virion. Hundreds of viruses are made in each infected cell.

5. *Translation of viral-directed mRNA.* Cellular ribosomes, *t*RNA, amino acids, energy, etc. are used in this step to bring about the synthesis of the proteins needed for the synthesis of new viral particles.

6. *Replication of viral nucleic acid.* One or more proteins produced under the direction of the viral genome function as enzymes for directing the synthesis of new viral nucleic acid molecules. The original viral nucleic acid molecule must serve as a template.

7. *Assembly of virus particles.* Viruses do not replicate by dividing as cells do but are assembled from pools of the viral nucleic acid and protein structure units. Many copies of a virus may be forming simultaneously within a single cell. Assembly may occur in the nucleus or cytoplasm, or partly in one and partly in the other area, depending on the type of virus. Assembly of the protein structure units into capsomers and then into capsids was described earlier. As the capsid forms, it encloses the viral nucleic acid. This process is not efficient, however, and often the capsid forms without enclosing the nucleic acid. It is called an empty virus particle. Often enough viral building blocks are produced to make 10,000 to 20,000 new virus particles per infected cell. Because of the inefficient assembly, however, only 200 to 300 particles will be properly assembled. Yet the entire process may only take an hour or two and several hundred offspring in this time provide an effective means of reproduction.

8. *Release of viruses.* Some viruses are released when the cell disintegrates as a result of the damage produced by the replication process. These viruses would have no envelopes. Other viruses migrate to a cell membrane and bud out through the membrane. The membrane pinches off and remains attached to the virus, thus forming the envelope. With some viruses, viral-directed proteins are formed and become embedded in the cell membrane and thus incorporated into the envelope.

SUMMARY

1. Viruses are submicroscopic structures containing both nucleic acid and protein. These structures are not capable of self-replication but require living host cells for synthesis and development. Hundreds of viruses have been identified, but it is possible that thousands exist. They are known to be responsible for many human, plant, and animal diseases and yet also appear to exist as commensals without harming their host cells.

2. Viruses have specific host cells that they infect. This specificity is determined by viral protein surface structure and corresponding host cell receptors. For convenience in studying viruses, they are frequently cultivated in in vitro organ or cell culture systems.

Introduction to
Viral Diseases

32

The outcome of the multiplication of viruses in an animal host may vary from rapidly progressing destruction of tissues with resulting disease and death to a completely inconsequential relationship in which the viruses multiply at a low level or are dormant and cause no damage or disease. Some general effects of viruses on individual cells and the general characteristics of viral infections are discussed in this chapter.

EFFECTS OF VIRUSES ON CELLS

Cell Destruction

Many viruses enter the host cell and promptly rearrange the cellular components into those needed for the assembly of viruses. These viruses are often able to turn off the metabolic pathways of the cell. The result is a rapid degradation of the cellular components with the resultant disintegration of the cell. This process may require 15 minutes for some viruses to several hours for many others. During this process changes may be observed in the infected cells. Aggregates of viral materials or cell debris may collect in areas of the cell and are called *inclusion bodies*. Characteristic inclusion bodies occur with some viral infections and serve as useful diagnostic aids (Figure 32-1). Usually within a few days these cell-destroying viruses have caused enough damage that symptoms of the clinical disease begin to appear in the host. The common acute viral diseases are caused by these cell-destroying viruses.

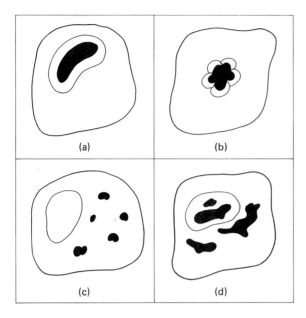

Figure 32-1 Some examples of the types of inclusion bodies formed when different viruses infect cells. (a) Intranuclear inclusions from a herpesvirus infection. (b) A rosette-type intranuclear inclusion from an adenovirus infection. (c) Intracytoplasmic inclusions (Negri bodies) from rabies virus infection. (d) Both intranuclear and intracytoplasmic inclusions in the same cell from a measles virus infection.

Cellular Alterations

Some viruses enter the host cells and replicate without significantly interfering with normal cellular functions. Only about 1% of the cellular components is "pirated" for the production of new viruses. These viruses are gradually released from the cell by budding through the cell membrane without causing apparent damage. With such infections, a balance may be maintained for years between the host cell and the infecting virus. Because of the lack of observable changes, this type of virus–cell relationship has been difficult to study. There is evidence, however, that after many years the host's immune mechanisms may react against these *latently* infected cells. The immune reaction or other effects of the virus may lead to the slow degeneration of the infected tissue. It has now been determined that several chronic degenerative diseases of humans may be caused by such infections, which are called *slow virus infections.* Only two such diseases of humans have been shown to be caused by slow viruses: *Creutzfeldt-Jakob* disease and *Kuru.* Both are rare; Kuru is found only in one tribe of natives living under primitive cannibalistic conditions in New Guinea. There is some indirect evidence that such diseases as multiple sclerosis and muscular distrophy may also be caused by yet-unidentified slow viruses.

Certain DNA viruses are able to enter a cell and their DNA becomes integrated into the DNA of the host cell. This integrated DNA may impart new characteristics to the cell but will not direct the formation of new viruses. This phenomenon has been well studied in bacteriophages and is called *lysogeny.* In some cases, the bacteriophage carries a gene for an important cellular product. The ability to produce diphtheria toxin in the bacterium *C. diphtheriae* is made possible by the presence of a genome from a bacteriophage. The phenomenon of lysogeny is not well documented with animal viruses; however, such DNA viruses as herpes (Chapter 34) and adeno (Chapter 33) seem able to insert their DNA into that of the host cells, where the viral genome may be carried in a latent form for many years. At a later time, when the viral genome is released from the cellular DNA, it may then direct the formation of new viruses with the resultant cell destruction and disease.

Cellular Transformation

A special type of alteration, called *transformation*, may occur following the insertion of viral nucleic acid into host cell DNA. Transformed cells are cancer cells that multiply rapidly and do not respond to the normal mechanisms that control cellular proliferation. The causes of many types of cancer are not known, but animal experiments have shown that certain types are caused by viruses. Well-documented studies have demonstrated that a number of ds-DNA viruses are able to produce tumors in animals. The papovaviruses (Table 32-1) are primarily tumor-producing viruses and certain strains are able to produce tumors in mice, rabbits, and other experimental animals. These tumors are most effectively produced when the papovaviruses are

TABLE 32-1 CLASSIFICATION OF ANIMAL VIRUSES

NA	Symmetry	Envelope	Size (nm)	No. of capsomers	Virus group or family
DNA	Cubical	−	18–24	32	Parvoviruses[a]
		−	45–55	72	Papovaviruses
		−	70–90	252	Adenoviruses
		+	100	162	Herpesviruses
		−	42	?	Hepatitis B
	Complex	−	230 × 300	−	Poxviruses
RNA	Cubic	−	25–29	?	Hepatitis A
		−	20–30	32	Picornaviruses
		−	60–75	32 + 92	Reoviruses[b]
		+	40–60	32	Togaviruses
	Helical	+	80–120	−	Orthomyxoviruses
		+	150–300	−	Paramyxoviruses
		+	60 × 180	−	Rhabdoviruses[c]
	Unknown or unsymmetrical	+	100	−	Retroviruses
		+	50–300	−	Arenaviruses
		+	80–130	−	Coronaviruses

[a] ss-DNA
[b] ds-RNA
[c] Bullet shaped

injected into newborn animals. The only tumors known to be induced in humans by a papovavirus are common warts.

Some human adenoviruses (Chapter 33) have been shown to produce tumors when injected into baby rodents, but there is no evidence of adenovirus-induced cancer in humans. Herpesviruses (Chapter 34) are able to produce cancer in their specific animal hosts. Some herpesviruses of humans are suspected of causing cancer.

At present, there is much interest in the cancer-producing capabilities of the RNA-containing retroviruses (Table 32-1). Retroviruses are the members of replication Class 6 described in Chapter 31. They contain ss-RNA and the reverse transcriptase enzyme. The ability to carry out reverse or *retro* transcription from RNA to DNA is the basis for the current name of this group of viruses. These viruses have also been called leukoviruses and oncornaviruses in recent years. As early as 1910 it was shown that a retrovirus, called *Rous sarcoma virus*, could produce cancer in chickens. In the past few decades retroviruses that cause cancer in mice, cats, baboons, and other experimental animals have been found. At first the induction of cancer by these ss-RNA viruses presented a dilemma, for it is impossible for the ss-RNA molecule to become inserted into the ds-DNA molecules of the host cells. This dilemma was resolved when the phenomenon of reverse transcription was discovered in the 1960s and showed how it is possible to change the genetic information in a ss-RNA molecule into genetic information in a ds-DNA molecule. The ds-DNA molecule is able to insert into the host cell DNA to induce the cellular transformation. Evidence in recent years suggests that certain forms of cancer in humans, primarily leukemia and breast cancer, may be caused by retroviruses.

INTERFERON PRODUCTION

Considering the rapid multiplication of cell-destroying viruses, it would seem that massive numbers of cells of the infected host could be destroyed in a relatively short time. Along with host defense mechanisms, such as phagocytosis and antibody formation, cells have a special built-in defense mechanism that produces a substance called *interferon* that limits the proliferation of viruses. When a virus infects a cell, besides directing the cell to produce more virus, it also induces the cell to produce interferon. The mode of interferon production and action is outlined in Figure 32-2. Interferon is a protein that readily diffuses out of the cell in which it is produced. When it reaches adjacent cells, it attaches to their cell membrane and induces a series of reactions that block the replication of viruses in these cells. Various theories as to how interferon induces resistance to viruses have been proposed, but as yet the exact mechanisms are not known. Interferon induces protection against all viruses, not only the type that stimulated its production, and is thus nonspecific in its action. It has little if any effect on normal cellular activities. Thus interferon may prove an effective antiviral chemotherapeutic agent and, in fact, much effort has been made to

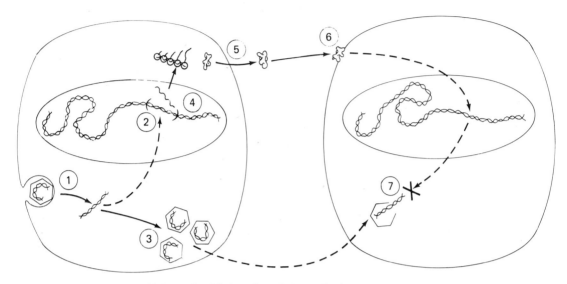

Figure 32-2   A simplified outline of the production and action of interferon. (1) Viral or chemical inducer of interferon enters the cell. (2) The virus induces derepression of the interferon-producing gene. (3) New viruses produced and released from cell. (4) *m*RNA for interferon synthesized. (5) Interferon produced and secreted from cell. (6) Interferon binds to wall of adjacent cells. (7) The binding triggers secondary reactions that induce mechanisms that interfere with the replication of any viruses that might enter this cell.

use interferon in treating viral infections. A major limitation is the species specificity of interferon; that is, interferon produced by human cells will induce protection only in other human cells. Therefore it has not been possible to produce interferon in such hosts as experimental animals or embryonated eggs for use in treating humans. In the 1970s methods were developed for producing some interferon in human white blood cells and fibroblasts grown in cell culture systems. This interferon was effective in treating some human viral infections, but only small amounts could be produced, which made treatments very expensive. Most applications were limited to research trials. Another limitation is the short duration of protection offered by interferon, which is about 2 weeks.

Certain chemicals are also able to induce interferon production in intact hosts. The most efficient stimulator is ds-RNA molecules; artificial ds-RNA molecules that appear to be nontoxic can be produced. When injected into animals, this ds-RNA stimulates the production of interferon and the animals are made more resistant to viral infections for several weeks. It is also possible to inhale aerosols of ds-RNA and stimulate the production of interferon along the mucosal tissues of the respiratory tract. Such a procedure may be able to give temporary protection against a wide variety of viral respiratory infections. If applied to a large segment of the population in advance of a respiratory disease epidemic, it may be possible to dampen or abort the epidemic.

It is now possible to insert human interferon genes into microorganisms, using recombinant DNA procedures. These genetically engineered microbes are able to produce relatively large quantities of human-specific interferon. It is hoped that the interferon from this source will provide an effective and economically feasible means of treating the numerous viral infections of humans. Some evidence from research studies indicates that interferon might also be helpful in treating certain forms of cancer.

SIGNIFICANCE OF VIRAL DISEASES

Most infectious diseases of humans are caused by viruses. Fortunately, many are not serious; that is, they are not life threatening and they do not require hospitalization. Still, they cause discomfort and incapacitation and are disruptive overall to normal human activities. Many serious problems still result from viral infections; however, several more serious viral diseases have been either eradicated or greatly reduced through active immunization programs. Smallpox, once the greatest killer of all viral diseases, has been completely eradicated. Such diseases as poliomyelitis, measles, and rubella, which up until the past few decades caused many deaths and left thousands crippled or impaired, have been greatly reduced in number.

Most viral diseases are unresponsive to antibiotics or other "wonder" drugs that are so effective in treating bacterial infections. And most treatments are symptomatic—that is, use procedures that reduce the discomfort and maintain the proper physiological functions of the body. Recovery results primarily from the patient's own natural defense mechanisms. Procedures or activities that would weaken the host, such as malnourishment, lack of sleep, and immunosuppressive drugs, should be avoided. Vaccines are very effective in preventing some viral infections. Viral infections may cause sufficient tissue damage to predispose a patient to secondary bacterial infections. In such cases, chemotherapy to combat the bacterial complications would be appropriate.

The impact of viral diseases on humans is most apparent with infections of the respiratory tract. It is estimated that about 75% of all infectious diseases are of the respiratory tract and about 80% of them are caused by viruses. A great majority of these viral infections are of the upper respiratory tract and cause such clinical diseases as common colds (rhinitis) and sore throats (pharyngitis). A fair number of infections, however, involve the lower respiratory tract and may cause serious problems, particularly in infants and small children. Approximately 150 different viruses are associated with these respiratory infections and it is estimated that, on the average, each person will experience about six such infections per year. Because of these infections, approximately 100 million work days are lost per year in the United States. In addition, they are responsible for 50% of the absences from school and a third of all patient visits to general practitioners or clinics. Most of these common respiratory infections occur during the cooler months with peak incidences in the winter, al-

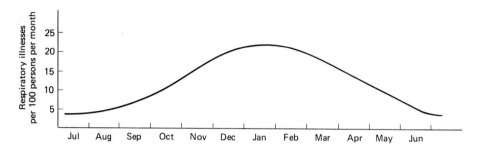

Figure 32-3 An approximate representation of the number of respiratory illnesses during each month of the year in persons living in the United States.

though some are seen year-round (Figure 32-3). The second most prevalent type of viral disease involves the gastrointestinal tract. Well over 50% of the cases of gastroenteritis in humans are caused by viruses; and viral gastroenteritis is a major cause of death of undernourished infants. Should the interferon produced by recombinant DNA procedures prove effective in treating these common viral diseases, it would constitute one of the major medical advances in the history of mankind.

CLASSIFICATION OF VIRUSES

It is possible to classify viruses into groups or families of related members according to chemical and morphological characteristics. Table 32-1 shows the major groups or families of animal viruses based on the following characteristics: type of nucleic acid, symmetry of capsid, presence or absence of an envelope, size of virion, and number of capsomers if the symmetry is cubical. The use of binomial Latin names for species is not well established in virology and attempts to introduce Latinized names have met with varying degrees of success. The Latinized ending *viridae* is becoming accepted for the families of viruses. At the genus level, "un-Latinized" names that are descriptive of the disease caused by the virus or some other feature of the virus are generally used. The species or subspecies level is usually designated by a letter or number after the genus level name. Thus viruses might be referred to as adenovirus 4 or 7, and influenza A or B, and so on.

Some species of each group listed in Table 32-1 cause diseases in humans. The papovaviruses and retroviruses are primarily associated with cancer and their possible role as causative agents of cancer in humans is still under investigation.

The viruses causing important diseases of humans will be discussed in the following chapters. The diseases caused by DNA viruses are presented first, followed by those caused by RNA viruses.

SUMMARY

1. Infection of cells by virus particles may lead to a variety of cellular responses ranging from latent infection through cell transformation to cellular destruction. Whatever the relationship, it seems to favor the development and survival of the viral species.

2. Viral infection of mammalian cells results in the production of a viral inhibitor called interferon. This host defense mechanism results in the reduction or even cessation of virus reproduction and is frequently responsible for initiation of recovery from or prevention of further viral attack.

Adenoviruses and Poxviruses

33

Viruses of both the adeno and pox groups contain ds-DNA. Adenoviruses cause some of the common respiratory diseases of humans. The major disease caused by poxviruses is smallpox, a disease that has been eradicated as a result of extensive immunization efforts.

ADENOVIRUSES

Adenoviruses are widespread in nature and currently 33 distinct serotypes have been isolated from humans. They are designated types 1, 2, etc. to 33. Different adenoviruses are also found in various avian and mammalian species. The adenoviruses were so named because they were first isolated from tonsils and adenoids. Many adenoviruses have been shown as the cause of some common upper respiratory infections of humans. Less frequently, they may cause infections in other tissues. The adenoviruses have the ability to remain sequestered in lymphatic tissues long after the primary exposure. About 50% of surgically removed tonsils and adenoids are found to contain some of these latent adenoviruses.

General Properties of the Viruses

Adenoviruses have a distinct appearance and can often be identified by direct observation with an electron microscope (Figure 33-1). The capsid is 60 to 90 nm in diameter, has cubical symmetry with 252 capsomers, and has no envelope. These viruses

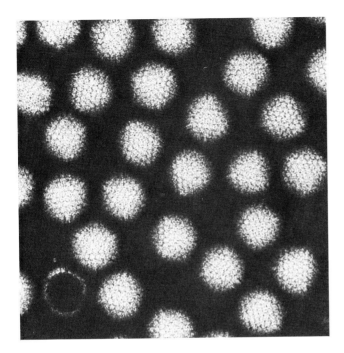

Figure 33-1 Transmission electron micrograph of adenoviruses magnified 150,000×. (Courtesy Robley C. Williams, University of California, Berkeley)

contain ds-DNA and can be cultivated in various types of cell cultures. Adenoviruses are quite stable and are able to survive for long periods once expelled from a host.

Pathogenesis and Clinical Diseases

Acute respiratory diseases

Close to 100% of the children living under crowded conditions become infected with adenoviruses early in life. The infectivity rates are less, but still 50% or more, in children living in less crowded conditions. About half the infected children develop definite clinical symptoms. The most common clinical disease is an acute respiratory infection with such common symptoms as sore throat, cough, runny nose (coryza), and headache. Tonsillitis and pneumonia may be seen occasionally. Adenovirus infections are also seen in adults but generally are less frequent and less severe.

A unique form of acute respiratory disease caused by adenoviruses is seen in military-recruit-training centers. Quite typically, military recruits begin to develop adenovirus infections after several weeks of training and during the next month or so more than 80% of the recruits may experience this respiratory disease syndrome. Symptoms may last up to 10 days; overall this disease may be quite disruptive to the recruit-training program. Typically outbreaks among the recruits are caused by type 4 adenovirus and less often by type 7. Paradoxically type 4 is rarely associated with disease in civilian populations. The reason for this unique epidemiologic pattern among military recruits is not known but may be associated with assembling large numbers of young persons from diverse backgrounds and subjecting them to the crowding and "stresses" of military life.

Pharyngoconjunctival fever and keratoconjunctivitis

Adenovirus-induced pharyngoconjunctival fever is a disease characterized by fever, conjunctivitis (inflammation of the eyelids), and sore throat. This disease occurs in sporadic outbreaks associated with swimming pools, summer camps, and small lakes. It usually involves children and young adults. All evidence indicates that transmission is by direct contact with contaminated water. Several outbreaks have occurred in swimming pools that were not properly chlorinated. The incubation period is 6 to 9 days.

Keratoconjunctivitis is an infection transmitted by adenovirus-contaminated instruments or medications in ophthalmological (eye) clinics. The adenoviruses are quite stable and often survive disinfection procedures that use alcohol and many other common chemical disinfectants. This syndrome starts with inflammation of the eyelid and spreads to the cornea. Damage to the cornea may lead to impaired vision. The incubation period is 8 to 10 days.

Besides their extensive multiplication in the respiratory tract, adenoviruses are also apparently able to grow in and are shed from the intestinal tract. Current evidence indicates that they are associated with gastroenteritis.

Transmission

Spread is from person to person by direct and indirect contact. The fecal-oral route is probably a major means of spread in children and the airborne route in all age groups. Contact with contaminated materials is the major route of transmission for eye infections.

Diagnosis

Adenoviruses can be isolated on a variety of cell cultures. Isolation should be correlated with a specific rise in antibody titer before an adenovirus can be considered the cause of a specific disease, for adenoviruses are frequently isolated from healthy persons. Adenovirus respiratory infections in the general population cannot be distinguished on clinical grounds from the many respiratory infections caused by a variety of other infectious agents. The specific laboratory tests required to identify an adenovirus infection are generally not done.

Treatment

No treatment is available other than measures taken to relieve symptoms.

Control and Prevention

Only in military-recruit-training centers are measures taken to prevent adenovirus infections. A live attenuated vaccine against types 4 and 7, when given by the oral route to military recruits, has successfully controlled the epidemics of acute respiratory disease syndrome caused by these viruses. This vaccine is not used in civilian populations.

Eye clinics should use proper methods of sterilization and asepsis to prevent the spread of adenoviruses.

CLINICAL NOTE

Adenovirus Type 7 Outbreak in a Pediatric Chronic-Care Facility: Pennsylvania, 1982

In July 1982, an outbreak of respiratory disease caused by adenovirus type 7 (Ad 7) occurred in a chronic-care facility in a pediatric hospital in Pennsylvania. On June 6, a physician, the presumed index case, developed infected conjunctiva; 2 days later, conjunctivitis; and on June 12, an acute upper-respiratory-tract illness [(URI) coryza and/or pharyngitis]. Between June 15 and July 9, four of the 14 children in the facility became ill with an acute respiratory illness characterized by either URI or lower-respiratory-tract illness [(LRI) fever and respiratory distress]. These four, and three other asymptomatic children, were culture-positive for Ad 7. Three of the four ill children had LRI and required mechanical ventilation; one with congenital heart disease and one with bronchopulmonary dysplasia died. In addition, three of the other 35 staff members (physicians, nurses, and play therapists) developed acute URI, and Ad 7 was isolated from cultures from two of them.

The chronic-care facility has a nurses' station, treatment room, playroom, and three patient rooms—with four, six, and seven beds, respectively. All 14 children remained in the facility throughout the outbreak. Culture-positive children resided in two of the three rooms.

The index case had contact with all 14 children on June 6 and 7 and from June 14 on. Both culture-positive staff members had contact with the first ill child as early as June 15. Ultimately, one of these staff members had contact with all seven culture-positive and three of seven culture-negative children. The other had contact with three culture-positive children and one culture-negative child. When these staff members became ill, they were excluded from patient contact. When the extent of the outbreak was recognized on June 22, children culture-positive for Ad 7 were moved into one room, and staff members with acute respiratory illness were excluded from contact with the children (*MMWR 32:*258, 1983).

POXVIRUSES

Poxviruses are large, 250×300 nm, brick-shaped, DNA-containing viruses. Many animal species have their own specific poxvirus infections, usually in the form of lesions (pocks) on the skin. The major poxvirus of humans is the variola virus that causes the disease of smallpox (Figure 33-2).

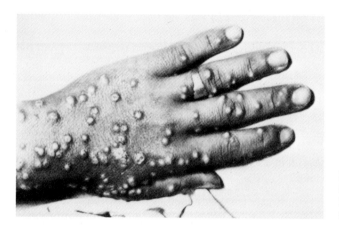

Figure 33-2 Lesions (pox) on the hand of a patient with smallpox. (Armed Forces Institute of Pathology, AFIP MIS #CA 44271-3)

Smallpox

Smallpox has been one of the most devastating diseases of humans. History is replete with reports of epidemics in which more than 50% of the inhabitants of a city or country developed smallpox, with as many as half the infected dying of the disease.

A new milestone in medical science was achieved with the eradication of smallpox from the world. It marks the first time that society has been able to eradicate a major infectious disease deliberately. Because future workers in medicine will not encounter smallpox, the pathogenesis transmission, diagnosis, and control of this disease will not be discussed. Instead a historical synopsis of the control of smallpox is presented with emphasis on those concepts that may be helpful in understanding the control of infectious disease in general.

The Control of Smallpox

Before the nineteenth century, smallpox was controlled in a limited way by purposely inoculating persons who had not yet contracted it with a mild form of the disease. The severe form of smallpox was called *variola major* and the mild form *variola minor* or *alastrim*. Recovery from either form conferred immunity against both forms. Inoculation with variola minor usually caused mild symptoms with a fatality rate of "only" 1 to 2%. Many considered it an acceptable risk compared to that of contracting and dying of smallpox. This practice of purposely inoculating persons with variola minor, called *variolation*, was pursued in Africa and Asia from ancient times and was used to a limited extent in some areas of North America during the eighteenth century.

The most significant contribution toward the eventual control of smallpox was the development of the vaccination procedure by Edward Jenner in 1796 (see Chapter 1), using the cowpox virus. Afterward the practice of vaccination against smallpox became widespread in most developed countries and a steady decline in the total number of cases occurred over the past 190 years. The last cases of smallpox seen in the

United States were in the lower Rio Grande Valley in 1949. The final struggle with smallpox began in 1966 when the World Health Organization embarked on a program of complete eradication of this disease. Much of the program's success was made possible by the development of a freeze-dried form of vaccine that was stable without refrigeration as well as effective, easy-to-learn, inexpensive methods of administering the vaccine. These developments made it possible to carry out effective vaccination programs in remote areas of the world. As a result of this concentrated eradication program, by 1972 all countries in North and South America were free of smallpox. By 1975 only Bangladesh, Ethiopia, and surrounding areas reported cases. After a slight reversal in early 1977, this eradication program has moved to its apparently successful conclusion. Based on current information (see Clinical Note), the last person to have a naturally acquired case of smallpox was a hospital cook in Somalia who came down with the disease in October 1977. After a 2-year waiting period in which no new cases occurred, the world was officially declared free of smallpox in October 1979 (see Clinical Note). Actually, the last known cases of smallpox occurred from accidental infections in a research laboratory in England in 1978. Now only four reference laboratories possess the smallpox virus and its use is stringently controlled.

Although smallpox was a severe and highly contagious disease, it possessed features that permitted its successful eradication. First, the disease was easily recognized and few if any subclinical cases occurred. This factor was a help in detection and diagnosis. Second, the virus did not remain in the body as a latent infection after the patient recovered from the clinical disease. Third, no regular nonhuman host could act as a reservoir of the virus. Fourth, an effective, easily administered vaccine was available, and, fifth, the virus does not readily mutate.

The most notable result of this eradication program in countries where smallpox was not normally found was the discontinuation of routine smallpox vaccination. The smallpox vaccination used a living virus and caused a mild infection in those vaccinated. In some persons, mostly young children with compromised host defense mechanisms, the vaccine might cause moderate-to-severe infections. Before smallpox vaccination was discontinued in the United States in 1971, about 500 children per year developed a serious vaccine-associated disease and about a dozen deaths would occur. Thus for many years in the United States and many other countries, many more children suffered or died from the ill effects of the vaccine than from the disease itself.

CLINICAL NOTE

Smallpox Certification: East Africa, October 26, 1979

Two years ago today the world's last known patient with endemic smallpox had an onset of rash. Ali Maow Maalin, a cook at the district hospital in Merka, Somalia, developed smallpox on October 26, 1977. Since then, intensive surveillance has failed to identify any additional cases of naturally transmitted smallpox.

Separate international commissions assessed campaigns in the last four countries requiring certification of eradication: Somalia, Kenya, Ethiopia, and Djibouti. In Nairobi the chairpersons of these commissions made their reports to the Director-General of the World Health Organization. The Horn of Africa is now certified as smallpox free. This meeting completed the documentation required to certify global eradication of smallpox (*MMWR 28*:497, 1979). (This documentation was reviewed by the Global Commission for Smallpox Eradication from December 6–9, 1979, in Geneva. The criteria for global eradication were met, and documentation was presented to the World Health Assembly in May 1980 for final global certification of smallpox eradication. To 1984, no new cases of smallpox have occurred.)

SUMMARY

1. Over 33 types of adenoviruses have been discovered. These DNA viruses are responsible for a variety of upper respiratory infections in humans that may be severe but are usually self-limiting.
2. Smallpox, a life-threatening infection of the DNA pox virus, has been eradicated from the ranks of human illness. Careful, thorough, and prolonged immunization efforts have apparently rid the world of this once dread disease.

Herpesviruses

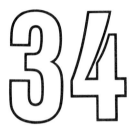

Members of the herpesvirus group are widespread in nature and infect many animal species. These viruses are usually host specific; that is, the human herpesviruses cause natural infections only in humans and not other animals and vice versa. On rare occasions, monkey herpesviruses have caused fatal infections in humans.

The common diseases of humans caused by herpesviruses are cold sores or fever blisters, chickenpox, and infectious mononucleosis. Exposure to these viruses generally occurs in the first decade of life and the resulting infection may be apparent or subclinical. An important characteristic of these viruses is their ability to remain sequestered inside certain cells long after the primary infection is resolved. These latent infections may persist for the life of the person with no further clinical symptoms or they may cause sporadic recurrences of clinical symptoms. Such latent infections allow these viruses to remain everpresent in a population, to be passed on to new susceptible individuals.

The four human herpes viruses—herpes simplex, varicella-zoster, cytomegalo, and Epstein-Barr—are discussed in this chapter.

GENERAL PROPERTIES OF THE VIRUSES

The capsid of the herpesviruses has cubical symmetry with 162 capsomers and is surrounded by an envelope (Figure 34-1). The capsid has a diameter of 100 nm. The herpesviruses are fairly unstable and become inactivated within hours, at room tem-

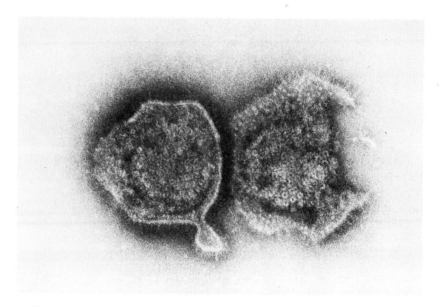

Figure 34-1 Transmission electron micrograph of herpesviruses showing icosahedral capsids (partially disrupted) surrounded by envelopes (magnified 160,000×). (Courtesy Robley C. Williams, University of California, Berkeley)

perature, after being shed from the body. The nucleic acid is double-stranded DNA and the viruses multiply in the nucleus of the host cell. This association of foreign DNA with the nucleus of host cells has provided theoretical evidence that herpesviruses may induce cancer. Some forms of cancer in lower animals are associated with these viruses and several lines of evidence associate herpes viruses, particularly the Epstein-Barr virus, with certain forms of cancer in humans.

Because cancer may be induced by the double-stranded DNA of the herpes viruses, there has been a reluctance to develop vaccines produced from the whole viruses, for the use of such vaccines would result in the introduction of relatively large amounts of this DNA into the tissues of humans. It has not been economically feasible in the past to produce herpes vaccines containing only the viral protein antigens. Yet theoretical and experimental evidence strongly suggests that antibodies against these protein antigens will offer protection against primary herpes infections. Because of advances in recombinant DNA technology, it is now possible to insert into bacteria or yeast cells the herpes virus genes that direct the formation of the viral antigens. These engineered microorganisms should be able to produce large amounts of inexpensive viral antigens that can be purified and used as vaccines. Using this technology, it is possible that effective vaccines against the major herpes virus diseases may soon be developed.

HERPES SIMPLEX VIRUSES

Two serotypes of herpes simplex viruses (HSV) have been identified. Type 1 is generally associated with infections of the upper half of the body and type 2 with infection of the genitourinary tract and surrounding tissues. Both types may cause generalized infections in infants and compromised patients.

Pathogenesis and Clinical Diseases

Cold sores or *fever blisters* (herpes labialis) are among the most common of all human infections and are caused by the type 1 HSV (Figure 34-2). The recurring lesions on the lips are the clinical manifestation of a complex chronic interaction between the virus and the host. Infants become susceptible to the primary infection after they have lost their passive immunity at about 6 months of age. They are then highly susceptible until about 18 months of age and have decreasing susceptibility to about 6 years of age; after this age, humans become relatively resistant to primary infection. Nevertheless, over 80% of the population has had a primary infection before reaching this resistant age. The primary infection is often asymptomatic or is not diagnosed as herpes. Symptoms are seen in 10 to 15% of the cases from 2 to 12 days after being exposed to the virus. The primary lesions may appear as small vesicles in the

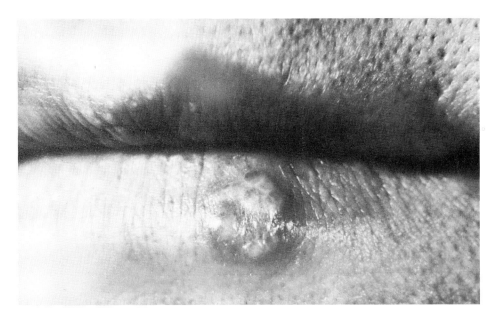

Figure 34-2 Herpes simplex fever blister on lower lip two days after onset (Centers for Disease Control, Atlanta)

throat, mouth, or nose and go relatively unnoticed. The most noticeable form of primary infection involves the lips, mouth, and gums (gingivostomatitis), in which the vesicles rupture and develop into ulcerative lesions. Fever, pain, and irritability usually persist for about 1 week, followed by gradual healing during the second week.

Recovery is associated with a rise in antibodies against the virus. During the primary infection, however, the virus apparently passes along nerve fibers to regional ganglia. In the case of gingivostomatitis, the trigeminal ganglion is commonly involved and the virus may become sequestered in a latent form in this tissue. While in this latent form, the virus cannot be detected by ordinary means during life. It causes no symptoms and is not affected by antibodies. Periodically, in from 20 to 30% of the general population, these latent viruses become activated and move down the nerve fiber to cause recurring skin lesions at the site of the original infection (Figure 34-3). The frequency of these recurring lesions varies from person to person, ranging from once every few years to about once a month. Various stressful stimuli, such as excessive sunlight, fever, cold winds, emotional stress, and hormonal changes, apparently trigger the reactivation of the virus. As the virus moves down the nerve fibers, it passes directly into the skin cells without becoming exposed to the host's antibodies. The antibodies do prevent the virus from spreading to other tissues of the body but are unable to prevent the recurring lesions.

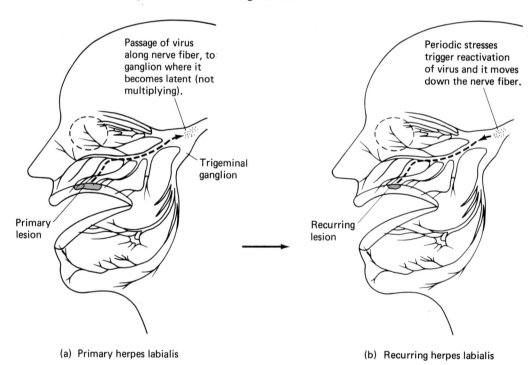

(a) Primary herpes labialis   (b) Recurring herpes labialis

Figure 34-3   Aspects of the pathogenesis of primary and recurring herpes infections of the lips.

Primary and recurring infections may also occur in the eyes, causing a disease known as *herpetic keratoconjunctivitis*. Lesions on the cornea are most serious, for the accumulating scar tissue may lead to vision impairment. This disease is a major cause of blindness in the United States today.

Occasionally almost any tissue of the body may become infected with these viruses. Primary and recurring infections may occur on any cutaneous area of the body. Traumatic injury may provide a portal of entry for primary infections that may develop in both children and adults. Such infections have been seen in wrestlers (herpes gladiatorum) due to skin abrasions, or in persons following burns, or on the thumb of a thumb-sucking child or the finger of a dentist (herpetic whitlow). Children with eczema may acquire a serious herpes infection over large areas of the body (eczema herpeticum). Herpes simplex viruses may also infect the central nervous system, causing a severe, and often fatal, infection (herpetic encephalitis).

A disseminated form of herpes occasionally occurs in newborns, particularly premature infants, and here the virus spreads throughout the body. These infections are usually fatal. Infections are acquired most often during birth as the infant passes through an infected birth canal. Disseminated herpes may also occur in patients of any age when they become immunosuppressed.

Today *genital herpes* is recognized as a very common sexually transmitted disease. Over 90% of these infections are caused by HSV type 2. In females the vesicles usually occur in the mucosal tissue of the vulva, vagina, or cervix, but any of the genital or surrounding tissues may be involved. These vesicles ulcerate, producing shallow lesions. The symptoms may include malaise, urinary retention, local pain, fever, vaginal discharge, and tender, swollen inguinal lymph nodes. In males the vesicles and subsequent ulcerations develop on the penis and surrounding tissues. These infections heal spontaneously in 1 to 2 weeks. Recurrent infections are common but are generally milder than the primary infection. All ages seem susceptible to genital herpes.

Transmission

HSV type 1 is transmitted by direct contact or by indirect contact on such objects as eating utensils. A typical mode of transmission is for an adult with an active recurring lesion to kiss or fondle a young child. Large numbers of viruses are present in the vesicular fluid and exudate from the ulcerative lesions. Transmission within family units is difficult to prevent. Some persons may be intermittent subclinical shedders of HSV, which further complicates attempts to prevent transmission of this agent. In general, transmission is much more efficient among persons living in crowded, unsanitary conditions.

HSV type 2 is spread among adults primarily by sexual contact and in the current sexually permissive societies the numbers of cases have increased alarmingly. HSV type 2 can be isolated from 10 to 15% of the patients who visit venereal disease clinics. Infected females may transmit this virus to infants during delivery. Such neonatally acquired HSV type 2 infections are generally serious and often result in death of the infant.

Diagnosis

Most diagnoses are made on the clinical appearance. Disseminated infections and atypical complicated cases often require a laboratory diagnosis. This diagnosis involves isolating HSV from the lesion during the first 5 days of illness or, in the case of encephalitis, direct fluorescent antibody determinations on biopsied brain tissue. HSV multiplies well in commonly used cell cultures. A correlation of antibody titers (a significant rise) is often needed to confirm a diagnosis, for these viruses may be found in normal-appearing tissues. HSV produces a characteristic inclusion body in the nucleus of infected cells; such intranuclear inclusions may be seen on microscopic examination of stained cells that are scraped from a suspected lesion.

Treatment

The herpetic infection of the cornea was the first viral infection to be routinely treated by chemotherapy. The chemical *iododeoxyuridine*, used in corneal infections, interferes with the replication of herpesviruses by inhibiting DNA synthesis. When applied to the surface of the cornea every hour or two, it may greatly reduce the severity of infection. This agent has been successfully used since the mid-1960s to prevent the scarring that leads to impaired vision. Questionable success has been obtained by treating herpes infections of other tissues with this chemical.

A second antiviral compound called *adenine arabinoside* is now licensed for use in the United States. This compound is also effective in treating eye infections when applied to the surface of the cornea; when given systemically (injected into the blood) early in the illness, it reduces the mortality from herpes encephalitis. A third compound called *acyclovir* is also available and appears to be an effective agent for treating genital herpes infections. While this compound reduces symptoms, it will not cure the infection or prevent reoccurrence. Many ointments and solutions are used to gain symptomatic relief from herpetic lesions but have no direct effect on the virus.

Prevention and Control

Whenever possible, persons with active herpetic lesions should avoid contact with young children. Children with primary lesions should be isolated from other children until the lesions have healed. Pregnant females with genital herpetic infections often have a Caesarean delivery to help avoid infecting the newborn.

Current evidence suggests that antibodies are able to prevent the primary infection but not the recurring lesions. This finding has stimulated research on a possible vaccine that could be given to young children before they lose their passive immunity.

If the primary infection were prevented in children, then it would follow that the recurring lesions later in life would also be prevented.

VARICELLA-ZOSTER VIRUS (V-Z VIRUS)

This herpesvirus is the causative agent of both chickenpox (varicella) and shingles (zoster), hence the double name. For many years it was thought that these two diseases were unrelated. Now it is known that chickenpox is the acute primary form of the disease complex whereas shingles is a delayed recurrent form of the same infection (Figure 34-4). Only a single serotype of the V-Z virus exists.

Pathogenesis and Clinical Diseases

Chickenpox
The V-Z virus enters the respiratory tract by the airborne route. The virus then apparently passes through the lymphatic system and is disseminated throughout the body via the bloodstream. The extent of viral multiplication and the tissues involved during the early stages of the incubation period have not been well documented. After an incubation period of 2 to 3 weeks, the virus is found to be multiplying in numerous foci of the deep skin and in the throat. General discomfort, together with a sore throat, may occur a day or so before the appearance of a macular (flat) rash on the skin. Within 24 hours the rash develops into vesicles. The vesicles form into pustules within the next 24 hours. The lesions next form scabs that fall off after a few days. Successive crops of vesicles develop and all stages of the lesions may be seen simultaneously (Figure 34-5). After about 5 days the lesions begin to disappear. Scarring usually does not result without secondary bacterial infection. The intense itching often causes scratching that, in turn, may lead to secondary bacterial infection with accompanying inflammation and scarring.

Chickenpox rarely has serious complications in otherwise healthy children. Occasionally a serious condition called *Reye's syndrome* develops during the recovery period and consists of diffuse metabolic and neurologic malfunctions. Chickenpox, however, can be severe or fatal in newborn infants, children with leukemia, or in other immunosuppressed patients. Infections in adults are more severe than in children, with varicella pneumonia being a much more frequent complication. Recovery confers lifelong immunity to reinfection. Nevertheless, the antibodies do not remove the viruses that become sequestered in the ganglia.

Shingles
Shingles is a recurrent clinical manifestation of a latent-dormant infection with the V-Z virus. Analogous to the latent infections with the herpes simplex virus, the V-Z virus is apparently able to become sequestered in neuroganglia following a typical

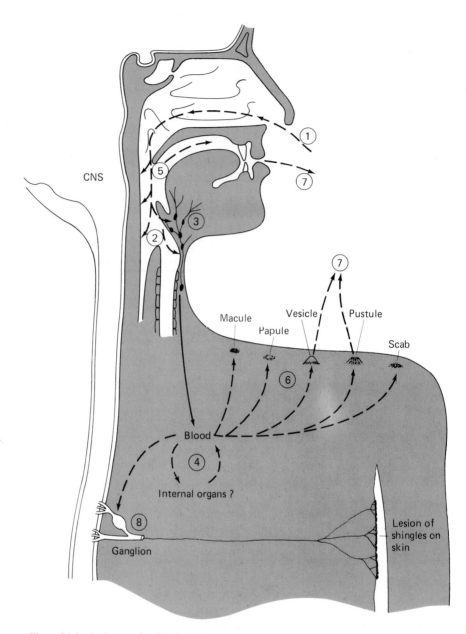

Figure 34-4 Pathogenesis of Varicella-Zoster. (1) Virus enters by airborne route. (2) Early viral multiplication in upper respiratory tract; no symptoms and patient not infectious. (3) Passage of virus into regional lymph nodes. (4) Passage of virus to blood and spread to various internal organs. (5) Several days before pock formation virus may be found in respiratory tract; patient may be infectious. (6) Virus deposited in the epithelial tissues with resultant pock formation; this occurs 14 to 21 days after exposure. (7) Virus shed from the respiratory tract and from the pocks. (8) Virus becomes sequestered in neural ganglia and remains latent. At a later time the virus may become active and moves along the sensory nerves to cause the localized lesions of shingles.

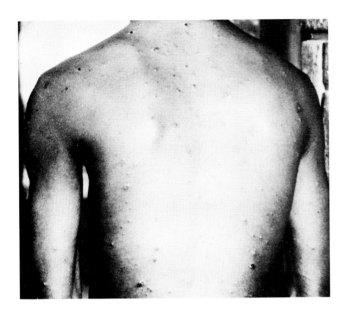

Figure 34-5 Chickenpox three days after onset of rash. Lesion in different stages of development can be seen. (Centers for Disease Control, Atlanta)

acute chickenpox infection. The V-Z virus may lie dormant for many years before it becomes reactivated. More than 65% of the cases occur in persons over 45 years of age; however, reactivation may occur at any age. Usually a person has only a single attack of shingles, but second episodes occasionally develop. The mechanisms of reactivation are not understood. One theory is that it may be associated with a waning of the acquired immunity. Shingles is much more common in persons who are immunosuppressed or who have irradiation or injuries to the spine. After the virus becomes activated, it moves down the sensory nerve leading from the infected ganglion. This step is accompanied by an abnormal sensation and/or pain over the area served by the involved nerve (dermatome). Several days later the eruption occurs (Figure 34-6) and is confined to the involved dermatome. The distribution is often in a band (*zoster* girdle) on one side of the body with an abrupt margin at midline (Figure 34-7). The skin involvement progresses through the rash, vesicular, pustular, and crusting stages, often fusing together into large lesions. Pain associated with the neurologic involvement may be severe for 1 to 4 weeks. Recovery occurs in 2 to 5 weeks with pain persisting (postzoster neuralgia) in some elderly patients for an additional period of time. The skin of the trunk and face are the areas most often affected.

Transmission

Chickenpox is one of the most communicable of all childhood diseases and most children become infected before the age of 10. The airborne route is the major means of transmission. Viruses are present in respiratory secretions, possibly a day or more before the appearance of a rash. Children are generally isolated after the rash ap-

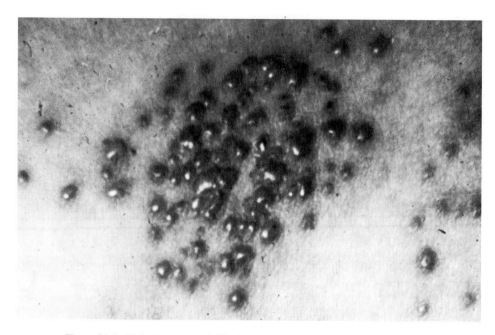

Figure 34-6 Vesicular lesions of shingles. (Centers for Disease Control, Atlanta)

pears; however, the V-Z virus may have already been spread by respiratory droplets to school mates and friends during the prodromal (onset) period. Viruses are also found in the vesicular fluid and pustular exudate during the first week of illness. Viruses are readily spread from this source by both direct and indirect contact and outbreaks are much more prevalent in the winter and spring (Figure 34-8).

Shingles is not transmitted from person to person; however, viruses are shed from the zoster lesions and susceptible children are able to contract chickenpox from this source. Thus the reactivation of the V-Z virus in zoster patients serves as a source that reintroduces the virus into a given population year after year.

Diagnosis

Chickenpox is usually diagnosed on clinical appearance. Occasionally an atypical case may require laboratory diagnosis. Clinically chickenpox resembles smallpox; when both diseases were present, it was important to make a rapid differential diagnosis. Since the eradication of smallpox, it is no longer important.

Diagnosis of zoster may be difficult in the early stages. Even in the later stages it may occasionally be confused with other skin infections. In such cases, it may be necessary to isolate and identify the virus by laboratory procedures.

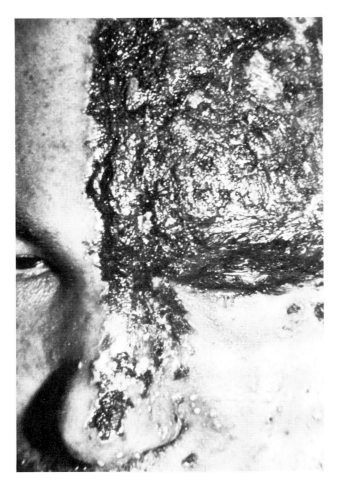

Figure 34-7 Shingles with extensive scab formation in a college-age student about 12 days after onset. Classical midline distribution is seen.

Treatment

No specific antiviral treatments are currently available; but based on clinical trials, acyclovir may be effective in treating disseminated infection in immunosuppressed patients. Symptomatic relief to relieve itching may be obtained with ointments. Secondary bacterial infections should be treated with antibiotic ointments.

Control and Prevention

No vaccines are currently available, but a living attenuated vaccine is in the testing stages of development and vaccines produced by recombinant DNA method may soon be developed. High-risk susceptible children, such as newborns or those who are immunosuppressed, who have been exposed to the V-Z virus may have the infection

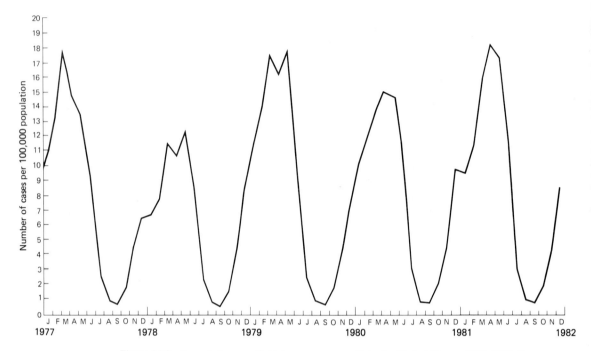

Figure 34-8 Reported cases of chickenpox per month in the United States, 1977–1982. Seasonal variations are consistently seen with peak incidence rates in March, April, and May. A total of 62,047 cases were reported in 1980 (modified from CDC annual summaries).

prevented or modified by receiving hyperimmune globulin obtained from the serum of patients who have recently recovered from herpes zoster.

Persons with chickenpox or zoster should be isolated for the first 5 to 7 days of illness to prevent further spread of the virus.

CYTOMEGALOVIRUSES (CMV)

The term *cytomegalo* means a cell of great size and describes the appearance of cells infected with this herpes virus. CMV multiplies slowly and causes the host cell to swell in size. Cells up to 40 μm in diameter with a large inclusion body in the nucleus are produced.

Pathogenesis and Clinical Diseases

Most CMV infections are inapparent and the virus is able to persist in the body for long periods. About 80% of adults have antibody against this virus, indicating that they have been or are still infected. The primary infection generally occurs early in life and the virus is shed for the next few years in the saliva and urine from many of these inapparent childhood infections.

Several clinical diseases are caused by the cytomegaloviruses. *Congenital infections* are acquired when the developing fetus becomes infected by viruses crossing the placental tissues from an infected mother. Some of these congenitally infected infants are born with severe deformities and die shortly after birth. About 1% of neonatal deaths are due to this virus. Some infants survive with serious physical and mental defects. Other congenitally infected infants survive without any obvious tissue damage. The second clinical form of this disease is an activation of an inapparent infection. It may be seen in both children and adults and is associated with prolonged immunosuppressive therapy for organ transplants or cancer. A third form of CMV disease is *posttransfusion mononucleosis* and is seen in recipients of massive blood transfusions who have received virus-contaminated blood. Normal adolescents may also develop a mononucleosis-type illness when exposed to this virus.

Transmission

About 1% of newborns are congenitally infected. Most infections occur early in life in children who are exposed to contaminated saliva and urine. Some infections are transmitted by blood transfusions. As with most diseases, transmission of CMV is more efficient in environments of poor sanitation.

Diagnosis

This virus may be cultivated from the infected tissues or secretions on cell cultures. Stained smears of cells taken from the site of infection may show the characteristic cytomegalic cells.

Treatment

No specific treatment is available.

Control and Prevention

Because of the large number of inapparent cases in the general population, no specific control measures are available. No vaccine currently exists, but developmental work on a vaccine is now underway.

EPSTEIN-BARR VIRUS (EB)

This widespread herpes virus has been incriminated as the possible cause of several forms of cancer, but all current evidence shows that it is also the long-sought-after cause of infectious mononucleosis.

Pathogenesis and Clinical Disease

The pathogenesis of infectious mononucleosis is not well understood. The best current evidence suggests that the natural infections are acquired by the oral route. The virus apparently passes from the throat through the lymphatic system and into the blood, resulting in wide distribution throughout the body. Lymphocytes seem to be the main cells that are infected. The EB virus is able to persist in the body for long periods and perhaps for the remaining life of some persons. Most infections are subclinical or so mild that they are not diagnosed as infectious mononucleosis. And most typical clinical diseases are seen in persons between 15 and 35 years of age. The incubation period may range from 2 to 6 weeks. The onset is gradual, lasting up to 1 week, and may consist of such general symptoms as malaise, headache, fatigue, and low-grade fever. The acute phase may last 1 to 3 weeks, but it is longer in some and is characterized by intermittent high fever, generalized weakness, severe sore throat, malaise, swollen lymph nodes, enlarged spleen, and a greatly increased number of abnormally appearing lymphocytes (mononuclear cells) in the blood. The last characteristic is the basis for the name infectious mononucleosis. The convalescent phase, with accompanying malaise and weakness, may be prolonged. Although antibodies develop and prevent reinfections, the virus may remain sequestered in the lymphocytes for the lifetime of the patient. Death or serious complications are rare.

It now appears that most people, particularly in areas where crowding and poor sanitation exist, contract this disease early in life and experience subclinical infections. The typical clinical disease usually occurs in adolescents and young adults who escaped infection earlier in life.

Transmission

About 90% of adults have been infected and the virus is found in the oral secretions of an estimated 20% of the general population.

The infection is widespread in young persons in tropical and subtropical areas as well as lower socioeconomic groups in temperate climates. People in such groups are frequently infected before school age and develop a subclinical or generalized infection that is not recognized as infectious mononucleosis. These persons may become lifelong carriers of the virus. The typical clinical disease is seen most often in adolescents and young adults; the highest incidence occurs in young persons who have had a more sheltered early life. When these individuals experience greater exposure during high school or college, they are prime candidates for the clinically recognizable form of infectious mononucleosis. Because the exchange of saliva by intimate oral contact is a most efficient means of transmitting this disease, the synonym "kissing disease" is appropriate; however, transmission may occur by other less direct routes. It is estimated that 100,000 college undergraduates contract infectious mononucleosis each year in the United States.

Diagnosis

The enlarged lymph nodes and increased number of mononuclear cells, along with the compatible generalized symptoms in persons of the appropriate age, strongly suggest infectious mononucleosis. The diagnosis is confirmed by showing a rise in antibodies. Tests are now becoming available to measure antibodies specifically against the EB virus. A nonspecific antibody test, called the *heterophile* antibody test, was helpful in diagnosing this disease for many years. This test uses sheep or horse red blood cells as the antigen and by the third week of illness 80% of the infectious mononucleosis patients develop antibodies that will agglutinate these red blood cells.

Treatment

There is no treatment other than supportive therapy. Bedrest is recommended during the acute phase and is usually spontaneous as a result of the generalized weakness of the patient. Contact-type physical activities should be avoided, for the swollen spleen could rupture if bumped.

Control and Prevention

No vaccine is available, but some are being developed. Isolation of patients is of little value. Due to the widespread distribution of this virus in asymptomatic carriers, only a recluse could purposely avoid being infected—a price most young people are not willing to pay to prevent this nonfatal disease.

SUMMARY

1. Infection due to the DNA herpesvirus group is of considerable attention and concern today. These viruses are responsible for a wide variety of disease conditions in both humans and animals. They cause benign, latent infections, such as cold sores, and extensive life-threatening infections, such as generalized herpes.
2. Herpes viruses are widely known because of current interest in their role as agents of a sexually transmitted disease caused by herpes simplex virus type 2 and because of infectious mononucleosis due to the Epstein-Barr virus.
3. Herpes viruses are among the few viruses for which a specific antiviral therapy has been developed.

Hepatitis Viruses

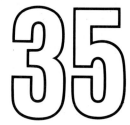

Although the clinical disease of hepatitis was recognized in ancient times, it was not until the early 1940s that sufficient evidence existed to distinguish at least two distinct types and to suspect that the etiologic agents were viral. One form of hepatitis was called *infectious*, for evidence indicated that it was passed from person to person by usual means, particularly the fecal-oral route. The other form was called *serum hepatitis* and was thought to be transmitted only by the injection of body fluids, such as blood, serum, and plasma, or the use of contaminated needles or syringes. Up until the late 1960s little progress was made in isolating and characterizing the viruses causing hepatitis by standard methods; however, since then new methods have yielded significant information on the nature of hepatitis. This new information is markedly changing our current understanding of these diseases; at present, our knowledge is expanding rapidly but is still incomplete. The disease previously referred to as infectious hepatitis is now called *hepatitis A* and serum hepatitis is called *hepatitis B*. This chapter summarizes our current knowledge of hepatitis A and B, and other possible types of viral hepatitis.

HEPATITIS A

Virus

For many years all attempts to grow this virus in cell cultures failed, but such propagation is now possible. Marmosets, monkeys, and chimpanzees can be experimentally infected, but, in general, experimentation has involved human volunteers. In

436

1973 virus-sized particles were observed via the electron microscope in the feces of patients with hepatitis A. These particles were 27 nm in diameter, possessed cubical symmetry, and specifically reacted with antibodies in the serum of patients who had recently recovered from hepatitis A. Currently evidence indicates that the suspect virus contains RNA. The hepatitis A virus is very stable and is not readily destroyed by many commonly used methods of disinfecting.

Pathogenesis and Clinical Disease

The hepatitis A virus enters the body orally. Most evidence indicates that the virus first multiplies along the intestinal epithelium and may result in anorexia (loss of appetite), malaise, intermittent fever, followed by nausea, vomiting, and diarrhea. In an undetermined percentage of infected persons the virus passes to the blood and spreads to the liver. Inflammation of the liver produces the classical signs of hepatitis, such as jaundice (yellowness of skin due to presence of bile pigments), dark urine, and pale, offensive feces. The signs of hepatitis appear about 1 week after the initial intestinal symptoms, recovery takes 4 to 6 weeks or longer, and the general weakness continues even longer. Death rates are less than 0.1%. The disease is mild in children and usually inapparent. It is now suspected that the hepatitis A virus might be widespread in tropical and underdeveloped areas, where most persons become infected early in life. In such environments clinical infections are most often seen in adult "outsiders" who enter the area. The extent of virus spread in countries with improved sanitation is difficult to determine at present. Clinical cases seem to increase, however, as living conditions improve, thus suggesting a condition similar to that seen with polio (see Chapter 38); that is, the lack of exposure early in life allows more susceptibles to accumulate in the adult population. An inexpensive serological test (ELISA) is now available to measure antibodies against the hepatitis A virus. Using this test, it is possible to study and gain a greater insight into the epidemiology of this disease.

Transmission

The fecal-oral route appears to be the major means of transmission. Outbreaks have been traced to contaminated water supplies and to food venders who are carriers. Outbreaks are common in mental institutions where sanitary practices are difficult to maintain. Over 30,000 cases of hepatitis A are reported each year in the United States.

Diagnosis

Routine serological tests are available to detect the virus and measure antibodies. Diagnosis is based on both serology and clinical signs associated with inflammation of the liver. Liver enzymes called transaminases, which are released into the blood during liver inflammation, can be measured as an indirect sign of viral hepatitis.

Treatment

Treatment is symptomatic and often prolonged rest is required before complete recovery occurs.

Control and Prevention

No vaccine is available. Maintenance of good sanitary conditions is the most effective control. Passive immunization with pooled human gamma globulin may offer some protection for several months. Such immunizations are recommended for military or other persons going into areas where poor sanitation exists.

CLINICAL NOTE

Outbreak of Food-borne Hepatitis A: New Jersey

An increase in the number of hepatitis cases In Monmouth County, New Jersey, was reported to the New Jersey Department of Health on June 15, 1981. Investigation by state and local area health departments revealed that 56 cases of hepatitis had occurred during the first 3 weeks of June in an area of Monmouth County where the usual average is 3-4 cases/month. Patients for whom appropriate laboratory tests had been done were confirmed to have hepatitis A.

Detailed food histories revealed that, within the appropriate incubation period for hepatitis A, 55 of the 56 patients had eaten at a Mexican style restaurant. Interviews of a control group matched for age, sex, and neighborhood of residence, showed that 10% of the controls ate food from this restaurant over a time period comparable with that for 90% of the patients. The restaurant agreed to close voluntarily pending further investigation.

Of the patients whose illness was related to the Mexican restaurant, 71% were male, 68% were between the ages of 15 and 29 years, and 4 were children under 15 years. A case-control study using 46 non-ill patrons revealed that patients were more likely to have eaten nachos, beans, and jalapeno peppers. Both beans and jalapeno peppers were used in preparing nachos.

Ten individuals including the two owners worked in the restaurant; all handled food at one time or another. Interviews on June 18 revealed that one employee who frequently ate food from the restaurant was ill with hepatitis at the time of the interview. Another employee had symptoms compatible with hepatitis on May 9. He had worked all day May 9, but felt too ill to work thereafter; the diagnosis of hepatitis A was confirmed for him on May 16. This employee prepared food—including grating cheese, shredding lettuce, and occasionally cutting meat; measured portions of meat, beans, jalapeno peppers, onions, cheeses, and lettuce into shells; and served the customers.

Because a food handler was recently ill with hepatitis and because the restaurant was implicated in the spread of hepatitis, immune globulin was offered to all individuals who ate in the restaurant from June 5 until it closed. A total of 1430 people were immunized at a 2-day clinic held June 19 and 20.

Editorial note: Hepatitis A virus (HAV) can be transmitted by food contaminated with feces from an infected food handler. If acute hepatitis A has been confirmed in a food handler by testing for IgM-specific HAV antibody, immunoglobulin prophylaxis (IG, gamma globulin) may be considered by patrons, depending on the probability of transmission of infectious virus and the probability of successful intervention in transmission by using IG. However, few food handlers actually appear to transmit disease via food, and IG prophylaxis of patrons is seldom warranted. Although for the past few years approximately 1000 food handlers with non-B hepatitis have been reported annually to CDC, an average of four outbreaks of food-borne hepatitis A have been reported each year (*MMWR 31*:150, 1982).

HEPATITIS B

Virus

The hepatitis B virus (HBV) differs from other known virus groups and possesses some unique characteristics. It cannot be grown in cell cultures and primates are the only susceptible experimental hosts. In spite of not being able to work with this virus by more conventional experimental methods, a significant amount of information has been obtained in the past decade. The complete virus is called a *Dane particle* (named after Dane who first characterized it) and is 42 nm in diameter with a double-shelled cubical capsid. The inner core is 27 nm and surrounds the nucleic acid, which is DNA. The outer shell is made of a different protein (called surface antigen) than the inner shell or core antigen. A unique feature of this virus is the excessive production of the surface protein antigen called *hepatitis B surface antigen* (HB$_s$Ag). This excess HB$_s$Ag forms into small spherical or filamentous particles that contain only the protein, are 22 nm in diameter, and are released from the cell into the blood. The presence of this HB$_s$Ag in the blood is a valuable diagnostic aid in the detection of persons who may be carriers of HBV. The structure of HBV is shown in Figure 35-1.

Pathogenesis and Clinical Disease

The clinical picture of hepatitis B is almost the same as for hepatitis A, but often it is more severe and death rates are higher, about 1% overall. For many years it was thought that hepatitis B was introduced into the body by the artificial inoculation of serum, transfusion of whole blood, or by contaminated needles and instruments. Indeed, a significant number of persons do become infected by these artificial routes, but today it is apparent that this infection is also spread by other routes, including sexual contact. The incubation period may take from 6 weeks to 6 months. Apparently the infection persists for months or years after the initial infection in some persons. These carriers contain a large amount of HB$_s$Ag in their serum, along with smaller amounts of the infectious 42-nm Dane particles.

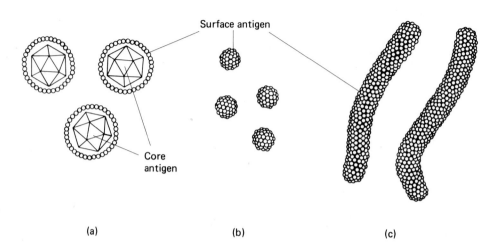

Figure 35-1 The various particles associated with HBV. (a) 42 nm complete virion (Dane particle); (b) 22 nm diameter spheres composed only of surface antigen; (c) 22 nm diameter filaments composed only of surface antigen.

Transmission

The most readily detected outbreaks of hepatitis B are usually transmitted by contaminated blood or blood products that are used in the treatment or immunization of patients. These cases are generally quite severe. The death rates may be from 10 to 20% in persons acquiring hepatitis B through blood transfusions, partly because of the large doses of virus received and partly because of the weakened or compromised conditions of the persons needing the transfusion. Contaminated needles, syringes, and similar items may readily transmit this virus and infectivity rates, as measured by the presence of HB_sAg in the serum, may exceed 50% among drug addicts who use and share unsterilized needles and syringes. The infection is also transmitted between sexual contacts and is a particular problem for homosexuals. About 16,000 cases of hepatitis B are reported in the United States per year.

With the development of serologic methods to detect the presence of HB_sAg in blood in the late 1960s and early 1970s, a better study of the epidemiology of hepatitis B was possible. The picture that is emerging indicates that this infection is widespread in certain cultures with most cases being subclinical. The infection is most widespread among populations in Asia, in primitive areas, in mental institutions, and in areas where sanitation practices are inadequate. The infectivity rates run from close to 100% in some groups, less (20–30%) in others with improving conditions, compared to about 0.1% in the United States. HB_sAg was originally discovered during a study of blood proteins of the Australian aborigines when it was thought that this protein was a common but unique component of their blood; so at first it was called the Australia antigen.

Control and Prevention

The major efforts to prevent hepatitis B in developed countries involve the avoidance of contaminated instruments when cutting tissues or injecting medication and transfusing blood that may contain HBV. Up until the discovery of HB_sAg in the late 1960s no reliable method was available to detect the presence of HBV in the blood of donors. Once the HB_sAg was isolated, it was possible to induce high levels of antibodies against this antigen in animals. These antibodies then became available for use in serologic tests to determine whether a given sample of blood contained the HB_sAg. Such sensitive serologic tests as radioimmunoassays have made it possible to detect and eliminate most HBV-contaminated blood products. Federal regulations now require that all blood samples used for transfusion, as well as blood products given by injection, must be tested for HBV.

Such serologic tests help to reduce the cases of posttransfusion hepatitis but are irrelevant to the control of HBV infections that are widespread in areas with low standards of hygiene. Until more is understood about the mode of transmission in such populations, specific control measures cannot be instituted.

Some progress has been made in the development of a hepatitis B vaccine. Even though the virus cannot be grown under experimental conditions, the HB_sAg can be obtained in significant amounts from the serum of chronic carriers of the infection. Thus many individuals who are not able to donate (or sell) their blood for blood transfusions because it contains HB_sAg can now sell their blood as a source of this antigen. The HB_sAg can be extracted, purified, and treated with formalin to kill any Dane particles and then used as an inactivated vaccine. Such a vaccine is relatively expensive, but it is useful in protecting high-risk individuals—for example, homosexuals—and those who must receive large numbers of blood transfusions. Recombinant DNA procedures are being used to produce hepatitis B surface antigens in yeast cells. Such antigens may serve as an effective vaccine in the future.

Hyperimmune gamma globulin may offer some passive protection to individuals who have been exposed to HBV-contaminated materials. Personnel working with hepatitis patients or blood products in the laboratory should be extra careful so as to reduce the chances of contracting hepatitis B.

Diagnosis

Diagnosis of hepatitis, in general, is made as described for hepatitis A. When the disease occurs in a patient who has received blood transfusions or other blood products, hepatitis B is suspected. Various serologic tests to detect the presence of hepatitis B antigens and antibodies in the serum are now available and are being used as specific tools in the diagnosis of this disease.

Treatment

Treatment is symptomatic.

OTHER TYPES OF HEPATITIS

One of the distressing discoveries in recent years has been the failure to eliminate posttransfusion hepatitis by eliminating blood that contains HB_sAg. It now appears that other hepatitis viruses may be present. Such hepatitis has been referred to as *hepatitis C* or *non-A, non-B hepatitis* (NANB). It is estimated that 90% of the posttransfusion hepatitis that does occur in the United States is not caused by hepatitis A or B.

A viruslike particle with cubical symmetry and a diameter of 27 nm has been associated with NANB hepatitis and may represent a newly discovered hepatitis virus.

SUMMARY

1. Hepatitis has long been one of the most common human diseases. Today the more widely known hepatitis A form has given way in interest to hepatitis B, which is transmitted through body excretions and is associated with increased health risks to hospitalized patients and personnel. A third hepatitis virus, non-A, non-B, appears to cause a disease similar to that of hepatitis B.

2. These viruses are not yet cultured effectively in in vitro systems. Some protection, however, is afforded to hepatitis A by passive immunization procedures and a recently developed hepatitis B vaccine offers some promise in reducing the incidence of this disease.

Orthomyxoviruses

36

The orthomyxovirus group contains the influenza viruses. Various animal species become infected with their own specific strains of influenza and, in some cases, the animal strains may produce mild infections in humans. The human strains of influenza viruses cause some of the more explosive and severe viral respiratory infections. The term "flu" is used in daily speech and may refer to a wide variety of infections, ranging from mild respiratory infections, such as the common cold, to various forms of enteritis (that is, "intestinal flu"). Yet when used correctly, the terms flu or influenza should describe a very characteristic disease that is discussed in this chapter.

INFLUENZA

Characteristics of the Viruses

Three general types of influenza viruses have been identified and are designated types A, B, and C. Type A causes the major influenzal epidemics of humans, type B causes moderate outbreaks, and type C is relatively insignificant. The following discussion is limited primarily to type A influenza.

The influenza virus has several features that need to be understood in any study of the unique epidemiologic patterns of influenza. Features of the influenza virus are shown in Figure 36-1. The inner core of the virion contains a helical capsid that surrounds a ss-RNA molecule. The RNA molecule is somewhat unique in that it is made up of seven or eight loosely connected or separate segments and each segment contains the genetic information for the formation of a specific viral component. Of

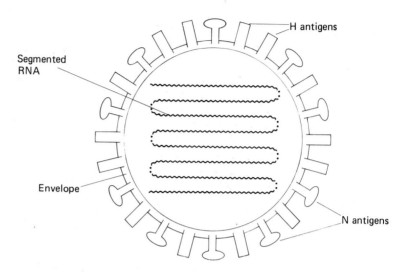

Figure 36-1 Schematic outline of an influenza virion. The H and N antigens are peplomers that protrude from the envelope. The RNA is in eight segments and is located inside a helical capsid.

importance to the following discussion are the two protein components (peplomers) that are embedded in the lipid envelope and project out from the virus. These protein peplomers are effective antigens and the antibodies that form against them provide immunity to the host. One peplomer serves as the attachment site between the virus and the host cells and also causes the clumping or agglutination of RBC (hemagglutination); thus it is called the *hemagglutinin* or simply the "H" antigen. The other peplomer is an enzyme that dissolves a component of mucus called neuraminic acid. This protein is thus called *neuraminidase* or the "N" antigen. The genetic controls over the H and N antigens are somewhat unstable, resulting in occasional minor changes in the configuration of the antigenic determinants and less frequent major changes in one or both antigens. The minor changes are called *antigenic drift* and the major changes *antigenic shift*. When the minor antigenic drifts occur, the antibodies in the general population are less effective in providing immunity and limited outbreaks of influenza develop. When a major shift occurs, the protective antibodies that are already in the population are of no further value, the virus is able to spread without restrictions, and a pandemic of influenza results.

Pathogenesis and Clinical Disease

Humans are infected by the airborne route. The viruses specifically attach to the ciliated epithelial cells of the respiratory tract for the initiation of the infection. As viruses are released from the few cells that are initially infected, many adjacent cells become infected and the infection spreads along the epithelium of the respiratory tract. Widespread inflammation results. Usually the infection is limited to the upper respiratory tract, but, in severe cases, the lower respiratory tract may also be involved. The influenza virus rarely spreads to the blood or deeper body tissues; however, toxic products from the virus are absorbed into the blood and are responsible for the generalized symptoms of influenza. Influenza has a distinct clinical picture with an onset of 1 to 3 days after exposure. A sore throat, cough, possible hoarseness, and nasal discharge are the localized signs. The systemic manifestations caused by the toxic materials include headache, fever, chills, generalized muscular aches, and, in severe cases, prostration. Gastrointestinal symptoms may also be present. Recovery is usually spontaneous after 4 to 7 days. Deaths are rare in otherwise healthy individuals, but increased death rates are noted among the very young, elderly, and chronically ill when an epidemic of influenza is in an area. Influenza weakens the natural defense mechanisms of the respiratory tract and so secondary bacterial pneumonia is a common complication during influenzal outbreaks and is responsible for many of the resulting deaths. Reye's syndrome (p. 427) occurs in a very small portion of children during the late recovery phase of influenza.

Epidemiology

There are few if any parallels today to the epidemiology of influenza. When major antigenic shifts occur in virulent strains, a worldwide pandemic occurs and may involve hundreds of millions of persons. Such pandemics are accompanied by significant increases in the overall death rate. Often such outbreaks force the closing of schools and factories and generally disrupt the normal flow of human activities. Fortunately, such major outbreaks only occur every 10 to 15 years; less extensive outbreaks occur every 2 to 4 years as a result of antigenic drift.

Figure 36-2 shows the general epidemiological patterns of influenza during the past century. The most devastating pandemic occurred in 1918–1919. This strain of influenza virus was highly virulent, particularly in young adults, for some yet unexplained reason and approximately 20 million deaths occurred throughout the world. As the world population developed antibody immunity to this virus, the rate of disease decreased. The technology of 1918 was not able to isolate the virus responsible for this great pandemic and its identity is still not known. In 1931 the first influenza virus was isolated from swine. It was noted, however, that serum taken from persons who had recovered from the 1918 influenza pandemic did contain antibodies that specifically reacted, to a limited extent, with the swine influenza virus. Whether any further relationship existed between these viruses could not be determined. The next pandemic occurred in 1932–1933 and at that time the first influenza virus of humans was isolated. This virus was antigenically different from the 1918 strain and is now designated A/London/33 (H_0N_1). In this designation the A stands for type A influenza, London stands for the location where the virus was first isolated, 33 stands for year 1933, and H_0 (zero) and N_1 stand for the major H and N antigens. Some antigenic drifting occurs after each pandemic and every 2 or 3 years limited epidemics of influenza are seen. When a pandemic occurs because of a major antigenic shift, the previous strain of influenza seems to be crowded out or becomes very scarce. After

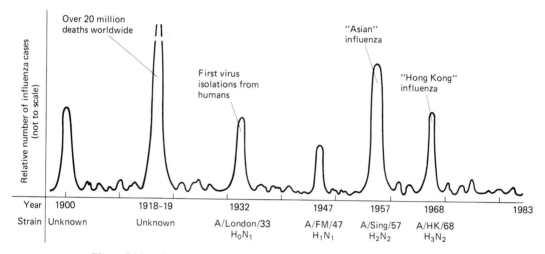

Figure 36-2 Time line showing when some of the major outbreaks and antigenic shifts occurred associated with type Λ influenza during the 1900s. Minor outbreaks occurred between the major outbreaks.

1933 the next antigenic shift occurred in 1947, when the H antigen underwent a major shift; this strain is designated A/Fort Mommoth/47 (H_1N_1). The following pandemic took place 10 years later when both the H and the N antigen underwent major shifts to produce the strain known as "Asian" influenza, which is designated A/Singapore/57 (H_2N_2). Because no antibody immunity was present in the world population against either the H or the N antigen, this strain of influenza spread most effectively and within 8 to 10 months was reported in most parts of the world. In 1968 a major shift occurred in the H antigen, creating strain A/Hong Kong/68 (H_3N_2), known as "Hong Kong flu." Like its predecessor, this strain spread rapidly from Asia to most parts of the world. From 1968 to 1983 no new major shifts have been reported. To-day's increased technology of analyzing influenza viruses, however, has provided more effective means of detecting the minor antigenic changes and a steady array of new influenzal strains are now being identified, such as A/New Jersey/76, A/Texas/77, A/Bangkok/79, and A/Philippines/82. The strain A/New Jersey/76 deserves special mention, for this strain is apparently the same or closely related to the swine influenza virus. The strain was first isolated from recruits at a military camp in New Jersey in January of 1976. Because it was first detected in young adults and was re-lated to "swine flu," there was a great deal of concern that it might be a return of the same strain that caused the great pandemic of 1918. In order to prevent a possible recurrence of such a devastating pandemic, with the possibility of millions of deaths, a massive immunization program was undertaken. By late summer and early fall of 1976 large segments of the population of the United States were being vaccinated. Fortunately, the A/New Jersey/76 strain was not the deadly strain of 1918; it was probably a random transmission of the flu from infected swine to humans.

Diagnosis

Preliminary diagnosis is made on the basis of clinical and epidemiological observations. The diagnosis is confirmed by demonstrating the presence of the virus in throat washings. The virus can be grown in cell cultures or in embryonated eggs. Changes in antibody levels can be readily demonstrated by hemagglutination inhibition tests.

Treatment

Unlike most viral diseases, early therapy of type A influenza can be accomplished with *amantidine hydrochloride*. This compound prevents the uncoating of the virus in host cells and so restricts its replication. Unfortunately, the compound is not effective against either type B or C and is therefore not commonly used as an antiviral agent. In all cases of influenza, supportive treatment of the symptoms may be helpful in comforting the patient and antibacterial chemotherapy may be needed to treat secondary bacterial infections.

Prevention and Control

Because of the increased mobility of today's world population, the influenza virus is apparently able to spread most effectively from country to country. Quarantine measures seem of little value. The major means of controlling outbreaks is through a killed vaccine. This type of vaccine is moderately effective in that it confers protection to about 70% of those who receive it; this protection lasts from 6 months to a year. The vaccine contains the toxic products of the virus and often induces mild systemic symptoms of influenza, such as headache, fever, and muscle aches. Currently purified vaccines having only the H and N antigens are being used to a limited extent and do not contain the toxic by-products. The most important aspect of influenzal immunization is to use the proper strain of virus for the production of the vaccine. When an antigenic shift occurs, the vaccines then in stock are of no value. Continual worldwide surveillance programs monitor for the appearance of new strains. When a new strain is found and is determined to be of significant virulence, a race begins between humans and virus with the goal being to produce large amounts of vaccine and vaccinate a significant proportion of the population before the viral pandemic arrives. The first time this race was run was with the advent of the Hong Kong flu of 1968. Unfortunately, delays occurred in the production of the vaccine and the pandemic had circled the earth before the vaccine became available. The next attempt was during the "swine flu" episode of 1976. In this case, the vaccine was prepared in time, but this strain of virus was of low virulence and no significant outbreak occurred. Whether this stratagem will work in aborting a major pandemic in the future due to an antigenic shift of a virulent strain remains to be determined.

In the United States information is collected each week from about 120 selected cities on the deaths due to pneumonia and influenza (Figure 17-4). When deaths exceed the expected range in a given area, an investigation is undertaken to determine if an influenza epidemic is occurring and what strain might be present. Frequent updates are reported in the *Morbidity and Mortality Weekly Reports*; an example is given in the following clinical note.

CLINICAL NOTE

Update: Influenza Activity: United States, Worldwide, April 15, 1983

United States: Morbidity reports collected weekly by each state indicate a continuing decline in influenza outbreaks. For the week ending April 9, 1983, two states (Kentucky and New Mexico) reported regional activity, and no state reported widespread activity. In recent weeks, reports of influenza virus isolations from collaborating laboratories have also indicated a decline in influenza activity. Most isolates (89%) continue to be type A (H_3N_2) virus, despite increases in influenza B and type A (H_1N_1). For the week ending April 9, 1983, an excess in the ratio of pneumonia and influenza deaths to total deaths were reported from 121 cities for the thirteenth consecutive week. The observed ratio was 5.2 and the expected ratio was 4.1

Worldwide: Influenza activity during the 1982–83 season has generally been moderate and largely associated with influenza type A (H_3N_2) viruses, which have been reported from all five continents since October 1982. A (H_3N_2) has been the type most frequently isolated in all areas of the world and has been associated with outbreaks in all age groups. Influenza type A (H_1N_1) isolates have been associated with sporadic cases and with outbreaks among schoolchildren. Influenza type B isolates, generally associated with sporadic cases, have been identified in several European countries. During late March and early April, influenza activity appeared to be declining in most European countries (*MMWR* 32:191, 1983).

SUMMARY

Influenza is the most common disease due to orthomyxoviruses. This disease while common in occurrence may prove serious in its consequences. An unusual genetic arrangement in the genome of this virus facilitates the repeated development of viruses with altered antigenic structures. These "new" viruses are the basis of periodic pandemics of the influenza. Vaccines are available against the influenza virus and consist of the most recent and common antigenic variations of the virus.

Paramyxoviruses

37

The paramyxoviruses are a group of related viruses that cause some common diseases of mankind. These viruses are structured somewhat like the orthomyxoviruses, but, compared to the influenza viruses, they are genetically stable so that new mutant serotypes do not periodically develop. Many common viral respiratory diseases, as well as such distinct clinical diseases as mumps and measles, are caused by paramyxoviruses. The parainfluenza, respiratory syncytial, mumps, and measles paramyxoviruses are discussed in this chapter. Rubella, which is caused by a togavirus, is also described here because its clinical manifestations are much like measles.

CHARACTERISTICS OF PARAMYXOVIRUSES

The paramyxoviruses contain ss-RNA and have helical symmetry. The helical capsid is wound in a loose sphere that is somewhat irregular in shape and ranges from 100 to 300 nm in diameter. They possess an envelope and N- and H-type peplomers. Paramyxoviruses are unstable and do not survive long outside the host.

PARAINFLUENZA VIRUSES

Four serotypes of parainfluenza viruses infect humans. The infections are seen primarily in infants and young children. Illnesses range from subclinical to mild upper respiratory infections to croup or pneumonia. The viruses do not spread to the blood.

449

Most cases are seen during the "respiratory disease season" from late fall to early spring. Many children are infected during the first years of life so that by age 10 most (over 80%) children have antibodies against the four types of parainfluenza viruses. Reinfections may occur at all ages, but they are much milder than the primary infection and present symptoms of the "common cold." These viruses cause about 15% of the acute respiratory diseases seen in children under 10 years of age. Treatment is symptomatic; no vaccines are available.

RESPIRATORY SYNCYTIAL VIRUS (RSV)

These viruses are a major cause of respiratory illness in infants during the first few months of life. About 50% of bronchiolitis cases and about 25% of all pneumonia occurring in infants up to 2 months of age are caused by the RSV. Deaths may result from these infections.

The infection is mild in older children and is limited to the upper respiratory tract (rhinitis and pharynigitis). No vaccines are available.

CLINICAL NOTE

Nosocomial Respiratory Syncytial Virus Infections in an Intensive Care Nursery: California

An outbreak of upper respiratory infection and pneumonia involving 9 infants and caused by respiratory syncytial virus (RSV) occurred in a 16-bed intensive care nursery (ICN) of a hospital and medical center in San Francisco, California, from February 25 through March 19, 1978.

On February 25 an 18-week-old premature infant with hyaline membrane disease and bronchopulmonary dysplasia developed fever with respiratory distress and had a convulsion. A nasopharyngeal viral culture taken then was subsequently positive for RSV. Two days later 2 other premature infants (aged 13 and 35 weeks) developed sneezing, cough, and rales. The 13-week-old was in isolation for a previously documented cytomegalovirus infection. Nasopharyngeal viral cultures from both infants were reported positive for RSV on March 2.

At that time the following procedures were instituted:

1. RSV fluorescent antibody (FA) screening and viral cultures were performed on nasopharyngeal swabs from all ICN patients.
2. All positive patients were isolated in a separate room.
3. Strict handwashing, gowning, and gloving procedures were required before contact with all ICN patients (masking was not required).

4. Certain nursing staff were assigned exclusively to infected infants.

5. All nursing staff with upper respiratory symptoms were considered infected with RSV. If well enough to work, they were allowed to care only for already-infected infants.

On the basis of direct FA screening, 2 additional infants were found positive for RSV on March 2 and were isolated. One had a collapsed right upper lobe; a culture was positive for RSV. The other patient had no respiratory symptoms; two of three FA studies were borderline positive for RSV, and none of eight viral cultures was positive.

FA screening was repeated March 6 on the remaining 11 patients in the unit, but no new cases were identified. The following day 2 patients, both aged 6 weeks, developed mild upper respiratory symptoms. Repeat FA testing was positive on both; cultures taken at this time subsequently grew RSV.

On March 19 a 6-day-old infant who had been in the ICN since birth developed nasal congestion. FA studies were negative and he was discharged from the hospital 2 days later. Viral cultures taken before discharge were later positive for RSV.

One additional infant developed RSV infection in association with this outbreak. The child, born on February 28, remained in the newborn nursery, a room adjoining the ICN, for 6 days because of neonatal hyperbilirubinemia. She was discharged on March 7 but was readmitted to another hospital ward on March 15 because of rhinorrhea and cough of 5 days' duration. FA studies and viral culture were both positive for RSV at the time of readmission. The child had had no direct contact with ICN babies during her first hospitalization. The nursing staffs of the intensive care and newborn nurseries are separate, but patients in both units are cared for by the same house staff members.

Routine viral screening of nursing and house staff members was not performed. However, from March 7 to March 21 FA studies and viral cultures were performed on 2 pediatric house officers, 11 ICN nurses, 1 nursery x-ray technician, and 1 phlebotomist, who regularly bled patients in the ICN. All 15 reported upper respiratory illnesses with onset occurring from 1 to 13 days (mean 4.9 days) before viral testing. The RSV FA test was strongly positive in 1 nurse and weakly positive in 4 additional nurses and the phlebotomist. None of the adults was positive by culture, perhaps owing to the delay in obtaining cultures after onset of symptoms (*MMWR* 27:260, 1978).

MUMPS

Mumps is one of the common communicable diseases of children and young adults. It is not as contagious as measles or chickenpox and outbreaks are generally limited to fewer cases. Along with the well-recognized swelling of the salivary glands, mumps may also involve other glands or the CNS.

Virus

The mumps virus is a typical paramyxovirus and is inactivated quite readily (within hours) once expelled from the body. Only one serotype is known and humans are the only natural host. This virus can be grown in a variety of different cell cultures and in embryonated eggs. Primates can be experimentally infected. Various serologic tests are available to measure antibodies against the mumps virus.

Pathogenesis and Clinical Disease

Humans are infected by inhaling infected droplet nuclei that contain the virus. This disease has an incubation period of 16 to 18 days and during this time the virus passes from the site of entry in the respiratory tract into the lymphatic system and then into the blood. The virus is deposited from the blood into the meninges and various organs, such as the salivary glands, ovaries, testes, mammary glands, and pancreas. Several days to a week before the onset of symptoms, and for about an equal length of time after the onset of symptoms, the virus may be found in the saliva, urine, stool, and blood. In about a third of these patients the infection remains subclinical or at least the infected person experiences none of the classical symptoms of mumps. In the other two-thirds the most readily recognizable sign is the swollen salivary glands (parotitis) (Figure 37-1). Swelling occurs only on one side (unilateral) in 25% of the cases. Several days to a week or more following the onset of parotitis, involvement of other glands may become apparent. Inflammation of the testes (orchitis) is rare in prepubertal males (under 11 to 13 years of age) whereas 20 to 30% of males over this age may experience orchitis. Usually orchitis is unilateral and all current evidence

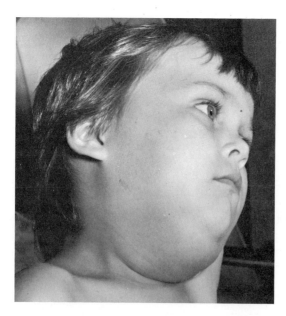

Figure 37-1 Child with diffuse swelling as a result of mumps infection. (Centers for Disease Control, Atlanta)

indicates that sterility is rarely caused by this infection. Inflammation of the ovaries and mammary glands is seen in a similar percentage of infected females and permanent damage rarely, if ever, occurs. The most serious complication from mumps results from infection of the central nervous system. Mumps is one of the most common causes of aseptic (nonbacterial) meningitis and encephalitis. Most patients with CNS involvement recover without permanent complications. Deafness may result in a small percentage of cases and death occasionally occurs.

Transmission and Epidemiology

Mumps is transmitted by the airborne route and by direct contact with saliva. No documentation of transmission by virus-infected urine or mothers' milk has been observed. Those with subclinical cases, however, are able to transmit the disease. Transmission is not as effective as with diseases like measles, chickenpox, or influenza. Epidemics occur every few years in the winter or spring, but cases tend to be more sporadic and occur throughout the year. It is quite easy for a person to go through childhood without contracting this disease and about one-fourth of the cases are seen in adolescents or young adults. About 20% of U.S. residents reach adulthood and have no antibodies against mumps. Because of this group of susceptible adults, mumps infection often occurs in recruits during the military mobilization of large numbers of persons. Since the introduction of a living vaccine in the late 1960s, the overall incidence of mumps has decreased. Recovery from mumps generally confers lifelong immunity. Reported second attacks of mumps are probably based on the assumption that any infection involving swollen salivary glands is mumps. When two attacks of mumps are reported in the same person, this assumption is not correct and one of the illnesses with parotitis would be assumed to be caused by an agent other than the mumps virus. The number of cases of mumps reported in the United States is shown in Figure 37-2.

Diagnosis

Typical cases of mumps with swelling of the salivary glands can be readily diagnosed on the basis of clinical appearance. Atypical cases require laboratory tests to confirm that they are mumps. The virus can be isolated from the throat, saliva, urine, or spinal fluid through cell cultures or embryonated eggs. Various serologic tests are available to measure specific mumps antibodies.

Control and Prevention

Children with mumps should be kept from school or other association with other children for about 2 weeks. A living attenuated vaccine has been available since 1968 in the United States. This vaccine is quite effective and induces immunity in over 95% of the recipients. The vaccine has no side effects. But because mumps is generally not a serious disease, vigorous campaigns to administer the vaccine have not been carried

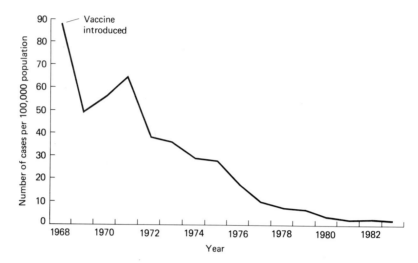

Figure 37-2 Reported cases of mumps per year in the United States, 1968–1983. In 1968, the year the vaccine was licensed, 152,209 cases were reported (modified from CDC annual summaries).

out. The vaccine should be given as part of the routine childhood vaccination series at about 1 year of age. It is usually given as part of a triple vaccine known as MMR, which stands for measles, mumps, and rubella. Mumps vaccines have been used effectively in military-recruit-training centers to control troublesome outbreaks in that environment. Significant decreases in mumps have been observed in areas where the vaccine has been widely used.

MEASLES

Measles is one of the most contagious diseases of mankind and before the development of an effective vaccine in the mid 1960s 98% of the population of the United States would have contracted it by the age of 18. Even though measles was considered a disease that everyone had to get and "get it over with," it is a serious disease and a leading cause of death in many undernourished children in developing countries where vaccination is not carried out. Cases of measles have declined significantly the past 10 to 15 years in countries where vaccination programs were applied.

Virus

Only one serotype of measles virus exists. This virus can be adapted to grow in cell cultures and embryonated eggs. It has a short survival time outside the body but does remain viable for a long enough time in a droplet nuclei to be spread effectively by the aerosol route.

Pathogenesis and Clinical Disease

The measles virus enters by the airborne route and is taken up by the draining lymph ducts of the respiratory tract. The virus passes into the blood and is deposited throughout the body. The incubation period is 9 to 12 days before the onset of prodromal symptoms of fever, cough, runny nose (coryza), and conjunctivitis. At this stage of the disease red macules or ulcer-type lesions, called *Koplik spots*, appear on the inside of the cheek. After about 3 days the rash appears on the skin and continues to spread and intensify over the next 1 or 2 days (Figure 37-3). General symptoms may be severe and such complications as secondary bacterial infections may occur. The CNS is infected and in about one out of every 1000 cases the encephalitis is severe enough to cause noticeable signs. About 15% of those with severe symptoms of encephalitis die; others may have permanent effects, such as epilepsy, hearing loss, and personality changes.

A rare degenerative neurological disease with the formidable name of subacute sclerosing panencephalitis (SSPE) develops in a few children or adolescents several years after a measles infection. All current evidence indicates that this disease is caused by measles viruses that have remained latent in the CNS.

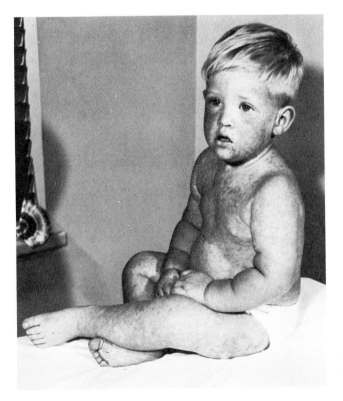

Figure 37-3 Measles rash on a child three days after onset. (Centers for Disease Control, Atlanta)

In the mid-1970s a new dimension in the clinical picture of measles appeared. The immunity of some children who had been vaccinated waned or their vaccinations were of insufficient potency to produce full immunity; consequently, a significant number of cases of atypical measles occurred. These atypical cases resembled various other diseases and it was necessary to use serologic tests to confirm that they were measles.

Transmission and Epidemiology

Transmission is by droplet nuclei expelled from the respiratory tract, often a few days before to a few days after the onset of the rash. The disease is highly infectious. When measles is introduced into an isolated population that has not had this disease, and no acquired immunity is present, almost 100% of the inhabitants contract it. In such cases, the mortality rate is high and may reach 10% if local health care is not available and the general nutritional state of the population is poor. Such an epidemic occurred on the Hawaiian Islands during early colonization by whites.

Before the introduction of vaccination, measles epidemics would occur every 2 to 5 years in a given area, with most cases happening during the winter and early spring. This epidemiologic pattern of measles has changed significantly since the introduction of vaccines in the mid-1960s. Within a few years after initiation of vaccination programs the total number of cases in the United States decreased 90%. Through the 1970s, however, the number of cases remained about the same, at around 20,000 to 30,000 cases per year. During this time the age distribution of cases shifted, with more outbreaks occurring in teenagers and college-age persons. Such a shift was attributed to the vaccination programs that had decreased the spread of measles among young children and, in turn, allowed more susceptibles to accumulate in the older age groups. Increased efforts were initiated in 1979 to immunize a larger proportion of the children as they entered their first year of schooling. This program has been successful and during 1982 the number of measles cases dropped to about 1600. This was less than one-fifth the number from 1980 and less than one-tenth the number seen in any year of the 1970s (Figure 37-4). The current goal, which seems within reach, is to reduce the number of cases of measles contracted in the United States to zero.

Diagnosis

Because of its characteristic appearance and epidemiology, measles is usually diagnosed clinically without laboratory tests. The appearance of Koplik spots is useful in diagnosing measles during early stages of the disease. But laboratory tests are needed to make a specific diagnosis in the cases of atypical measles in partially immunized children. Virus isolation can be made during the acute phase of the disease; however,

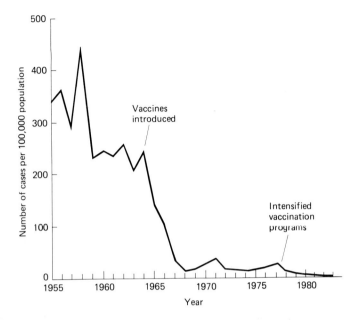

Figure 37-4 Reported cases of measles by year in the United States, 1955–1983. In 1958, 763,094 cases were reported compared to 2905 in 1981 (modified from CDC annual summaries).

most laboratory diagnoses are made by showing a significant increase in antibodies to measles virus between the acute or convalescent sera.

Treatment

No specific antiviral treatment is available. Antibiotics may be given to treat secondary bacterial infection.

Control and Prevention

The control of measles at present relies almost entirely on the use of an attenuated vaccine. This vaccine is given subcutaneously to young children after they have lost all passive immunity from their mothers, usually at about 1 year of age. The measles vaccination is normally administered as part of the MMR triple vaccine and gives prolonged protection. Whether more than one vaccination is needed for lifelong protection is currently under investigation. As a precaution to protect children who may not have received adequate protection from the first immunization, it is being recommended that a second immunization be given as the child enters school at 5 or 6 years of age. All current evidence indicates that effective vaccination programs directed at preschool-age children can control measles.

CLINICAL NOTE

Imported Measles with Subsequent Airborne Transmission in a Pediatrician's Office: Michigan

An outbreak of seven cases of measles was reported in Muskegon County, Michigan; rash onsets occurred from November 14 through December 10, 1982. The outbreak began with an international importation in a 7-month-old baby who arrived in the United States from Korea on October 29 for adoption. She infected four other children in a pediatrician's office; two additional measles cases occurred subsequently in family members of these four children.

The index patient (Patient A) had onset of rash on November 14 and visited a pediatrician's office on November 16. She was in the office waiting room from 11 A.M. to noon and in a single examination room from noon to 12:30 P.M. After measles was diagnosed, the pediatrician reviewed the immunization records of all children known to have been in the office at the same time and offered immune globulin (IG) to the three unimmunized children, all of whom were less than 15 months of age. Two received IG, while the third, a 6-month-old infant did not. No cases occurred among these children. However, cases did occur in patients not known to have been in the office at the same time as Patient A. One child who was subsequently infected arrived approximately 5 minutes before Patient A left the office, but did not have face-to-face contact with her; the other three arrived in the office 60 to 75 minutes after Patient A left. Only one of these four children used the same examining room as Patient A, but all four shared the same waiting room. None of the children were in contact with any other persons who had rash illnesses. No other common activities or contacts with individuals or shared objects could be identified to account for these cases. The last-known measles cases in Muskegon County had been reported in February 1981.

The patients with secondary cases ranged in age from 4 months to 2-1/2 years; none had been immunized. Two of these children transmitted measles to family members—a 14-year-old with a history of measles vaccination at 11 months and 5 years, and a 24-year-old, whose immunization status was unknown.

Of 29 children who were in the office when Patient A was present or who arrived within 90 minutes of her departure, 19 were 15 months of age or older, the recommended age for routine measles vaccination. Two of these children had not been vaccinated; both developed measles. None of the 17 vaccinated children developed measles. Of 10 children less than 15 months of age, all unvaccinated, two were infected, two received IG, and six remained well. Four of the six well patients were 6 months of age or less (*MMWR 32*:401, 1983).

RUBELLA

Rubella is a mild disease that is of little direct concern in children or adults, but it may have disastrous effects on the developing fetus should the mother become infected early in pregnancy. The term *German measles* is also used for this disease; however, this term often leads to confusion with regular measles and it would be better to use the name rubella consistently when referring to this disease.

Virus

The virus that causes rubella defied isolation by standard procedures during the 1940s and 1950s but was finally isolated in the early 1960s. The feature that made isolation difficult was the inability of this virus to cause observable changes in cell cultures (cytopathic effect) or death in embryonated eggs even though the virus will proliferate in these systems. Only a single serotype of rubella has been found. All current information indicates that the rubella virus is morphologically similar to the togaviruses (Chapter 40).

Pathogenesis and Clinical Disease

This disease has the same pathogenesis as many other diseases; that is, the virus is inhaled into the respiratory tract, followed by passage through the lymphatic system into the blood. After an incubation period of around 14 days, the symptoms produced are usually trivial and include swollen lymph nodes, mild fever, and often a slight rash lasting for 2 to 3 days.

When a pregnant female is infected, the rubella virus may infect the developing fetus and cause a disease known as *congenital rubella syndrome*. This syndrome may include any of the following effects: cataracts with partial or complete blindness, loss of hearing, heart defects, mental retardation, or generalized tissue damage. The chance that the developing baby will develop serious damage due to congenital rubella is much greater if infection occurs during the first trimester of pregnancy. Severe damage results in about 50% of the fetuses infected during the first month; serious effects on the fetus are rare if the mother contracts rubella after the fourth month of pregnancy.

It is theorized that the rubella virus has such damaging effects on the fetus because of its mild nature. More virulent viruses, if they infected the fetus, would cause severe damage that would result in fetal death and lead to spontaneous abortion. On the other hand, the rubella virus, because of its mild effect, simply slows cell growth, which, in turn, leads to malformation of the tissues as they differentiate during early fetal development.

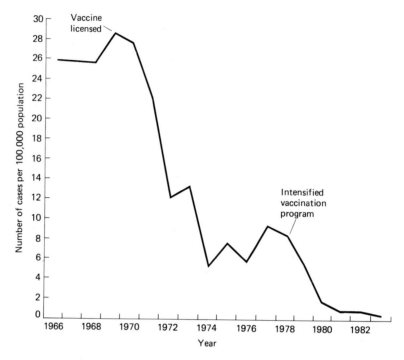

Figure 37-5 Reported cases of rubella by year in the United States, 1966–1983 (modified from CDC annual summaries).

Transmission and Epidemiology

Rubella is primarily transmitted by the respiratory route with the patient being infectious several days before to about a week after the onset of the rash. Before the widespread use of the vaccine, moderate epidemics of rubella would occur every 6 to 9 years and major epidemics at greater intervals of up to 30 years. The last major epidemic in the United States was in 1964 when about 500,000 cases occurred. Because of this epidemic, thousands of children were born with congenital rubella syndrome.

Rubella babies present a special problem in transmission, for they continue to shed virus in saliva, urine, and other body secretions for 1 month to 6 years after birth. The reported cases of rubella per year in the United States are seen in Figure 37-5.

Diagnosis

The major problem in diagnosing rubella centers around the concern of exposure or potential exposure of females during the early stages of pregnancy. The expense and time involved in a laboratory diagnosis are not warranted in routine cases. When a susceptible female in the first trimester of pregnancy has been exposed to a possible rubella patient, however, it is important to know whether the exposure was indeed to rubella. Laboratory serologic tests and viral isolation can determine if the infection is caused by the rubella virus. Routine serologic tests are available to determine whether females of child-bearing age have antibodies against rubella. In some states rubella serologic tests are required when obtaining a marriage license.

Treatment

No direct treatment is available.

Control and Prevention

Once discoveries in the early 1960s showed that the rubella virus could be grown in cell cultures or embryonated eggs, rapid progress was made in developing a rubella vaccine. A living vaccine was first licensed in 1969 and appears to induce a high degree of immunity after a single dose. Mild infection sometimes results from the vaccine, but in nonpregnant persons it is of little consequence. Because it is not known if this living vaccine causes damaging infections in the developing fetus, conception should be delayed until at least 3 months after a female has been vaccinated and pregnant females should not be vaccinated.

Two general approaches have been used in rubella vaccinations. One is to immunize preschool-age children, thus limiting the spread of the virus within a community and reducing the chance of exposure to expectant mothers. The other approach is to immunize girls in their early teens and older females of child-bearing age who have no antibodies against rubella. It has as yet not been determined which approach is more effective in preventing the congenital rubella syndrome. Since the introduction of wide-scale vaccination, the overall incidences of rubella and congenital rubella syndrome have decreased significantly.

CLINICAL NOTE

Rubella Outbreak on a College Campus: Wisconsin

In the period October 12 to November 9, 1977, 45 cases of rash illness consistent with rubella were reported to the Student Health Service of Marquette University, Milwaukee, Wisconsin. Rubella virus had been isolated from the pharynx of eight students and another student had a fourfold rise in hemagglutination inhibition (HI) antibody titers to rubella.

Signs and symptoms in the reported cases were: rash (100%), adenopathy (19%), pharyngitis (76%), fever 37.4°C (99°F) (71%), headache (51%), conjunctivitis (47%), and photophobia and joint complaints (44% each). Males and females experienced the joint signs and symptoms with equal frequency. Two males noted bilateral testicular tenderness. Five of 30 students complained of itching at the onset of rash.

Of the 45 cases reported, 44 occurred in undergraduate students, an attack rate of 6/1000. Rates were equal in males and females and were not significantly different among the four classes. The attack rate in students living in campus dormitories, however, was twice as high as for those living off campus (8/1000 versus 4/1000).

More than 1000 students were vaccinated in a rubella immunization program prompted by these cases. Vaccine was given to all males requesting it. However, because previous testing of the university's junior and senior nursing students had revealed a 90% prevalence of antibodies to rubella, initially all women were not vaccinated. Instead, vaccine was offered only to those found to be serologically negative. When it became apparent that the outbreak was continuing and that only 70 to 85% of the women who had come to the clinic had detectable antibodies, all female students requesting it were vaccinated after appropriate counseling on the need to avoid pregnancy. Each woman's blood specimen was frozen in the event that serologic tests might later be useful.

Editorial note: Because college campuses are recognized potential sites of rubella outbreak, ideally all susceptible females should be identified and vaccinated before they enter college. Colleges and universities should consider requiring serologic screening of all incoming female students at the time of preadmission physical examinations. Susceptible, nonpregnant females should be vaccinated against rubella at a time when pregnancy will be avoided for the ensuing three months (*MMWR* 26:392, 1977).

SUMMARY

1. The RNA-containing paramyxoviruses are responsible for several of the more commonly known childhood diseases. These infections include croup (epiglotitis), mumps, measles and a not uncommon pneumonia in newborns caused by respiratory syncytial virus.

2. Disease due to these viruses has been so widespread that although any given infection may be mild in its symptoms, the small percentage of infections with serious consequence were, in fact, quite common. This situation has spawned the development of excellent vaccines that should be used to limit the occurrence of rubella, measles, and mumps.

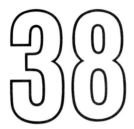

Picornaviruses

The picornavirus family includes large numbers of viruses that infect humans and animals. They are among the smallest viruses and contain ss-RNA, hence the name *pico* (small) plus RNA (Figure 38-1). Two genera of picornaviruses are found in humans: the rhinoviruses, which primarily inhabit the nasal cavity, and the enteroviruses, which are found mainly in the alimentary tract. The rhinoviruses can only proliferate in the superficial tissues of the upper respiratory tract and are one of the frequent causes of the common cold. The enteroviruses are further subdivided into the poliovirus, coxsackievirus, and echovirus groups. Generally they produce mild or asymptomatic infections of the intestinal tract but may also cause respiratory or systemic infection. Enteroviruses are also responsible for infections of the central nervous system.

The picornaviruses are stable and able to survive for long periods in sewage, water, and foods.

RHINOVIRUSES

Rhinoviruses grow best at 33°C and have thus adapted to grow in the cooler superficial tissues of the nasal cavity, thereby inducing the infections referred to as coryza or the common cold. These infections do not spread beyond the nasal cavity and tissue damage is usually slight to moderate. Much of the symptomatology of the common cold is due to the release of histamine from the patient's mast cells—a reaction stimulated by virus-induced tissue damage. The released histamine induces such symptoms

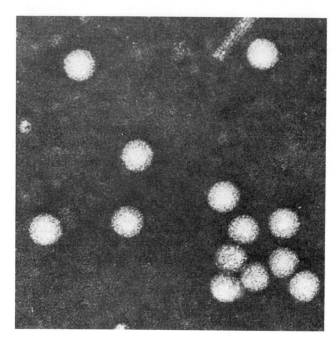

Figure 38-1 Transmission electron micrograph of polioviruses magnified 300,000×. (Courtesy Robley C. Williams, University of California, Berkeley)

as increased mucous secretions, watery eyes, and sneezing. About 100 different rhinovirus serotypes have been identified.

Common colds are most frequent during the winter and it has been postulated that such factors as crowding in buildings, low relative humidity, and chilling may increase the rate of infection. Attacks of the common cold occur repeatedly, partly because of the large number of serotypes of rhinoviruses. Another factor is the relatively short duration (about 3 to 6 months) of immunity that is conferred to the superficial mucosal tissues by the IgA antibody response. Various other viruses are also able to cause common colds.

No specific treatment for the common cold is available; antihistamines and other medications, however, may be used to relieve symptoms. The possible role of vitamin C in treating and preventing colds is debatable; as yet it does not appear to provide either protection or therapy. Vaccines are not available.

POLIOVIRUSES

Three serotypes of polioviruses have been identified and at present the diseases caused by these viruses constitute minor problems in developed countries. The widespread use of effective vaccines has reduced the number of cases of poliomyelitis, or just polio, in the United States to fewer than a dozen per year. The conquest of polio is one of the great success stories of modern medical research. Although the disease of paralytic polio is no longer a threat in the developed countries, persons involved in health fields need to understand both the principles involved in the "rise and fall" of this disease during the first 65 years of the twentieth century and how these principles may still apply in underdeveloped countries. It is also important to understand why continued emphasis on immunization is needed to prevent possible future recurrences of the disease.

Pathogenesis and Clinical Diseases

The poliovirus generally enters the body via the oral route. The virus first proliferates in the throat and small intestines and then passes through the draining lymph nodes and enters the blood, thus becoming widely disseminated (Figure 38-2). On occasion the virus passes into the CNS but infects only certain motor nerve cells of the spinal cord or brain. Varying degrees of paralysis may result, depending on the location of the destroyed nerve cells. Paralysis of lower limbs results from infection of the anterior horn cells of the spinal cord whereas infection in the brain stem, called *bulbar poliomyelitis*, may cause death due to respiratory or cardiac failure. It is now known that less than 1% of those infected with polio virus show signs of CNS involvement. In over 99% of the cases the infection is limited to tissues other than the CNS and the infected persons may experience only minor nonspecific symptoms of a respiratory or intestinal tract infection. The presence of circulating antibodies is very effective in preventing the spread of the virus through the blood to the CNS.

Epidemiology

The epidemiology of paralytic polio is closely associated with the sanitary conditions of a population in a paradoxical way. That is, paralytic disease is rarely seen in populations living under conditions of poor sanitation and the paradox is explained in the following manner. Polio viruses are widespread in populations where poor sanitary conditions prevail and all persons possess specific polio antibodies. An infant born into such a culture possesses sufficient passive immunity to prevent the virus from passing through the blood to the CNS. These circulating IgG-type antibodies, however, will not prevent infections of the intestinal tract; under unsanitary conditions the infants are invariably infected with the polio viruses before they lose their passive immunity. The natural intestinal infection then stimulates lifelong natural active immunity. Only when sanitary conditions begin to improve is it possible for infants to avoid the primary infection long enough for the passive immunity to disappear. Yet these infants will generally contract the natural disease fairly early in life and about 1% will develop the paralytic disease. The change from poor sanitary conditions to improved conditions began to occur during the latter part of the nineteenth century in the United States and in some European countries. At that time paralytic polio was first recognized as a specific disease; and because it occurred mainly in young children, it was called *infantile paralysis*. As sanitary conditions continued to improve, it

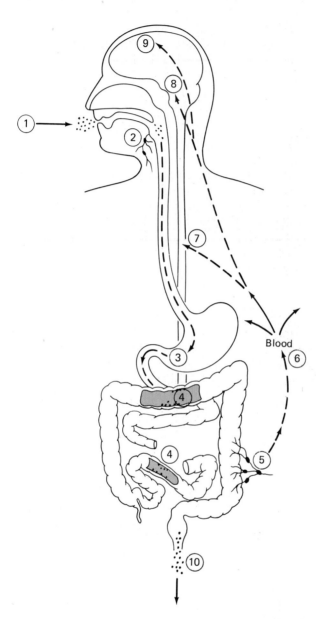

Figure 38-2 The pathogenesis of poliomyelitis. (1) Ingestion of virus. (2) Some multiplication may occur in tonsils and lymph nodes of upper respiratory tract with common cold type symptoms. (3) Virus resistant to stomach acids and digestive fluids. (4) Multiplication of virus in Peyer's patches and other lymphoid cells along the intestinal tract with clinical symptoms of enteritis. (5) Viruses drain into regional lymph nodes which stimulates antibody response. (6) Viruses may pass into blood. (7) In a small percentage of infections, the viruses may cross the blood-brain barrier into the CNS. Motor nerves (anterior horn cells) are specifically infected and result in paralysis of certain muscles. (8) Lower brain centers may be infected causing bulbar polio. (9) Motor cortex may be infected causing widespread paralysis. (10) Large amounts of virus shed in feces.

became possible for more and more children to avoid primary exposure for longer and longer periods and in the first decades of the 1900s more and more paralytic polio occurred in progressively older persons. The annual polio rate in the United States reached its highest level in the early 1950s and then dropped sharply after the introduction of the killed vaccine (Figure 38-3).

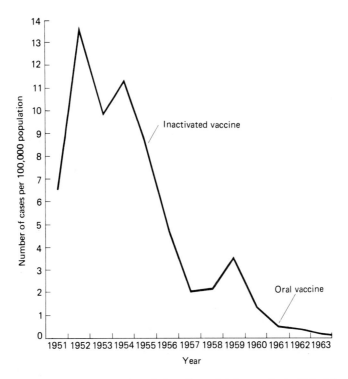

Figure 38-3   Reported cases of paralytic poliomyelitis by year in the United States, 1951–1963. The case rates since 1963 have been less than 0.06 per 100,000 population. In 1952, 57,879 cases were reported compared to 7 cases in 1974 (*CDC Annual Summary*, 1980).

Prevention and Control

Polio has been controlled through the development of effective vaccines. A killed vaccine, containing all three serotypes, was first introduced in 1955 and induced adequate immunity when given as a series of three injections over a 3- to 6-month period, followed with booster injections every 2 or 3 years. By the early 1960s a living attenuated vaccine became available and has completely replaced the use of killed vaccine in the United States and many other countries. The living vaccine provides long-lasting immunity after one administration and it can be taken orally, thus saving time and money and avoiding the discomfort of hypodermic injections.

Even though a small risk is involved with the use of the living vaccine, in that one out of approximately every 8 million receiving it may develop paralytic disease, the overall success of the polio vaccines has been phenomenal. Cases were reduced from 28,985 in 1955 to between 7 and 20 cases a year since the late 1960s. The few vaccine-associated cases may be further reduced by not administering the living vaccine to immunosuppressed children.

CLINICAL NOTE

Poliomyelitis: Pennsylvania and Maryland

The first paralytic poliomyelitis case in the United States with onset in 1979 was reported in a 22-year-old unvaccinated, female resident of a small Amish community in Franklin County, Pennsylvania. The patient, who had been hospitalized in Maryland, became ill on January 5 with headache, fever, and generalized myalgias. On January 6 and 7 she developed right and then left lower-extremity weakness and decreased deep tendon reflexes. She had no sensory abnormalities. On January 17 the Maryland State Department of Health and Mental Hygiene reported that type 1 poliovirus had been isolated from a stool specimen collected from the patient on January 10.

An epidemiologic investigation revealed that the patient had no known exposure to other individuals with clinical poliomyelitis or to recent recipients of the live virus vaccine. In addition, there was no history of recent travel to known polio-endemic areas. At least three Amish weddings had taken place during the period of November through January, resulting in extensive interactions among the Amish communities in Franklin and eight other Pennsylvania counties and other Amish communities in Maryland, Ohio, Vermont, New York, and Ontario, Canada. The patient's most recent out-of-state travel had been to an Amish community in St. Marys and Charles counties, Maryland, in late November. Stool specimens were collected on January 18 and 19 from 17 asymptomatic members of this community; 12 were positive for type 1 poliovirus. In addition, stool specimens collected on January 18 through 20 from 32 individuals in the patient's own community revealed that 16 were positive for poliovirus.

Surveys by Pennsylvania and Maryland health departments revealed that few individuals had been completely immunized in the two affected Amish communities. It was strongly recommended that all members of the affected Amish communities and all non-Amish persons who have had close association with these communities be vaccinated with the trivalent oral poliovirus vaccine. Vaccination clinics have been set up in Pennsylvania and Maryland. Approximately 67% of the target population in Maryland was vaccinated by January 31.

Surveillance for paralytic illness and aseptic meningitis possibly due to poliovirus infection has been intensified in Pennsylvania and Maryland as well as in Amish communities in other states (*MMWR 26*:49, 1979).

COXSACKIEVIRUSES AND ECHOVIRUSES

The coxsackieviruses are so named because they were first isolated in 1948 from children living in the town of Coxsackie, New York. The children were thought to have mild cases of polio. The first echoviruses were discovered several years later during field trials of the killed polio vaccine. It was customary in these trials to examine many vaccinated children to determine if they were shedding the polioviruses. Besides finding some polioviruses and coxsackieviruses, a group of previously unidentified viruses was discovered. Because these new viruses were isolated from the intestinal tract, produced a cytopathic effect in cell cultures, were isolated from humans, and were not associated with any apparent diseases, they were given the name *ECHO*, which is an acronym for *E*nteric, *C*ytopathic, *H*uman, *O*rphan viruses. Since that time, however, many of the echoviruses have been shown to cause a variety of diseases.

About 30 different serotypes of coxsackieviruses and 33 serotypes of echo viruses are identified. Differences between these two groups of viruses are slight and the current procedure is not to classify new isolates into either of these groups but simply call them enteroviruses and give them a numerical designation—for instance, *enterovirus 70*.

These viruses are transmitted by both the fecal-oral and the airborne route. Generally the enterovirus infections are subclinical or mild with generalized symptoms. Occasionally symptoms may be more severe. Such clinical diseases as common colds, fevers with skin rashes, pharyngitis, pneumonitis, meningitis, encephalitis, carditis, and diarrhea may be caused by coxsackieviruses or echoviruses. The highest rate of infection tends to occur in late summer.

CLINICAL NOTE

Echo 9 Outbreak: New York

During July 1975 an outbreak of illness caused by Echo 9 virus occurred in a vacation colony in Dutchess County, New York.

All residents of the colony were surveyed and blood, stool, and throat cultures were obtained on 15 individuals with recent illness. Results of this survey revealed that from June 30 through July 23, 88 (37.6%) of the 234 colony residents became ill. Typical symptoms and signs were headache (59%), fever (53%), stiff neck (36%), and rash (36%). Other less frequent manifestations included vomiting (18%), diarrhea (16%), and sore throat (13%). Age-specific attack rates were highest in the 0 to 4 (18%) and 5 to 9 (46%) year groups. Attack rates were similar for both sexes in persons under 21 years of age, but were significantly higher for females (41%) than males (17%) in the 21 or older age groups. The dates of onset suggested person-to-person-spread as the mode of transmission in this outbreak.

Analysis of the intervals between primary and secondary household cases suggested an incubation period of 2 to 4 days. Echo 9 virus was isolated from 9 of 15 throat cultures and 11 of 13 stool specimens submitted to the New York Department of Health laboratory. Control measures taken to interrupt further transmission consisted of closure of the day camp, restriction of swimming pool use to postconvalescent persons, and temporary confinement of children to their quarters (*MMWR 25*:32, 1976).

SUMMARY

The small RNA viruses are best known for their role as the causative agents of the disease polio. Use of polio vaccines has made this disease almost nonexistent in the United States. Other picorna viral diseases occur with regular frequency and produce symptoms ranging from diarrhea or the common cold to meningitis and carditis.

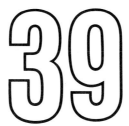

Rhabdoviruses

Rhabdoviruses infect various vertebrate and invertebrate hosts; they contain RNA and have helical symmetry. The helix is wound in a rod shape with one end tapered, which gives the virion a "bullet" shape (see Figure 31-2). Rabies is the only serious widespread disease of humans caused by a rhabdovirus.

RABIES

The rabies virus appears capable of infecting and causing serious disease in most mammals. Most die, but some are able to carry and shed the virus for prolonged periods. The disease of rabies in humans was recognized and reported in ancient times as a disease transmitted by the bite of a mad (rabid) dog. Once signs of rabies begin to appear in humans, indicating infection of the central nervous system, the disease almost invariably progresses until death results.

Pathogenesis and Clinical Disease

Generally humans are infected by the bite of an infected animal that introduces the virus into the tissues. The virus remains localized for several hours at the site of the bite, where some local multiplication may occur. The virus then spreads slowly from the local site of entry, apparently moving along nerve fibers to the regional ganglia and the CNS. The incubation time—that is, the period between the time of the bite and the onset of signs of the disease in the CNS—varies greatly, depending on the site and the severity of the bite as well as other host factors that are not well defined. The incubation period is a reflection of the rate of spread of the virus and may range from a week to months and even a year or more. The incubation period is usually longer when the bite occurs on an extremity, such as an arm or leg, and shorter when occurring about the neck and head.

The virus fails to progress from the site of entry to the CNS in approximately half or more of the persons bitten by an infected animal. Once the virus enters the CNS, however, it spreads rapidly throughout these tissues and may also be present in other tissues. When this stage is reached, the overt signs and symptoms of the disease begin with fever, headache, and loss of appetite. Then they progress to convulsions, excessive flow of tears and saliva, insomnia, anxiety, muscle spasms triggered by swallowing, and sometimes maniacal behavior. Ascending paralysis may be seen and death sometimes results after 2 to 6 days because of respiratory or cardiac failure. In other cases, patients lapse into a coma, followed by death. Clinical rabies has invariably resulted in the death of the patient except in three known cases.

The pathogenesis of rabies in animals has many similarities and some differences from the disease in humans. The route of infection in animals is often by the bite of another infected animal, but disease may also result from eating a diseased animal. In many animals the virus passes to the CNS during the long incubation period. In dogs, cats, and related animals the virus appears in various excretory glands, especially the salivary glands, several days before the onset of signs of CNS involvement. Once signs of the CNS infection occur, the animal usually dies within a relatively short time. A small percentage of these animals have been found to shed rabies virus in their saliva for up to 2 years without developing the clinical disease. Bats are often infected with rabies virus and appear to tolerate the infection much better than most other animals. Some evidence indicates that bats are able to carry and shed the rabies virus for prolonged periods without showing signs of the disease.

Transmission and Epidemiology

Normally the route of transmission is by the bite of an infected animal (Figure 39-1). This route works extremely well, for the irritation of the infection on the CNS drives the animal into a frenzy that results in the biting of other animals. Such biting occurs at the time when high concentrations of virus are found in the saliva. Rabies in humans and in animals like cows or horses is usually a dead end because the infection is not conveniently transmitted to other hosts by biting. Although only a few cases of rabies are seen in humans each year in the United States (Figure 39-2), many wild animals are infected (Figure 39-3).

Rabies may be transmitted orally through eating infected meat and may be an important means of transmission among wild carnivores. Airborne transmission in bat caves, while rare, has occurred. Four cases have been documented in persons receiving corneal transplants from donors who had died of undiagnosed rabies. Rabies in cattle is a major economic problem in Latin America and is transmitted by the bite of infected vampire bats. Bats, in general, probably serve as the most important reservoir of the rabies virus.

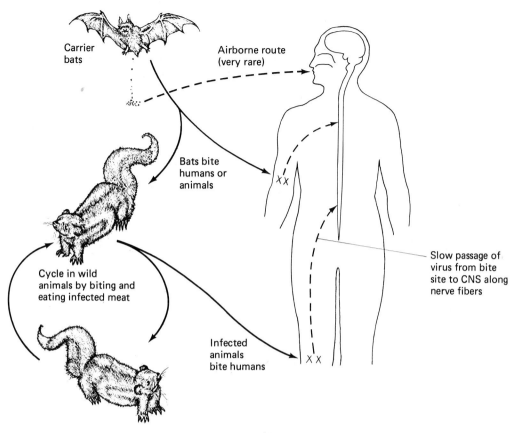

Figure 39-1 Modes of transmission of rabies viruses among animals and to humans.

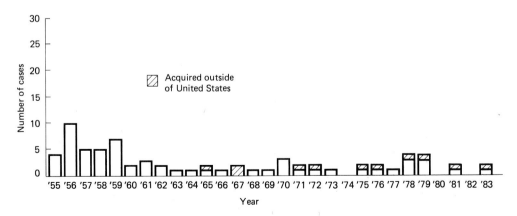

Figure 39-2 Reported rabies cases in humans by year in the United States, 1955–1983 (modified from CDC annual summaries).

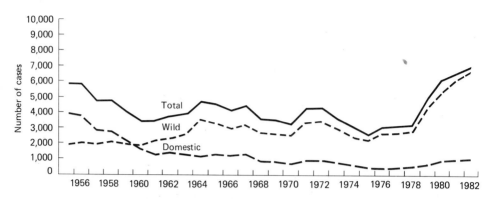

Figure 39-3 Reported rabies cases in wild and domestic animals by year in the United States, 1955–1982 (modified from CDC annual summaries).

Diagnosis

The most important priority is the rapid detection of rabies in an animal that has bitten a person. Whether the biting animal is infected directly determines the type of treatment that the bite victim should receive. Whenever possible, an animal that bites a person should be apprehended or killed. If domestic animals like dogs or cats do not show definite signs of rabies, the animal should be placed under observation at the public health laboratory for 8 to 10 days and monitored for the appearance of clinical signs of rabies. Wild animals or domestic animals showing signs of rabies should be killed and either the intact animal or the head taken immediately to a public health laboratory. The animal should be wrapped in a plastic bag to prevent possible contamination and kept cool if possible.

The laboratory worker examines the brain cells for the appearance of clusters of viral materials (inclusion bodies) in the cytoplasm called *Negri bodies*. Negri bodies are rapidly and specifically identified by using specific fluorescent antibodies. A positive diagnosis can be made on most infected animals within a few minutes via this procedure. As a backup test, brain tissue is injected into suckling mice that will develop rabies within the next 1 to 3 weeks if the virus is present.

Diagnosis in humans is based on clinical signs and symptoms and on a possible history of exposure to rabies. Diagnosis is confirmed after death by demonstrating the presence of rabies virus in the brain tissue by the fluorescent antibody method and by mouse inoculation.

Treatment

Treatment of clinical rabies has generally been unsuccessful. A few exceptions have occurred. The most notable was a 6-year-old boy in Ohio who was bitten by a rabid bat in 1970. He went through the Pasteur treatment but still developed clinical rabies. Through close medical supervision and such standard medical interventions as a tracheotomy to control respiration, drainage of cerebrospinal fluid to prevent excessive pressure on the brain, anticonvulsive drugs, and monitoring of heart rhythm, this patient was able to survive complications that killed most other known rabies patients. Apparently his own defense mechanisms were able to fight off the rabies virus infections and his recovery was complete.

Prevention and Control

A great deal of effort and resources go toward preventing and controlling rabies and in most countries these programs have been highly successful. Cases of human rabies in the United States have been reduced to only a few a year. Still, those who may be exposed to rabies each year number approximately 30,000.

Prevention and control of rabies are carried out in the following areas:

1. Control in domestic animals by vaccination and quarantine
2. Vaccination of persons who have a high risk of being exposed
3. Postexposure prophylaxis (the Pasteur treatment)

Before the initiation of strict control measures, most human rabies were contracted by the bite of domestic cats or dogs. Leash laws, licensing of dogs, and vaccinations have reduced the cases of rabies in these animals to an insignificant number in many countries and eliminated rabies completely in such regions as Great Britain, Scandinavia, Australia, New Zealand, Hawaii, and Taiwan. Rabies is prevented from reentering these rabies-free countries by the strict quarantine of imported animals. Still, in many parts of the world rabies is widespread in wildlife and no effective methods are available to control or eliminate this reservoir of the virus. The major animal reservoirs in the United States are bats, skunks, foxes, and raccoons; yet virtually any wild animal may be infected and so any animal exhibiting abnormal behavior should be suspect.

Several vaccine varieties for both humans and animals are available. A living attenuated vaccine is generally used to vaccinate dogs and cats. Vaccination is recommended for veterinarians, animal control officers, campers, and similar people who are in frequent contact with wild animals. For many years an inactivated vaccine produced in embryonated duck eggs was used for the vaccination of humans in the United States; production of this vaccine was discontinued in 1981. In 1980 a purified killed rabies vaccine, produced in human diploid cell cultures, became available. This new vaccine seems much more effective than the older vaccines and is now the only vaccine available in the United States for rabies vaccinations or postexposure prophylaxis. A killed vaccine called the Semple vaccine, which is prepared from a 10% emulsion of rabies-infected rabbit CNS, is still used in some countries for human vaccinations and postexposure prophylaxis. It will probably be replaced by the human diploid cell vaccine in the future.

The prevention of rabies primarily concerns how people are handled following their exposure to rabies. Possibly because of the long incubation period, rabies is the only disease in which the initiation of active vaccination after exposure is successful. This procedure was developed by Pasteur in 1884 when he prevented the development of rabies in a boy who had been severely bitten by a rabid wolf. Pasteur injected progressively more potent preparations of rabies-infected rabbit spinal cord extracts into the boy daily over a 21-day period. The treatment worked and was referred to as the Pasteur treatment. Some modifications were made in the Pasteur treatment over the years, but no controlled studies were carried out to determine the optimum dosage schedules to use. All programs today use only killed vaccines.

Local treatment of the wound is helpful in preventing rabies. The wound should immediately be cleansed thoroughly and flushed with soap and water. The patient should then be taken to a physician to receive antiserum treatment. Hyperimmune antirabies human gamma globulin is now available and should be instilled in the depths of the wound and infiltrated around the wound. Next, the Pasteur treatment should be initiated. Up until 1980 either the duck embryo or Semple vaccine was used for the Pasteur treatment and was administered via 14 or 21 daily injections. Major side reactions often resulted from these injections, causing great discomfort and sometimes permanent neurologic damage. The purified human diploid cell rabies vaccine was licensed for use in the United States in 1980. The first dose of this new vaccine is followed by doses 3, 7, 14, and 28 days later. Some minor discomfort may be experienced with the new vaccine, but none of the major side reactions associated with the older vaccine has been seen.

The treatment regimen should be correlated with the diagnostic program on the animal that inflicted the bite. If tests show that the animal is not infected, the Pasteur treatment should be stopped to avoid further discomfort and possible danger to the patient. For this reason, it is important to apprehend the biting animal. If the animal is not apprehended, the victim usually has little choice but to go through the Pasteur treatment. About 30,000 Pasteur treatments are given in the United States annually.

CLINICAL NOTE

Imported Human Rabies

The first case of human rabies in the United States since August 1981 has been reported to CDC. The patient, a 30-year-old American architect from Waltham, Massachusetts, was exposed to rabies from a dog bite in Ososo, Nigeria, West Africa. He died on January 28, 1983, 28 days after onset of symptoms.

On October 8, the patient, who worked in Nigeria, was bitten on the right wrist by his pet Doberman pinscher while attempting to free it from a trap. The dog died later that day and was buried without laboratory examination for rabies. The patient sought medical attention at a nearby clinic and received tetanus immunization, but because the dog had recently been immunized against rabies, it was decided that postexposure prophylaxis was unnecessary.

Eleven weeks later, the patient returned to the United States and remained well until January 1, 1983, 85 days after the bite, when he developed numbness and tingling at the healed bite-site. During the next several days, the patient developed low back pain, a temperature of 38.9°C (102°F), sore throat, anorexia, and malaise. On January 5, he complained of difficulty breathing, mild chest discomfort, excessive salivation, and occasionally gagging when attempting to drink. He was examined by a physician, who noted that he had nonspecific ST-T changes on an electrocardiogram. He was admitted to Waltham Hospital, Waltham, Massachusetts, for further evaluation.

On admission, the patient was anxious and was producing a large volume of saliva, which he refused to swallow. He suggested that a milk deficiency caused his illness, and exhibited unusual fear of some medical procedures. His pharynx was slightly erythematous, and his neck or throat structures contracted when touched with the hands or examining instruments. The remainder of the physical examination was unremarkable. Laboratory tests revealed a white blood count of 9900, with a normal differential, normal serum electrolytes and calcium, and normal chest x ray. On January 6, the patient exhibited marked hyperactivity and refused to swallow barium for a radiologic examination. On the evening of January 6, he had respiratory arrest and a generalized seizure, and an endotracheal tube was inserted. Following the respiratory arrest, his temperature rose to 41.1°C (106°F). A chest x ray showed diffuse pulmonary infiltrates. A diagnosis of rabies was considered, and the patient was placed in strict isolation. A skin biopsy, taken from the back of his neck above the hairline, was sent to CDC for direct immunofluorescent antibody (FA) testing for rabies.

On January 7, the biopsy was reported positive. The patient was able to communicate rationally with hospital staff by writing notes. He demonstrated marked pharyngeal and laryngeal spasms when his face or neck was stimulated by either a wet sponge or a draught of cool air. Bacterial cultures of cerebrospinal fluid (CSF), blood, urine, and sputum were negative. Computerized tomography and electroencephalogram were normal. The patient continued to require ventilatory support and a dopamine infusion to maintain adequate blood pressure. On January 8, he was started on systemic interferon treatment. He was given human leukocyte interferon, 10 million units twice daily intramuscularly, and 5 million units once daily intraventricularly into a Rickham reservoir connected by a cannula to a lateral ventricle of his brain.

During the next 10 days, the patient became progressively less responsive and was in a deep coma by January 18. He had numerous medical complications during the course of illness, including *Pseudomonas* sepsis and keratoconjunctivitis, recurrent seizures, hypo- and hyperthermia, anemia, hypotension, abnormal blood clotting, and acute renal failure. The interferon therapy was discontinued on January 25, 17 days after the first dose was administered. The patient developed adult respiratory distress syndrome refractory to ventilation and died of cardiovascular collapse on January 28. Serum collected daily from the patient and tested at CDC for rabies antibody turned positive 1:12 on the 16th day of illness and remained minimally positive at 1:25 or less until his death. At postmortem, many tissues were positive for rabies virus, including specimens from brain and spinal cord, skin and nerve from the bite site, pancreas, liver, bladder, periaortic lymph node, pericardium, adrenal gland, and salivary gland.

A total of 132 persons were evaluated for potential contact with infectious secretions from the patient. Twenty-eight persons received rabies postexposure prophylaxis, including seven physicians, 14 nurses, three respiratory therapists, one microbiologist, two friends and relatives of the patient, and one other hospital contact. In addition, three pathologists received pre-exposure prophylaxis before the patient's death (*MMWR 32*:78, 1983).

SUMMARY

A bullet-shaped, helical RNA rhabdovirus is responsible for the disease rabies. This is a common disease among lower animals and in humans in foreign countries, but its occurrence is limited in people living in the United States. The disease is unusual in its mode of transmission and devastating in its consequences. Control of rabies is best accomplished by the immunization of domestic animals and individuals at high risk. Vaccines with risk of serious side effects have largely been replaced by a more useful diploid cell vaccine.

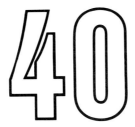

Other Viruses

This chapter discusses unrelated groups of viruses that cause a variety of significant diseases of humans.

TOGAVIRUSES

The togaviruses are a group of about 250 related viruses. They contain RNA, have cubical symmetry, and possess an envelope. The presence of the envelope is the basis for the name *toga*, which means an outer garment or mantle. The togaviruses constitute a major portion of a group of viruses called the *arboviruses*, which stands for arthropod-borne viruses. Arboviruses are able to multiply in such blood-sucking arthropods as mosquitoes, ticks, and gnats, as well as in many different vertebrate hosts that include mammals, birds, and reptiles. These viruses are passed from vertebrate hosts to arthropods and vice versa during the taking of blood meals by the arthropods. Mosquitoes are the main vector involved in transmission. Most togaviruses are arthropod borne, but also included as arboviruses are some members of the rhabdovirus, reovirus, and bunyavirus groups. The rubella virus is morphologically similar to the togaviruses, but its pathogenesis and epidemiology are similar to that of the paramyxoviruses and so this virus was discussed with the paramyxoviruses in Chapter 37.

Pathogenesis and Clinical Diseases

Many togaviruses are maintained in nature with only slight or no observable effects on their natural arthropod or vertebrate hosts. Humans are accidently infected when

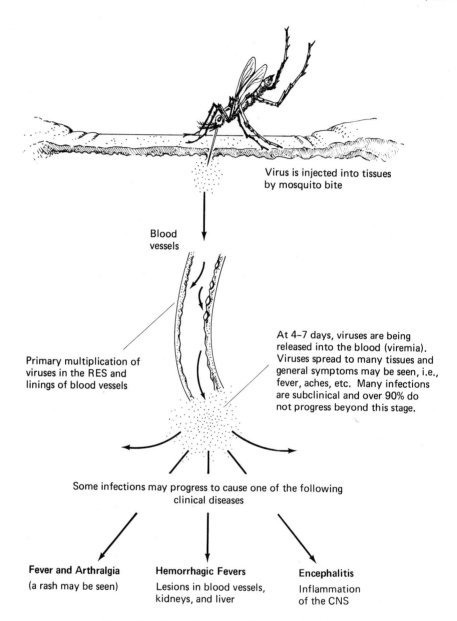

Virus is injected into tissues
by mosquito bite

Blood
vessels

Primary multiplication of
viruses in the RES and
linings of blood vessels

At 4–7 days, viruses are being
released into the blood (viremia).
Viruses spread to many tissues and
general symptoms may be seen, i.e.,
fever, aches, etc. Many infections
are subclinical and over 90% do
not progress beyond this stage.

Some infections may progress to cause one of the following
clinical diseases

Fever and Arthralgia

(a rash may be seen)

Hemorrhagic Fevers

Lesions in blood vessels,
kidneys, and liver

Encephalitis

Inflammation
of the CNS

Figure 40-1   The pathogeneses of togavirus infections.

bitten by an infected insect and are usually a dead end in the transmission chain. Most
human infections are mild or subclinical; some togaviruses, however, are able to
cause serious disease. Figure 40-1 shows an outline of the pathogenesis and general
categories of togavirus diseases. The viruses first multiply in the cells lining the blood

vessels (endothelial cells) and the cells of the RES. In 4 to 7 days viruses are being released into the blood. Most human infections are subclinical or relatively mild with generalized symptoms of fever, aches, and chills. Moreover, most do not progress beyond this mild or subclinical stage. A dozen or so togaviruses, however, are able to cause serious diseases that progress beyond the generalized symptoms to produce the syndromes listed next.

Fever and arthralgia

These diseases are characterized by the sudden onset of fever, headache, swollen lymph nodes, conjunctivitis, and excruciating pains in the back, muscles, and joints. A rash may or may not occur. Diseases of this category are primarily seen in subtropical and tropical areas. Deaths are rare. Dengue fever is the most frequently experienced disease of this type and increased numbers of cases have been seen in Mexico and the Caribbean islands in the 1970s and 1980s. Limited outbreaks that occurred in southern Texas in 1980 were the first cases reported in the United States since 1945.

Hemorrhagic fevers

A few togaviruses damage the blood capillaries, resulting in subcutaneous hemorrhaging and bleeding from body openings. This type of hemorrhagic disease is found in many parts of the world but not in the United States. A second type of hemorrhagic fever causes lesions of the liver and kidney: it is the serious disease of yellow fever. Yellow fever was once one of the major diseases of mankind, with devastating outbreaks occurring in crews of sailing ships in tropical areas, among military troops, or in construction crews. Work on the Panama Canal was stopped in the late 1800s because of yellow fever. Walter Reed, a U.S. medical officer studying yellow fever in Cuba during the Spanish-American War, first demonstrated that this disease was transmitted by the *Aedes aegypti* species of mosquito. Control of the *Aedes aegypti* mosquito led to a control of yellow fever, although the disease is still prevalent in some tropical areas. An effective vaccine is available and persons traveling in endemic areas must be vaccinated. Death rates from yellow fever are about 10%.

Encephalitis

Various togaviruses are able to cause encephalitis. This disease begins with generalized symptoms and then after several days develops into encephalitis. The symptoms of encephalitis include drowsiness and stiff neck; severe cases may progress to confusion, paralysis, coma, and death. The term *sleeping sickness* is sometimes applied to these diseases but should not be confused with the protozoan disease of African sleeping sickness. Some residual effects, such as mental retardation, deafness, and blindness, may result. These infections occur in all parts of the world and several thousand sporadic cases are seen in the United States during the summer months. Rates are highest when large numbers of mosquitoes are present, as during extra wet summers. Mosquito-borne encephalitis is the only type generally found in the United States. Tick-borne, as well as mosquito-borne, cases appear in other countries. The major types seen in the United States are Eastern, Western, St. Louis, and Venezuelan equine encephalitis. Eastern equine encephalitis is the most severe and causes frequent deaths. The others are less severe in humans, death rates being around 1%. The term equine is attached to the name of these viruses because these diseases were first recognized in horses. Horses are often infected and the disease may be quite severe with relatively high death rates. Equine encephalitis can be a major problem to the equine industry because it forces the cancellation of races, rodeos, and horse shows and results in the death of valuable animals.

Transmission and Epidemiology

Togaviruses, as well as the other arboviruses, are transmitted in a complex ecosystem that involves the blood-sucking arthropod vectors and animal reservoirs. The viruses are usually passed in these natural hosts with few consequences. Problems result when these infections "spill over" from these natural hosts into humans and horses. This spillover occurs when environmental conditions permit a large buildup in the numbers of insect vectors and natural animal hosts and when the viruses are introduced into this environment. Such conditions frequently occur in swampy areas and in other areas that have extra wet summers. The reported cases of encephalitis from all causes are shown in Figure 40-2; the marked increases during the summer are due to togavirus infections.

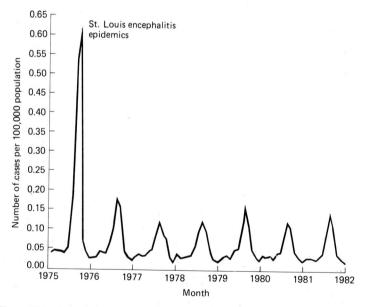

Figure 40-2 Reported cases of encephalitis from all causes in the United States per month, 1975–1982. The marked increases during the summer months were due primarily to togavirus infections (modified from CDC annual summaries).

Diagnosis

The generalized nonspecific infections usually go undiagnosed. The severe infections are tentatively diagnosed on clinical and epidemiological findings. Confirmed diagnoses are made by viral isolations and/or showing specific increases in serum antibody levels.

Treatment

No specific treatment is available.

Prevention and Control

The major control methods are to prevent exposure to mosquitoes or ticks. Eradication or reduction in the number of mosquitoes is routinely carried out in many areas during the summer. Immunization is required for persons traveling to areas where yellow fever is present. Vaccines against other togavirus encephalitides have been developed but are not licensed for human use in the United States. Such vaccines, however, are widely used for the immunization of horses.

CLINICAL NOTE

Western Equine Encephalitis: Minnesota and North Dakota, 1975

In the early summer of 1975 the Red River flooded into the valley area of eastern North Dakota and northwestern Minnesota. Subsequently health officials initiated a mosquito surveillance program that indicated an unusually high mosquito-population density in the area. Of 96 mosquito pools collected in three North Dakota counties in mid-July, nine yielded isolations of Western equine encephalitis (WEE) virus. Because of the predominance of the mosquito vector and the resultant increased risk of virus transmission, officials intensified disease surveillance in horses and humans.

Horse surveillance.   Cases of equine encephalitis were first observed in early June and a total of 192 cases of clinical encephalitis were reported through August 9, 1975. Of the 192 ill horses, 24 unvaccinated ones had sera collected, and 17 of these horses had high hemagglutination inhibition (HI) and serum neutralization (SN) antibody titers to WEE and no titers to Eastern equine encephalitis. Paired sera from 2 of the 192 ill horses showed a fourfold rise in HI antibody titer to WEE. Of 165 ill horses, 3 (1.8%) were known to have been vaccinated more than 2 weeks before the onset of clinical encephalitis.

Human surveillance.   Surveillance in North Dakota and Minnesota uncovered 27 cases of acute, febrile central nervous system (CNS) disease, with onset dates from July 10 to August 6, 1975. All cases were associated with an increased number of cells in the cerebrospinal fluid and most were reported from hospitals in the Red River Valley. Of the 27 cases, 15 were diagnosed as aseptic meningitis and 12 as clinical encephalitis. Four deaths from suspected encephalitis have occurred, all in North Dakota. In 3 cases, including 2 of the deaths, the diagnosis of WEE infection was serologically confirmed by fourfold or greater HI antibody titer rises.

In addition to intensive local and state mosquito control measures that began in Minnesota on July 26, aerial spraying of ultra-low-volume malathion over population centers was begun August 1. Twelve counties in eastern North Dakota received two applications of insecticide; spraying of 11 western Minnesota counties began August 12. The gradual natural reduction of breeding sites in the postflood period, combined with spraying, resulted in a substantially decreased mosquito population, but levels remained greater than normal.

Other states reporting seropositive cases of WEE in horses are: Colorado (20), Kansas (18), South Dakota (16), Oklahoma (13), Nebraska (11), Oregon (2), Montana (1), and Iowa (1). To date, no cases of WEE in humans have been reported from these states (*MMWR 24*:270, 1975).

ARENAVIRUSES

In the late 1960s accumulated evidence demonstrated that some previously unclassified viruses shared a common morphology. These viruses are pleomorphic with diameters ranging between 60 and 350 nm. They contain dense, ribosome-sized (20 nm) particles that give the appearance of sand particles when viewed by the electron microscope (Figure 40-3). This is the basis for the name of this virus group (*arenosus* = sandy).

These viruses are normally found in various wild rodents where they cause persistent, lifelong infections, usually without acute clinical signs. The viruses are shed in the feces and urine of the rodent and contaminate food or water. Humans coming in contact with the contaminated materials may contract an acute viral infection. The major arenavirus infections of humans are discussed next.

Lymphocytic Choriomeningitis

The lymphocytic choriomeningitis virus is widespread in domestic house mice throughout the world. In rural areas about 1% of the human inhabitants show serologic evidence of having been infected. The illness is usually nondescript or asymptomatic and rarely is a specific diagnosis made.

Argentinian and Bolivian Hemorrhagic Fevers

Argentinian and Bolivian hemorrhagic fevers occur in limited geographic areas of the respective countries and are caused by closely related arenaviruses. Most outbreaks occur in farmworkers during the harvesting of crops when they apparently come in contact with contaminated urine and feces of infected rodents. These diseases are quite severe in humans, causing widespread damage to the linings of blood

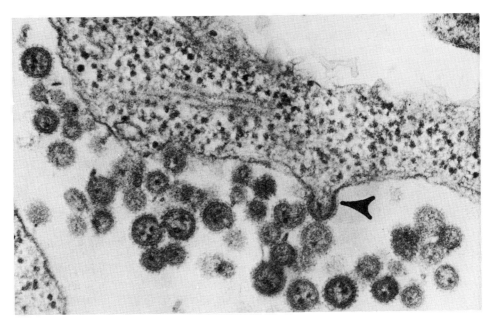

Figure 40-3 Transmission electron micrograph of granule-containing arenaviruses. Arrow points to a virus budding from the infected cell. (Centers for Disease Control, Atlanta)

vessels and capillaries. The result is internal hemorrhaging and death rates between 15 and 20%.

Lassa Fever

Lassa fever was first characterized in 1969 when this disease was dramatically brought to the attention of the world through extensive press coverage of an outbreak among American missionaries in Nigeria, Africa. The first case was reported in a missionary nurse and the disease was transmitted to two attending nurses. The index case and one of the attending nurses died. Clinical specimens were flown to the United States, where two laboratory personnel working with this specimen contracted the disease. One died and the other was saved by receiving passive immunization from serum taken from the original attending nurse, who had recovered from Lassa fever. Lassa fever rapidly developed the label of a severe new West African killer virus disease. In the intervening years this disease was studied in greater detail, using stringent safety precautions, and was found to be present in a variety of wild rodents in Nigeria, Liberia, and Sierra Leone. Both mild and severe cases occur among humans. The mild cases usually go undetected whereas those severe enough to require hospitalization have a death rate of 30 to 66%.

No vaccines are available against any of the arenavirus infections. Proper sanitation and antirodent measures are the most effective means of prevention.

CORONAVIRUSES

The human coronaviruses were first discovered in the mid-1960s and were shown to be a frequent cause of common cold-type infections. The structure of these viruses resembles that of the paramyxoviruses except that the projections (peplomers) are more prominent with knoblike structures on the ends. When viewed by the electron microscope, these projections give the appearance reminiscent of the solar corona—hence the name *coronaviruses*.

Usually the human viruses cannot be isolated on regular cell cultures but require a more difficult procedure that uses organ cultures of tracheal ciliated epithelium. Consequently, the amount of research that can be carried out on these viruses is limited. All current evidence indicates that the coronaviruses cause about 15% of the mild upper respiratory tract infections, such as the common cold. All ages are infected and immunity seems to be short lived; a person can be reinfected with the same serotype throughout life. At least three different serotypes have been identified.

REOVIRUSES

The reoviruses (Figure 40-4) are a group of viruses that contain a ds-RNA molecule as the genome. These viruses also possess a double-layered protein coat. The first reoviruses of humans to be discovered were found in both the respiratory and intestinal tracts but were not associated with a specific disease and the name "reo" is an acronym of *r*espiratory *e*nteric *o*rphan viruses. A second type of reovirus, now called oribivirus, is widespread in insects and may be transmitted to humans or animal by the bite of the virus-carrying tick. Colorado tick fever virus is the only known oribivirus to cause disease in humans. The symptoms are much like those of dengue fever except that no rash is produced.

Rotaviruses, a third type of reovirus, were discovered in 1973. The double-layered protein coat of these viruses gives a characteristic appearance of a wheel when viewed with an electron microscope—hence the name rotavirus (*rota* = wheel). Initially rotaviruses were detected only by electron microscopic examination of tissues and feces. Only in the past decade has it been possible to show limited growth of these viruses in cell cultures. Rotaviruses are now recognized as causing 50% of the cases of diarrhea in infants and young children in all countries. To put this picture in perspective, it is estimated that in Asia, Africa, and Latin America alone over 400 million episodes of diarrhea from all causes occur each year in children under 5 years of age and result in 10 to 15 million deaths. Although diarrhea is also a frequent disease in children in developed countries, death rates are much lower because of a greater number of children who are better nourished and who receive proper medical treatment and supportive therapy. Rotavirus illness is characterized by vomiting, diarrhea, and dehydration. Treatment is directed primarily at replacing body fluids and electrolytes that are lost from vomiting and diarrhea. Often hospitalization is required. Diagnosis can be made by serologic tests that are able either to detect the presence of the ro-

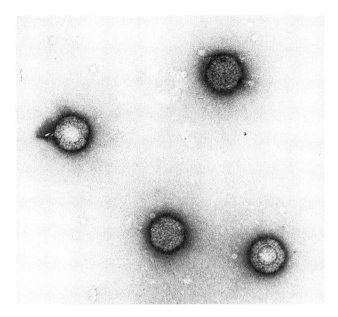

Figure 40-4 Transmission electron micrograph of reoviruses magnified 110,000×. (Courtesy Robley C. Williams, University of California, Berkeley)

tavirus antigen in feces or measure an increase in antibody levels between acute and convalescent sera. Diagnosis can also be made by demonstrating the presence of the characteristic wheel-shaped virus particles in fecal samples examined with an electron microscope. No vaccine is available; the best control measure involves good sanitation to reduce transmission by the fecal-oral route.

NORWALK GROUP OF VIRUSES

The Norwalk group of viruses has not been well characterized but appears similar to the parvoviruses in size, shape, and other physical characteristics. Some studies have suggested that these viruses may be associated with about one-third of all outbreaks of viral gastroenteritis in some population groups. Infections are associated more with gastroenteritis in older persons and less with infections in infants and young children.

ACQUIRED IMMUNE DEFICIENCY SYNDROME (AIDS)

This disease, of considerable public interest, has been shown to be caused by a virus related to the cancer producing retroviruses (p. 409). Currently this virus is referred to by the dual names of human T-lymphotropic virus type III/ Lymphadenopathy-associated virus (HTLV-III/LAV). This disease has had an interesting history that began during 1981 when there were several reports from Los Angeles and New York City of a rare form of tumor known as Kaposi's sarcoma. The disease was most unusual in that it occurred in young adults and was found in persons not usually thought to develop Kaposi's. The reports, few in number at first but growing in frequency, also noted that many of these patients also suffered from an unusual form of pneumonia due to a protozoan known as *Pneumocystis carinii*. Although other common features of the infection gradually came to light, the most striking was the markedly higher incidence of the disease among homosexuals, particularly homosexual males, and persons who are of Haitian ancestry.

As the incidence of this disease increased, it became possible to describe its features more accurately. One striking characteristic was that patients with this disease had an almost complete absence of certain types of immune response. This lack of immunity actually contributed the name of the disease, which is now known as *acquired immune deficiency syndrome*, commonly referred to as AIDS. A careful examination of the lymphocytes found in AIDS patients has shown that there are more T cells with an immune repressor function than T cells with an immune helper function. This condition leaves the patient highly vulnerable to certain opportunistic infections. A better description of the disease is now known and contributes to the syndrome (collection of symptoms) commonly associated with AIDS. These patients frequently have severe diarrhea, pneumonia, fungal infection, dark reddish-purple areas on the body, swollen lymph nodes, and, not uncommonly, a generalized form of tuberculosis caused by *Mycobacterium avium*.

As reports of this disease continued to be received by the Centers for Disease Control in Atlanta, Georgia, a number of epidemiologic patterns arose. Most patients were male homosexual or intravenous drug abusers, lived in major metropolitan areas of the United States, or were Haitian in origin. Most alarming was the death rate, which exceeded 40% of the cases first diagnosed over one year previously and is even higher for cases first diagnosed two years earlier. No cause or cure has been discovered. Patients are treated for their opportunistic infections, but the underlying immunodeficiency is not yet curable.

The transmission pattern of AIDS seems to parallel that seen with hepatitis B (p. 439). It has been transmitted heterosexually through blood transfusions (persons with hemophelia A are at increased risk), *in utero* to unborn infants, and via the common use of hypodermic needles. Control of this disease in general is difficult as the incubation period between exposure and illness may be as long as 2 years. Control measures to reduce transmission by blood transfusions are now in use. These include refraining from using blood from members of groups at increased risk for AIDS and the testing of blood for the presence of antibody to the HTLV-III/LAV virus. Certainly caution must be exercised by all health care personnel who may be exposed to body fluids from active patients or persons in the incubation period.

SUMMARY

Various unrelated viruses and a suspected viral disease are discussed in this chapter.

1. Togaviruses are widespread in nature and some cause important diseases of humans and animals.

2. An arenavirus causes Lassa fever, a killer disease found in Africa.

3. Coronaviruses cause about 15% of the common colds.

4. Rotaviruses are a frequent cause of severe infantile diarrhea.

5. Norwalk viruses are associated with gastroenteritis in older persons.

6. Acquired immune deficiency syndrome (AIDS), a serious disease of certain population groups, is thought to be caused by a retrovirus.

Infection Control in Hospitals

41

The hospital constitutes a special environment with relationship to microbial infection. Within this single complex environment are many patients who have compromised host defense mechanisms against infections, patients who are subjected to procedures that could introduce microbes into the deep body tissues and still other patients admitted to the hospital suffering from an infectious disease who may be shedding large numbers of pathogenic microbes. This chapter describes some problems associated with the spread of microorganisms within the hospital environment and the role of hospital personnel in preventing or minimizing such spread.

COMPROMISED PATIENTS

Many patients admitted to hospitals have an illness or other medical problem that may impair one or more of their basic defense mechanisms. These patients are much more susceptible to diseases than healthy persons and special precautions must be taken to protect them from harmful microorganisms. Often microbes of low virulence, those that are usually unable to cause diseases, can cause serious infections in these compromised patients. These low-virulent microbes may be from either exogenous or endogenous sources.

Some more common causes of compromise in patients are diabetes, kidney diseases, chronic heart or lung diseases, cancer, and extensive burns or other wounds. Generally recipients of organ transplants are given immunosuppressive drugs to prevent rejection of the organ and such drugs usually render the patient highly susceptible to infectious agents. Corticosteroids and radiation used in treating various diseases are also immunosuppressive. Therefore the possible benefits given through these procedures must be weighed against the increased risk that the patient will develop a serious infection, such as pneumonia. Some tumors and most anticancer treatments increase the susceptibility of these patients to infection. Most elderly patients also have reduced resistance to infections; at the other age extreme, neonates and premature infants are highly susceptible to infections, too. Such patients should receive special attention to protect them from infecting microbes, but all hospital patients should be considered compromised in one way or another and continual efforts should be made to protect them from disease-producing microbes.

MEDICAL PROCEDURES

Many modern medical procedures increase the chance that infections will occur. Such procedures as total hip-replacement operations, open-heart surgery, and brain surgery may expose susceptible deep tissues to the external environment for prolonged periods. Various forms of catheterization, punch biopsies, and bone marrow aspirations are additional procedures that may introduce microbes into deeper body tissues. Blood transfusions and hemodialysis treatments with artificial kidney machines may introduce microorganisms directly into the blood. All medical procedures, particularly those that penetrate the epithelial barriers, must be carried out in such a way as to minimize or completely prevent the introduction of microbes into the body.

INFECTIOUS PATIENTS

The relative number of patients admitted to hospitals for treatment of infectious diseases is much less today than in the period before chemotherapy. Yet many patients with infectious diseases are still admitted. Patients with pneumonia constitute 10% of all current hospital admissions and next to cancer, cardiovascular diseases, and accidents, infectious diseases are the leading cause of deaths in the United States. Over 300 million infectious diseases that are serious enough for medical attention occur per year in the United States. Most, however, are handled in outpatient clinics.

Hospital personnel and visitors may also carry infectious agents into hospitals. A constant responsibility of hospital personnel is to develop and follow procedures that will minimize cross infections among patients who come together in the common hospital environment.

HOSPITAL-ACQUIRED INFECTIONS

Hospital-acquired infections are, of course, those contracted by patients after they enter a hospital. The term *nosocomial*, which means hospital associated, is frequently used when referring to hospital-acquired infections. Various studies have shown that

about 5% of the patients who enter a hospital in the United States contract a nosocomial infection (Table 41-1). This percentage amounts to about 1.5 million infections
per year and results in or is a contributing factor in about 30,000 deaths. The added
costs in treating these patients are estimated at $1 billion annually. Postoperative
wound infections, the most common nosocomial infections, develop in from 3 to 8%
of surgical patients.

Although it may not be possible to eliminate all nosocomial infections, they can
be significantly reduced if medical personnel conscientiously follow procedures that
are designed to prevent the spread of infectious agents. Some of these procedures are
discussed next.

Direct Contact

Contact between patients is a potential source of nosocomial infection. The most
hazardous contact would be between highly compromised patients and any infected
patients who are shedding large numbers of virulent microorganisms. Hospital personnel may serve as symptomatic or asymptomatic carriers of pathogens that may be
transmitted to patients (see clinical note on p. 218). Conversely, patients with infec-

TABLE 41-1 NOSOCOMIAL INFECTION RATES
These figures represent national averages gathered by the National Nosocomial
Infection Survey and issued in 1982. The figures represent the percent of patients
infected and percent of organisms recovered.

Nosocomial infections by service and hospital

	Medical service				
Hospital	Surgery	Medicine	Obstetrics	Pediatrics	All combined
University	5.9	4.8	2.9	3.2	4.4
Federal	3.8	4.0	3.8	1.2	3.7
Community	3.5	2.4	1.6	0.7	2.5
All hospitals	4.6	3.4	2.1	1.6	3.3

Nosocomial infections by site of infection and pathogen

	Site of infection				
Pathogen	Blood	Surgical wound	Respiratory	Urinary tract	All
E. coli	14.4	13.4	6.8	31.9	18.3
S. aureus	13.7	14.8	9.9	1.9	9.9
Enterococcus	6.8	9.2	1.5	14.2	9.2
P. aeruginosa	4.8	5.9	9.5	11.4	8.4
Klebsiella species	13.7	5.2	11.2	9.4	7.9
All pathogens	4.3	24.7	15.3	37.0	—

tious diseases may transmit an infection to attending medical personnel (see clinical note on p. 233). Moreover, housekeeping personnel or visitors may be involved in an exchange of potentially dangerous microbes with patients.

Various means are used to reduce person-to-person transmission of infections in hospitals. First, patients who are compromised and those who have infectious diseases should be isolated from each other and from other patients. In order to do so, a rapid diagnosis of the patient's illness is necessary. Whenever possible, particularly when dealing with a patient who might have a communicable disease, the patient should be isolated at least until a specific diagnosis is made. Once it is determined which patients are infectious and which are compromised, appropriate methods of separation are applied. The infectious patient should be placed in a room that is designed to prevent any microorganisms from escaping—a situation called *regular* or *forward* isolation. Various levels of isolation may be used. Strict isolation is necessary for patients who have highly contagious diseases. The conditions of isolation are modified, depending on the type of infections; that is, a respiratory infection would be handled differently from an enteric infection. Isolation rooms should be posted with a sign giving instructions on the procedures to follow when entering or leaving the room (Figure 41-1 and Table 41-2). For strict isolation, gowns, masks, and shoe covers must be worn by all persons entering the room. Gloves must be worn when examining the patient and all articles used in the room, such as thermometers and stethoscopes, must be left in the room or placed in a container to be sterilized before being reused. When personnel leave the room, items like gown, mask, and gloves must be placed in a receptacle that will later be sterilized. Disinfectant-impregnated mats may be placed in the entrance to remove contaminants from the bottom of shoes. Hands should be washed with a disinfectant soap before leaving the room. The isolation room should have negative air pressure relative to the corridor so that no air flows out. Exhaust air should be passed through absolute filters that remove all airborne particles.

Compromised patients should be placed in *protective isolation*, also called *reverse isolation*, to protect them from microbes that might be transmitted from other patients or hospital personnel. These rooms should be under positive air pressure so that no air from the corridor can flow into the room. The same gowning, masking, and other procedures used for strict isolation should be applied. For severely compromised patients, such as those with extensive burns, completely enclosed canopies may be placed around the patient to isolate them more effectively from microbial contaminants. Visitors should preferably be restricted from isolation rooms; if admitted, they should follow the same gowning procedures as medical personnel. Housekeeping personnel, as well as all others who enter these rooms, must also follow the same procedures.

Medical personnel with infections, including respiratory diseases or such skin lesions as cellulitis, should be excluded from duty until their infections are resolved. Persons working in surgery or with highly compromised patients may periodically have their nares cultured to determine if they are carriers of antibiotic-resistant *Staphylococcus aureus*. If found to be positive, they should be relieved from duty

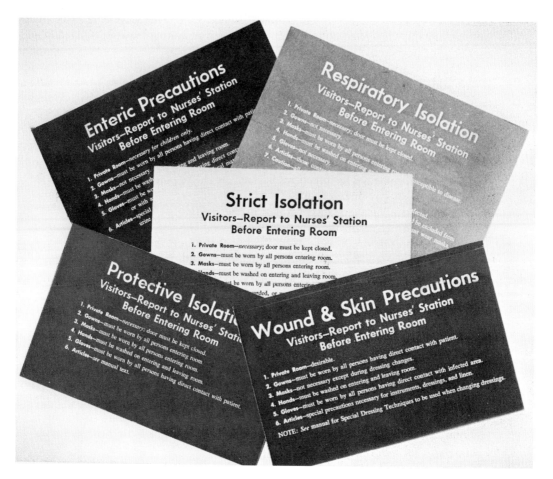

Figure 41-1 Standard warning and instructional signs that are posted at the entrance to different types of isolation rooms in hospitals.

with these patients until their carrier state is resolved. Similarly, visitors with infections should not be permitted to visit patients. Many hospitals do not allow children under 14 years of age to visit because, among other reasons, they are frequently carriers of a variety of infectious agents and are themselves more susceptible to others.

Contaminated Objects

Any object that comes in contact with an infected patient or that patient's surroundings may become contaminated with pathogenic microbes. If the same object later comes in contact with another patient, some microbes may be successfully transmitted. Such items as bedding, books, and toys may indirectly transmit infections. Medical paraphernalia, such as stethoscopes, bronchoscopes, and thermometers, as well

TABLE 41-2 A LISTING OF THE INFORMATION GIVEN ON THE FRONT AND BACK OF THE WARNING SIGNS POSTED BY ISOLATION ROOMS IN HOSPITALS

Enteric Precautions

Visitors—Report to Nurses' Station Before Entering Room

1. **Private Room**—*necessary for children only.*
2. **Gowns**—must be worn by all persons having direct contact with patient.
3. **Masks**—not necessary.
4. **Hands**—must be washed on entering and leaving room.
5. **Gloves**—must be worn by all persons having direct contact with patient or with articles contaminated with fecal material.
6. **Articles**—special precautions necessary for articles contaminated with urine and feces. Articles must be disinfected or discarded.

Diseases Requiring Enteric Precautions

1. Cholera.
2. Enteropathogenic *E. coli* gastroenteritis.
3. Hepatitis, viral (infectious or serum).
4. Salmonellosis (including typhoid fever).
5. Shigellosis.

Protective Isolation

Visitors—Report to Nurses' Station Before Entering Room

1. **Private Room**—*necessary; door must be kept closed.*
2. **Gowns**—must be worn by all persons entering room.
3. **Masks**—must be worn by all persons entering room.
4. **Hands**—must be washed on entering and leaving room.
5. **Gloves**—must be worn by all persons having direct contact with patient.
6. **Articles**—*see manual text.*

Conditions Requiring Protective Isolation

1. Agranulocytosis.
2. Severe and extensive, noninfected vesicular, bullous, or eczematous dermatitis.
3. Certain patients receiving immunosuppressive therapy.
4. Certain patients with lymphomas and leukemia.

Respiratory Isolation

Visitors—Report to Nurses' Station Before Entering Room

1. **Private Room**—*necessary; door must be kept closed.*
2. **Gowns**—not necessary.
3. **Masks**—must be worn by all persons entering room if susceptible to disease.
4. **Hands**—must be washed on entering and leaving room.
5. **Gloves**—not necessary.
6. **Articles**—those contaminated with secretions must be disinfected.
7. **Caution**—all persons susceptible to the specific disease should be excluded from patient area; if contact is necessary, susceptibles must wear masks.

Diseases Requiring Respiratory Isolation

1. Chickenpox.
2. Herpes zoster.
3. Measles (rubeola).
4. Meningococcal meningitis.
5. Meningococcemia.
6. Mumps.
7. Pertussis (whooping cough).
8. Rubella (German measles).
9. Tuberculosis, pulmonary—sputum-positive (or suspect).
10. Venezuelan equine encephalomyelitis.

Strict Isolation

Visitors—Report to Nurses' Station Before Entering Room

1. **Private Room**—*necessary; door must be kept closed.*
2. **Gowns**—must be worn by all persons entering room.
3. **Masks**—must be worn by all persons entering room.
4. **Hands**—must be washed on entering and leaving room.
5. **Gloves**—must be worn by all persons entering room.
6. **Articles**—must be discarded, or wrapped before being sent to Central Supply for disinfection or sterilization.

Diseases Requiring Strict Isolation

1. Anthrax, inhalation.
2. Burns, extensive, infected with *Staphylococcus aureus* or Group A streptococcus.
3. Diphtheria.
4. Eczema vaccinatum.
5. Melioidosis, pulmonary, or extrapulmonary with draining sinus(es).
6. Neonatal vesicular disease (Herpes simplex).
7. Plague.
8. Rabies.
9. Rubella (German measles) and Congenital rubella syndrome.
10. Smallpox.
11. Staphylococcal enterocolitis.
12. Staphylococcal pneumonia.
13. Streptococcal pneumonia.
14. Vaccinia, generalized and progressive.

Wound & Skin Precautions

Visitors—Report to Nurses' Station Before Entering Room

1. **Private Room**—desirable.
2. **Gowns**—must be worn by all persons having direct contact with patient.
3. **Masks**—not necessary except during dressing changes.
4. **Hands**—must be washed on entering and leaving room.
5. **Gloves**—must be worn by all persons having direct contact with infected area.
6. **Articles**—special precautions necessary for instruments, dressings, and linen.

Note: *See manual for Special Dressing Techniques to be used when changing dressings.*

Diseases Requiring Wound & Skin Precautions

1. Burns, extensive, not infected with *Staphylococcus aureus* or Group A streptococcus.
2. Gas gangrene.
3. Impetigo.
4. Staphylococcal skin and wound infections.
5. Streptococcal skin infection.
6. Wound infection, extensive.

as equipment used for administering anesthesia or inhalation therapy, have been incriminated as transmitters of some nosocomial infections. Almost any items used in patient care have the potential to transmit infectious agents.

Much has been done in the past few years to prevent the transmission of infectious agents by inanimate objects. Individualized personal-care kits containing a water pitcher, thermometer, and other items for use of only one patient have reduced the need for repeated disinfection of these items and eliminated any chance for transmission of infections by these items. Many other disposable items, such as gloves, syringes, hypodermic needles, catheters, and tubes, have further reduced the chance of patient-to-patient transmission of microbes (Figure 41-2). Special care must be taken with items like bronchoscopes that are not disposable and that cannot be sterilized by autoclaving or ethylene oxide. Such items must be thoroughly cleaned and sterilized or disinfected with a liquid disinfectant, usually by soaking in 2% glutaraldehyde for 12 hours.

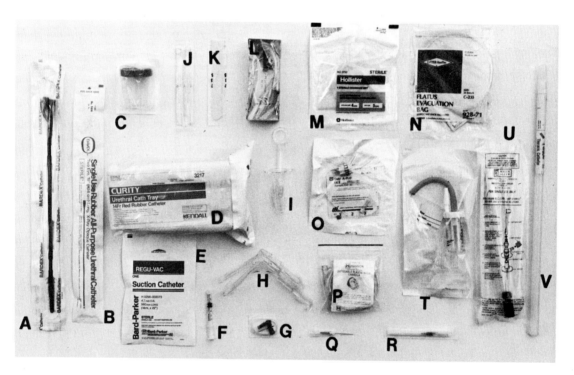

Figure 41-2   Some of the disposable items used in patient care that help reduce the chance for transmission of infections. A & B, urethral catheters; C, specimen cup; D, urethral catheter tray; E, suction catheter; F, hypodermic syringe; G, intravenous infusion needle; H, speculum; I, Rectal speculum; J, Cotton-tipped applicators; K, tongue depressor; L, intravenous kit; M, wound drainage set; N, Evacuation bag; O, intravenous tubes; P, nasal cannula; Q, intravenous needle; R, hypodermic needle; T, specimen trap; U, sigmoidoscopy kit; V, thoracic catheter.

Persons working directly with patients or who prepare materials to be used around patients must have a basic understanding of the possible modes of transmission of microbes and then be continually aware of how each procedure may either contribute to or prevent the spread of infection. Well-managed hospitals have outlined procedures designed to prevent the spread of microbes during routine activities involving patients. It is important that all medical personnel understand and follow these procedures. Yet not every procedure used to prevent transmission of microbes can be easily outlined and each person involved in patient care must use his or her own knowledge of microbiology to eliminate the possible spread of microbes while carrying out daily activities.

Endogenous Spread

The various routes of endogenous spread of microbes were discussed in Chapter 10. Special care must be taken when working with patients with wounds or burns to reduce or prevent cross contamination from one part of the body to another. Bandaging of open lesions is an effective method of preventing some endogenous spread. Education of the patient as to the modes of endogenous spread and how to reduce this spread is helpful.

Airborne Transmission

Droplet nuclei from coughing or sneezing and microbe-containing dust or fine particles may be carried in air currents from person to person or from one part of the hospital to another. Changing contaminated bandages or shaking contaminated bedding may send massive numbers of microbes into the air. Sweeping floors, walking, and various types of movements result in large numbers of microbe-containing dust particles being disseminated into the air.

Airborne contaminants can be greatly reduced by handling contaminated materials carefully. Such items as bandages should be carefully removed with forceps and placed in a plastic bag. All soiled bedding, linens, and trash should be placed in airtight plastic bags for transport to laundry or disposal areas. Care must be used in sorting soiled laundry to avoid creating clouds of pathogens that might cause infection in workers. Contaminated materials should be autoclaved before being sent to the laundry. Floors should be cleaned with wet vacuums or mops that prevent the generation of dust.

All properly designed hospitals should have air systems that prevent the recirculation of contaminated air from one area to another. The use of positive or negative air pressure in isolation rooms has been discussed. Air entering critical areas like surgeries (Figure 41-3), nurseries, and intensive care areas should be filtered or irradiated with ultraviolet light to remove or destroy the airborne microbes and the airflow should carry airborne particles away from patients (Figure 41-4).

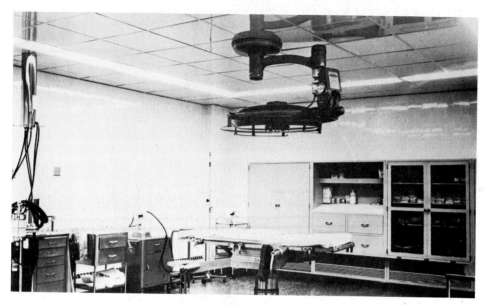

Figure 41-3 An operating room equipped with an aseptic air system. The ceiling is made of perforated panels through which filtered and ultraviolet light irradiated air passes. Air return ducts are located all around the base of the room. The air moves downward and out of the room at sufficient velocity to prevent airborne particles from drifting over and onto the surgical wound. (Courtesy Joseph R. Luciano)

INFECTION CONTROL PROGRAMS

Each hospital must have an effective infection control program. This program is under the direction of an *infection control committee*, which should include the following members:

1. The hospital epidemiologist, who is a physician or another person with knowledge of and interest in epidemiology and infectious diseases.
2. A representative from each of the major clinical departments—for example, medicine, surgery, and pediatrics.
3. A member of the pathology/microbiology laboratory.
4. The infection control nurse, who is an R.N. trained in the principles of epidemiology and infectious diseases.
5. The director of nursing and/or nursing supervisor.
6. A representative from the hospital administration.
7. Liaison members from various services, such as pharmacy, housekeeping, central supply, inhalation therapy, and local health departments.

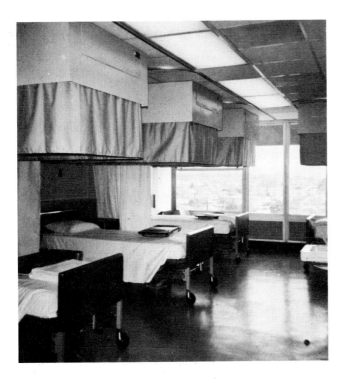

Figure 41-4   A hospital ward equipped with aseptic air canopies over each bed. A mass of microbial-free air moves down over each patient and is drawn out of the room through return ducts at the head of the beds. Such downward air movement prevents lateral movement of airborne microorganisms between patients. (Courtesy Joseph R. Luciano)

The functions of this committee are as follows:

1. Determine the methods to be used for effective surveillance of nosocomial infections.
2. Determine what control measures need to be taken when dealing with isolation procedures or other special procedures where highly susceptible patients are involved.
3. Make proper use of the microbiology laboratory for environmental surveillance and identification of isolated pathogens.
4. Delegate authority to the hospital epidemiologist and the infection control nurse.
5. Convey the infection control policies to those who must carry them out and assess the completeness and effectiveness of the implementation of these policies.
6. Meet once a month or more often to review infection control procedures and policies and so on.

The infection control nurse and hospital epidemiologist should be primarily responsible for directing the day-to-day implementation of the environmental surveillance, infection control procedures, and inservice training of other hospital personnel relative to infection control procedures.

SUMMARY

1. The control of infection in the hospital environment centers around two main factors: (a) the introduction of highly virulent, easily transmissable infectious agents into the hospital environment by patients, visitors, or hospital personnel and (b) the transmission of relatively avirulent normal flora-type organisms to compromised patients either through self-inoculation or routine hospital procedures.
2. Stringent control procedures have been adopted by most hospitals in order to reduce the occurrence of nosocomial infections.

Biochemical Pathways

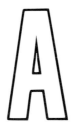

This appendix is included to give further details of some biochemical reactions outlined in Chapter 4.

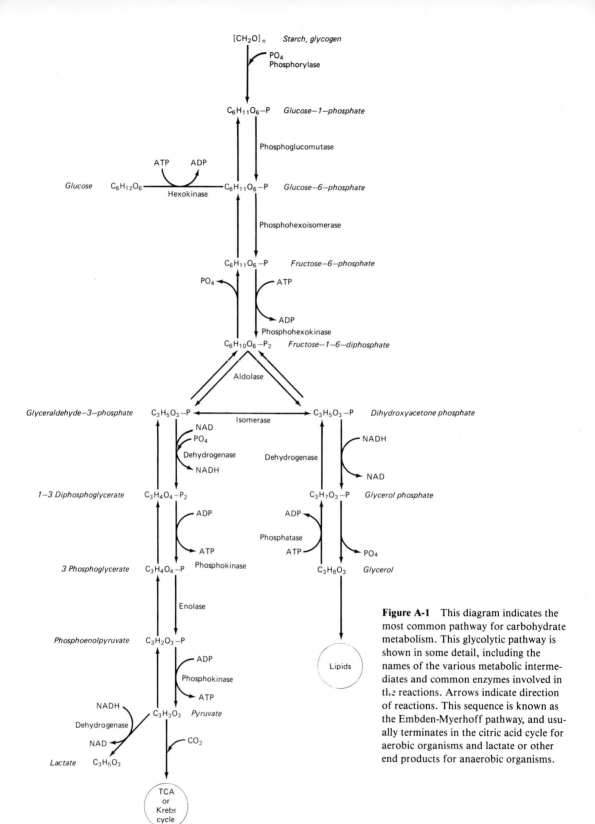

Figure A-1 This diagram indicates the most common pathway for carbohydrate metabolism. This glycolytic pathway is shown in some detail, including the names of the various metabolic intermediates and common enzymes involved in the reactions. Arrows indicate direction of reactions. This sequence is known as the Embden-Myerhoff pathway, and usually terminates in the citric acid cycle for aerobic organisms and lactate or other end products for anaerobic organisms.

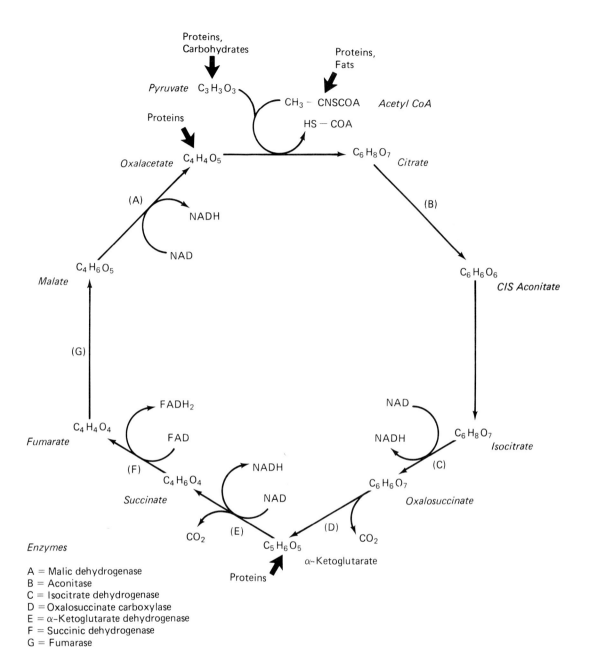

Figure A-2 The biochemical reactions associated with the citric acid cycle. This metabolic sequence is frequently called the Krebs cycle. A single passage through the cycle results in the loss of three carbon atoms from pyruvate. Therefore, two complete turns of the cycle will remove all the carbon from a glucose molecule entering into glycolysis. Enzymes associated with the cycle are shown.

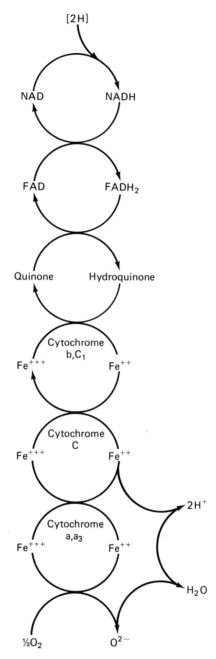

Figure A-3 Electron transport system or pathway of oxidative phosphorylation. The energy associated with the reduced carrier molecules NAD and FAD are brought to this sequence of reactions. Here, by removing the energy in a series of oxidation-reduction reactions, it is captured into ATP molecules. Most of the ATPs derived from the oxidation of glucose to CO_2 and H_2O are produced in this system.

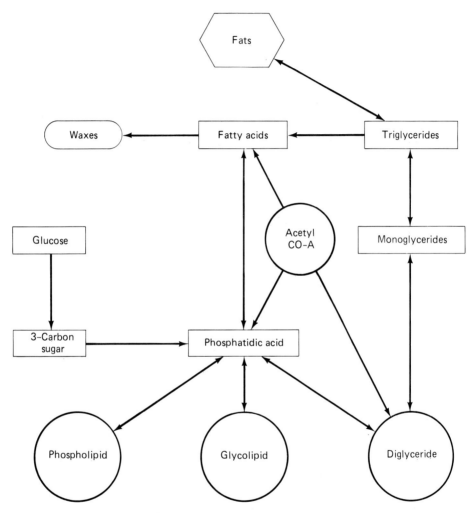

Figure A-4 This is a schematic diagram indicating the direction of catabolism and anabolism of lipids. While the details are not given, this system interlocks with most of the energy-storing systems in the cell. Note that acetyl CO-A and the 3 carbon sugar can be found in the diagram of the citric acid cycle—Figure A-2.

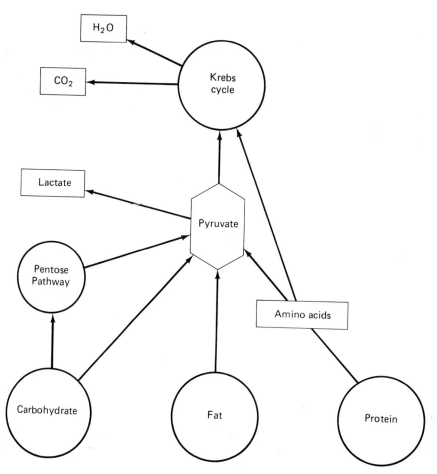

Figure A-5 A schematic diagram indicating the interactions among the major metabolic pathways and classes of macromolecules. This interrelationship allows the cell to convert a plentiful supply of a metabolite into a needed metabolite which may be limited in its availability.

Human Parasites

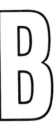

Here is a list of the most common parasitologic organisms found in humans. The list includes scientific and common names of the parasite or disease as well as the source from which infection is most commonly derived.

PROTOZOA

Type	Species	Relationship	Common name	Source
Amebae	*Entamoeba histolytica*	Intestinal pathogen	Amebiasis	Human feces
	E. hartmanni	Intestinal commensal		Human feces
	E. coli	Intestinal commensal		Human feces
	E. polecki	Intestinal commensal		Human feces
	Endolimax nana	Intestinal commensal		Human feces
	Iodamoeba butschlii	Intestinal commensal		Human feces
	Naegleria fowleri	CNS pathogen	Encephalitis	Freshwater swimming
	Pneumocystis carinii	Tissue pathogen		Unknown
Ciliate	*Balantidium coli*	Intestinal pathogen		Pig feces
Coccidia	*Isospora belli*	Intestinal pathogen		Human feces
	Sarcocystis bovicanis	Tissue pathogen		Poorly cooked meat
	Toxoplasma gondii	Tissue pathogen		Cat feces
Flagellates	*Dientamoeba fragilis*	Intestinal pathogen		Human feces
	Trichomonas hominis	Tissue commensal		Human
	T. vaginalis	Tissue pathogen		Human
	Chilomastix mesnili	Intestinal commensal		Human feces
	Giardia lamblia	Intestinal pathogen	Giardiasis	Mamalian feces
	Leishmania donovani	Tissue pathogen	Leishmaniasis	Sandfly bite

PROTOZOA (*cont.*)

Type	Species	Relationship	Common name	Source
Sporozoa	*L. tropica*	Tissue pathogen		Sandfly bite
	L. braziliensis	Tissue pathogen		Sandfly bite
	Trypanosoma gambiense	Tissue pathogen	Sleeping sickness	Fly bite
	T. rhodesiense	Tissue pathogen	Sleeping sickness	Fly bite
	T. cruzi	Tissue pathogen	Chagas disease	Bug bite
	Plasmodium falciparum	Tissue pathogen	Malaria	Mosquito
	Plasmodium malariae	Tissue pathogen	Malaria	Mosquito
	Plasmodium ovale	Tissue pathogen	Malaria	Mosquito
	Plasmodium vivax	Tissue pathogen	Malaria	Mosquito

METAZOA

Type	Species	Relationship	Common name	Source
Cestodes	*Diphillobothrium latum*	Intestinal pathogen	Tapeworm	Uncooked fish
	Dipylidium caninum	Intestinal pathogen	Tapeworm	Dog feces
	Echinococcus granulosis	Tissue pathogen	Tapeworm	Dog feces
	Hyminolepsis nana	Intestinal pathogen	Tapeworm	Human feces
	Taenia saginata	Intestinal pathogen	Tapeworm	Uncooked beef
	Taenia solium	Intestinal pathogen	Tapeworm	Uncooked pork
Nematode	*Angiostrongylus cantonensis*	Tissue pathogen		Mollusks
	Ancylostoma duodenale	Intestinal pathogen	Hookworm	Human feces
	Ascaris lumbricoides	Intestinal pathogen		Human feces
	Brugia malayi	Tissue pathogen	Elephantiasis	Mosquito
	Capillaria hepatica	Tissue pathogen		Rodent feces
	C. philippinensis	Intestinal pathogen		Raw fish
	Dipetalonema perstans	Intestinal pathogen		Midge bite
	Enterobius vermicularis	Intestinal pathogen	Pinworm	Human feces
	Loa Loa	Tissue pathogen	Eyeworm	Fly bite
	Mansonella ozzardi	Tissue pathogen		Fly bite
	Necator americanis	Intestinal pathogen	Hookworm	Human feces
	Onchocerca volvulus	Tissue pathogen	River blindness	Fly bite
	Strongeloides stercoralis	Intestinal pathogen		Human feces
	Toxocara canis	Tissue pathogen	Larva migrans	Dog feces
	Trichinella spiralis	Tissue pathogen	Trichinosis	Uncooked pork
	Trichuris trichiura	Intestinal pathogen	Whipworm	Human feces
	Wuchereria bancrofti	Tissue pathogen	Elephantiasis	Mosquito
Trematode	*Clonorchis sinensis*	Tissue pathogen	Liver fluke	Raw fish
	Fasciola hepatica	Tissue pathogen	Sheep liver flukes	Freshwater plants
	Fasciolopsis buski	Intestinal pathogen	Intestinal fluke	Human feces
	Metagonimus yokagawi	Intestinal pathogen		Raw fish
	Paragonimos westermani	Tissue pathogen	Lung fluke	Uncooked shellfish
	S. japonicum	Tissue pathogen		Water
	Schistosoma mansoni	Tissue pathogen	Bilharziasis	Water

Glossary

Abscess   Pus accumulated in a localized area, often associated with inflammation

Acid fast   A property by which some bacterial cells fail to decolorize when washed with an acid alcohol solution

Acute   A disease of short duration or exhibiting sharp clinical signs

Adjuvant   A compound (often lipid) added to an antigen to increase the antibody response

Agar   A polysaccharide extracted from algae that is used as a solidifying agent in bacteriological culture media

Agglutination   Clumping or bunching of particulate antigens resulting from the presence of a specific antibody

Albumin   A water-soluble protein commonly found in animal sera

Allergy   An altered (often damaging) reaction, the result of an antigen-antibody interaction in hypersensitive animals

Alveolus   A small air sac located in the lung

Amino acid   An organic compound with both amino and carboxyl groups as part of the same molecule. The monomeric components of protein

Anaerobe   A bacterium that does not use oxygen as a metabolic hydrogen acceptor. Often unable to grow in the presence of atmospheric oxygen concentrations

Anamnestic   A secondary or booster phenomenon observed following a primary immunologic response

Anaphylaxis   A severe, systemic hypersensitivity response to an antigenic challenge

Anorexia   Loss of appetite

Anti-   A prefix suggesting opposition or against. The use of this prefix in medicine relates to curative processes

Antibacterial   A compound or process detrimental to bacterial growth or survival

Antibiotic   A substance produced by a living organism or cell system which is useful for therapy of infectious diseases

Anticodon   A triplet nucleotide base sequence associated with transfer RNA that is complementary to the codon triplet of messenger RNA

Antigen   A substance capable of eliciting an antibody from an immunocompetent animal

Antigenic determinant   The portion of an antigen molecule that determines the specificity of antibody synthesis

Antimicrobial   A compound or process detrimental to microbial growth or survival

Antiseptic   Literally, against sepsis (infection). A compound that can be applied to animal tissues in order to reduce the likelihood of infection

Arbovirus   RNA virus, transmissable by insect vector, frequently associated with encephalitis

Arthralgia   Severe joint pain

Arthropod   An invertebrate having jointed legs, commonly acting as infectious disease vectors

Aseptic   Free from microorganisms

Aspirate   Material removed from a patient by suction

ATP   (Adenosine triphosphate) A molecule containing two high-energy phosphate bonds that act as an energy transport and exchange molecule in metabolic reactions

Attenuation   Reduction in virulence. Microorganisms that have lost virulence but have retained antigenicity are attenuated

Avirulent   Not virulent. Refers to microorganisms that are not capable of producing an infectious process

Bacteremia   A condition in which living bacteria are found to be present in the bloodstream

Bactericidal   A condition or compound that results in the killing of bacteria

Bacteriophage   Virus that infects bacteria

Bacteriostatic   A condition that prevents the growth of bacteria but does not directly kill these microorganisms

Bactiuria   A condition in which bacteria are found in urine

Balanced growth   Growth during which the number and composition of cells remain constant

BCG   (Bacille Calmette-Guerin) An attenuated mycobacterium used as a vaccine against tuberculosis

Beta lactamase   An enzyme that hydrolyzes the beta lactam ring structure essential to the antibacterial activity of penicillins and cephalosporins

Binary fission   The form of cellular division associated with bacteria, resulting in equal distribution of cellular content between the daughter cells

Bloom   The occurrence of a major outgrowth of algae

Botulism   Food poisoning; specifically that due to the toxin produced by *Clostridium botulinum*

Broad spectrum   Antimicrobial agents that are effective against a large number of different types of bacteria, usually including both gram-positive and gram-negative genera

Bronchi   Major air passageways that branch from the trachea

Broth   A liquid culture medium

B cell   A group of bone-marrow-derived lymphocytes that produce immunoglobulins

Capnophile   A microorganism requiring carbon dioxide for growth

Capsid   A viral protein coat

Capsomere   The subunit of a capsid. Capsomeres occur in repetitive sequence in order to form the capsid

Capsule   A polysaccharide or rarely a polypeptide layer surrounding bacterial cells peripheral to the cell wall

Carbohydrate   A sugar molecule

Carrier   Generally an individual who has recovered from an infection but who continues to shed the etiologic agent into the environment

Caseous   Having a cheeselike consistency. Associated with tuberculous lesions termed caseation necrosis

Catabolism   Metabolic breakdown of organic compounds

Catalyst   A molecule that lowers the energy of activation of a chemical reaction

Cellulitis   Inflammation or infection of connective tissue. Usually resulting in a typical inflammatory lesion

Chancre   A superficial ulcer generally occurring at the site of primary syphilis infection

Chemotaxis   The movement of cells toward or away from a chemical stimulus

Chemotherapy   The use of chemical compounds in the treatment of disease. Usually associated with cancer therapy

Chronic   Lasting for a long time. Such as the disease tuberculosis

Ciliated epithelium   Epithelial tissues containing numerous ciliated cells, such as the tracheal surface

Cistron   A structural gene. A unit of DNA that codes for a single function

Clone   A population of cells derived from a single progenitor cell. A bacterial colony

CNS   (Central nervous system) The brain and spinal cord

Code   Genetic information associated with the triplet base sequence of DNA

Codon   A base triplet found in messenger RNA that codes for a single amino acid

Coenzyme   A molecule involved in the transfer of small molecules between enzymic reactions

Colon   The large intestine

Colony   A visible accumulation of bacterial cells that are the progeny of one cell on solid culture media

Commensal   An organism that exists without rendering either harm or benefit to its environment

Communicable   An infectious disease that can be transmitted between susceptible individuals

Competitive inhibition   An enzymic reaction that can be stopped by the reversible interaction of an inhibitor with the free enzyme

Complement   A system of serum proteins, activated in sequence, which produce a variety of biological effects

Complement fixation   A serological reaction which depends on the binding of complement in an antigen-antibody complex

Compromised host   An individual with decreased resistance to infection

Conjugation   The process whereby bacterial DNA is transferred between individual cells through a pilus

Conjunctivitis   Inflammation of the conjunctiva (tissue surrounding the eyeball)

Contagious   See communicable

Cortex   The outer portion of an organ such as the brain

Croup   An upper respiratory obstruction, usually produced by swelling of the epiglottis or pharynx. Characterized by a hoarse cough

Cyst   A dominant life stage of some parasites. Cysts have increased resistance to environmental changes or antibiotic processes

Cystitis   An infection of the bladder

Cytopathic effect   Observable changes in in vitro cells resulting from viral infection

Dark field   A form of microscopy where light is reflected from an object such that it appears as a light against a black background

Delirium   A state of disordered mentality, often associated with high fever

Deoxyribose   The five-carbon sugar present in DNA

Desensitize   Reduction in the hypersensitivity state resulting from exposure to small repeated doses of antigen

Determinant group   The portion of an antigen that determines antibody specificity

Diffusion   The movement of molecules from an area of high to low concentration

Dimorphic   Having two structural or anatomical forms

Disease   An abnormal state of health

Disinfect   The removal of some or all microorganisms from an environment

Dissemination   The development of a generalized from a localized infection. The involvement of additional organ systems secondary to a primary focus of infection

DNA   (Deoxyribose nucleic acid) A polynucleotide consisting of four nucleotide bases in a random sequence. The informational molecule of chromosome

Electrolyte   A substance that readily conducts an electric current when dissolved. In medicine these substances are ions like K^+ and Na^+ in serum

Electron microscope   A microscope that uses an electron beam to illuminate the object under study

Electrophoresis   The separation in an electrical field of molecules having differences in electrical charge

Empirical   Not founded in experimental data

Encephalitis   An inflammation of the brain resulting in neurological changes

Endocarditis   Inflammation of the endocardial lining of the heart   ·

Endogenous   From an internal source. Associated with self

Endonuclease   An enzyme that will hydrolyse DNA

Endoplasmic reticulum   A reticular membrane formation found in cellular cytoplasm, often associated with protein synthesis

Endospore   A bacterial spore, associated with resistance to environmental inactivation

Endothelial cell   A cell lining a cavity or tube

Endotoxin   A lipopolysaccharide associated with gram-negative cell wall

Enterotoxin   A bacterial toxin that is absorbed by and acts primarily on the intestinal tract

Envelope   A lipid covering found peripheral to the viral capsid on some virions

Enzyme   A protein catalyst that facilitates biochemical reactions

Epidemic   The occurrence of a specific disease in greater than normal or expected numbers

Epidemiology   The study of disease, its occurrence, control, and effects on the environment

Epiglotitis   Inflammation of the epiglotis, frequently producing a severe croup

Erysipelas   A severe streptococcal infection of the skin

Eschar   A deep dark crust or scab that develops at the site of an injury, such as a burn

Etiologic agent   The cause of a specific infection

Eucaryotic   Refers to a true nucleus that is bounded by a nucleus membrane

Exotoxin   A powerful, proteinaceous toxin produced by any of several different genera and species of bacteria

Exudate   A fluid (cellular or acellular) that passes through blood vessels into surrounding tissues

Fastidious   Selective, usually refers to those bacteria requiring special nutrients for growth

Febrile   To have a fever

Fermentation   The anaerobic breakdown of carbohydrates

Fibrinous   A structureless, insoluble protein exudate, such as a blood clot, resulting from cellular injury

Fimbriae   A slender hairlike structure found on the surface of some bacteria that are used for attachment

Fission   To divide or split into two or more parts. An asexual reproduction process

Flagella   A relatively long proteinaceous projection extending from some bacteria that provides a mechanism for propelling the organism through its environment

Fomite   An inanimate object involved in the transmission of disease agents

Food poisoning   Illness resulting from consuming food that has been contaminated by a disease-producing microorganism

Gamma globulin   Serum proteins with antibody activity

Ganglion   A group of nerve cells located outside the central nervous system

Gangrene The process whereby tissues die because of a lack of blood supply

Gastroenteritis Infection of the intestinal tract, often accompanied by diarrhea

Generation time The time required for an organism to produce one new generation of progeny

Genetic code The genetic information contained in the nucleotide sequence of DNA. The code is based on triplet sets of nucleotide bases

Genetic engineering The intentional alteration of genetic structure through addition or subtraction of nucleotides

Genotype The genetic makeup or structure of a cell

Genome The nuclear content of a virion

Germacide A chemical compound that kills microorganisms

Glycolysis The metabolism of glucose to pyruvic acid

Granulocyte One of a series of white blood cells that contains granules in the cytoplasm. A polymorphonuclear leucocyte

Granuloma A nodule of fibrous tissue, resulting from an inflammatory reaction

Growth rate The number of generations produced in 60 minutes

Hapten A compound that can stimulate an antibody response and act as a determinant group when combined with a large molecular carrier molecule

Heavy metal Any of a group of elements found in periods 4, 5, or 6 of the periodic table constituting groups 1 to 8

HeLa cell Tumor cells taken in 1953 from Helen Lane and maintained in in vitro cell culture

Helix A spiral structure

Hemagglutination A serologic procedure that uses the agglutination of red blood cells as an indicator for a positive test

Hemolysis Breaking of red blood cells

Herbivore A plant-eating organism

Heterotroph A system of nutrition that requires preformed organic molecules as a source of energy

Histamine A small molecule found in some tissue cells that, when released, acts to produce a number of immunologic phenomena. A substance that will promote shock

Host An individual serving as a source of food for a parasite

Humoral Pertaining to body fluids

Hybridoma A clone of cells arising from an artificial combination of two cells into a single unit

Hydrophobic A compound that repels water

Hyperimmune sera Serum with a high antibody titer prepared by the repeated immunization of an animal

Hypersensitivity Being abnormally sensitive to antigens. Usually associated with allergic reactions to environmental antigens

Hypha A single filament of a fungal colony

Immune Possessing specific resistance to disease

Immunize To make immune, usually through the injection of antigen

Immunodiffusion A serologic procedure that determines the presence of either antigen or antibody by diffusing both materials through an agar or semisolid medium

Immunoglobulin Antibodies. Globulin proteins produced in response to an antigenic stimulus

Immunosuppressed A condition in which the normal immune response has been reduced or eliminated

Impetigo An infection of the skin characterized by a vesicular lesion that often breaks and crusts

Inclusion body Bodies or structures of high density, often stainable, and microscopically visible that occur in the cytoplasm or nucleus of cells infected by an intracellular parasite

Infectious A living agent capable of producing disease in a host

Inflammation A localized tissue response to injury or infection, characterized by redness, swelling, and an accumulation of phagocytic cells (pus)

Innate Naturally occurring

Inoculation Injection, often by needle, of material into a host. The process of placing bacteria on a culture medium

Interferon Protein produced by virus-infected or polynucleotide-stimulated cells that can inhibit viral development in other cells

Intravenous Located inside a blood vessel (vein)

In vitro Outside the host, without life

In vivo In life; specifically, inside a living host

Iodophore A carrier molecule complexed with iodine and used as an antiseptic

Ionizing radiation Radiation of sufficient energy to produce ionization of atoms when they are struck

Latent A hidden infection. One that is not manifest

Ligature A cord used to tie a vessel or tube

Lipid A fat. A water-insoluble compound generally soluble in chloroform, ether, or alcohol

Lipopolysaccharide A complex molecule containing both lipid and polysaccharide

Lipoprotein A complex molecule composed of both lipid and protein

Lymph A colorless, acellular fluid found in the vessels of the lymphatic system

Lymphatic A vessel that carries lymph

Lymphocyte A leukocyte with a large nucleus and small amount of cytoplasm, having a primary immunologic function

Lymphokine Any of a number of peptides that are produced by T cells and affect the behavior of target cells, such as B cells or other T cells

Lysogenic The state of a bacterium infected with a temperate virus

Lysosome A membrane-bound intracellular vacuole that is primarily filled with digestive and hydrolytic enzymes

Lysozyme An enzyme found in tears and other body fluids that can hydrolyze bacterial cell walls

Macromolecule A very large and often complex molecule. Usually associated with cell function and includes proteins, lipids, nucleic acids, and polysaccharides

Macrophage A large mononuclear phagocytic cell associated primarily with the reticuloendothelial system

Malaise The feeling of illness

Mantoux test The intradermal injection of antigen used to measure hypersensitivity to the tubercle bacillus

Mesophile A microorganism that grows best between 20 and 40°C

Mesosome An invaginated and convoluted area of bacterial cell membrane that carries out functions similar to the mitochondria of higher cells

Meningitis An infection of the meninges surrounding the brain

Metabolite A product of intermediary metabolism

Microaerophilic A microorganism that grows best at reduced oxygen concentrations

Monoclonal antibody Antibody produced in vitro by a clone of antigen-stimulated B cells. Having a single determinant specificity

Monolayer An in vitro cell culture forming a single cell layer on the surface of a container

Monomer A small molecule that forms the basic subunit of a polymer

Mucosa A mucous membrane

Mucus A thick, viscous liquid secreted by cells of the mucosa

Mutation A random alteration in the genetic structure of a cell

Mycelium The hyphal mat produced by growing mold (a mold colony)

Mycoses A fungal infection

NAD (Nicotinamide adenine dinadeotide) A coenzyme that acts to transfer hydrogen atoms

Necrosis The death of cells due to injury or disease

Neutralization A serological procedure used to detect the presence of antibody by inhibiting (neutralizing) growth of a pathogen

Neutrophile A granulocyte that is heavily involved in the inflammatory response and a major component of pus

Nosocomial An illness that is acquired incident to hospitalization

Objective lens The lens of a compound microscope that makes the first magnification of an object under observation

Ocular The lens of a compound microscope nearest the eye of the viewer

Oncogenic A tumor-inducing material

Opportunist An organism of low virulence that depends on a reduction in normal host defenses in order to produce disease. Frequently an organism of normal flora

Organic A molecule composed of one or more carbon atoms and one or more hydrogen atoms

Organelle A functional macromolecular structure that is subcellular but associated with a primary singular cellular activity

Osmotic pressure The pressure created across a semipermeable membrane by solvents containing differing concentrations of solute

Osteomyelitis   An infection of bone

Otitis   An infection of the ear. *O. media*, an infection of the inner ear

Oxidation   An increase in oxygen. The loss of a hydrogen atom (electron) from a molecule

Pandemic   An outbreak of infection involving more than one nation

Parasite   An organism that depends on some other organism to supply an essential nutrient. This relationship is gained at no expense to the parasite and no benefit to the host

Parenteral   The body spaces outside the intestine

Paroxysm   A spasmotic or sudden attack of symptoms

Pasteurize   A process of decontaminating liquids that uses heat at less than boiling temperatures. Most often used for milk

Pathogen   An organism that can cause a disease in its host

Pelvic inflammatory disease   A serious infection of the female involving the internal reproductive organs as well as peritoneal spaces

Penicillinase   An enzyme that will destroy the effectiveness of penicillin by breaking the beta lactam ring

Peptidoglycan   The rigid structural molecule of bacterial cell walls

Peptide bond   A covalent bond joining adjacent amino acids in a polypeptide

Peritoneal   Pertaining to the abdomen

Phagocyte   A cell that has the primary function of ingesting and destroying foreign matter found in the body

Phagosome   A membrane-bound vesicle containing material ingested by phagocytosis

Pharyngitis   An infection of the throat

Phenol   A chemical material used as the basis of a number of disinfectants (C_6H_5OH)

Phenol coefficient   The ratio of effectiveness of a disinfectant when compared to that of phenol

Phenotype   The actual expression of the information present in the genome

Pili   The same as fimbrae but also involved in bacterial conjugation with the exchange of DNA

Plasma   The liquid (noncellular) portion of the blood, primarily composed of water, proteins, and salts

Plasma cell   Lymphocytic cells that function to produce immunoglobulins

Plasmid   A dense, circular extrachromosomal DNA not essential to cell function, often found in those bacteria having antibiotic resistance

PMN   Polymorphonuclear leukocyte, a neutrophilic phagocyte

Pneumonia   An inflammation of the lungs resulting in an accumulation of exudate in the alveolar spaces

Polymer   A large molecule primarily composed by a number of similar subunit molecules

Polypeptide   A chain of amino acids, not as large as a protein

Polyribosome   (Polysome) A complex of ribosomes found on a single messenger RNA

Polysaccharide   A large, complex carbohydrate consisting of numerous smaller sugar monomers

Precipitin test   A serological reaction in which a soluble antigen combines with an antibody to produce a visible precipitation

Procaryotic   An organism with a rudimentary nucleus that lacks a membrane

Prostration   A loss of strength, exhaustion

Protein   A large polymer composed of amino acids

Protozoa   Microscopic, single-celled animals. Most are free living, but some are responsible for human disease

Pruritis   Itching due to irritation of sensory nerve endings

Psychrophile   An organism that grows best at temperatures less than 20°C

Purulent   Pus forming or pus containing

Putrification   The decomposition (usually bacterial) of organic matter with an attendant foul aroma

Pyelonephritis   An infection of the kidney

Quellung   The apparent increase in size of a bacterium caused by the interaction of the capsule with its specific antiserum

Radioactive   A compound that emits subatomic particles in the very short wavelength regions of the electromagnetic spectrum

Receptor   A chemical complex on the cell surface that is recognized by a corresponding chemical group, resulting in specific adherence between the two

Recombination   The process by which DNA from one chromosome is integrated into the DNA of another chromosome

Replication   The process of viral multiplication within a cell. The duplication of the DNA molecule

RES   (Reticulo endothelial system) A system composed of phagocytic macrophages present in sinuses and reticulum of various organs and tissues, such as the lung, spleen, and bone marrow. Important in prevention of and recovery from infectious diseases

Resistant   An organism that is not inhibited by an antimicrobial agent is said to be resistant

Respiration   The process of obtaining nutrient energy by breaking down sugar compounds

Restriction endonuclease   An endonuclease that hydrolyses DNA at points of specific nucleotide sequences

Rheumatic fever   A disease characterized by chorea, arthritis, and carditis resulting as a sequelae to streptococcal pharyngitis

Ribosome   An RNA-protein particlelike structure that serves as the site for mRNA-tRNA interaction and protein synthesis

RODAC   An acronym for replicate organism detection and counting (RODAC) plate—a petri dish with a raised agar surface for impression sampling of environmental surfaces or wounds

Salpingitis   Infection of the fallopian tube

Sanitation   The establishment of conditions that are favorable to health

Saprophyte   An organism that does not produce infectious disease

Sensitize   To develop specific antibody as the result of an antigenic stimulus

Sepsis   A toxic, febrile condition associated with bacterial infection and characterized by bacteremia

Septum   The dividing membrane structure between two cellular or body cavities

Serology   The study of serum. Usually associated with approaches to the diagnosis of present or past disease based on measurement of antibody content

Serum   The liquid portion of blood remaining after the clotting proteins have been removed from plasma

Sexually transmitted disease   (STD) Diseases normally transmitted by sexual intercourse

Shingles   A severe vesicular eruption resulting from latent viral infection of dorsal root ganglia by the virus that causes chicken pox

Shock   A condition manifested by a decreased blood pressure, circulatory insufficiency, and a weak pulse

Single-cell protein   Protein used as a nutritional source derived from microorganisms

Sinus   An anatomical space or cavity

Spectrum   The range of organisms inhibited by an antimicrobial agent

Spinal fluid   A clear, waterlike fluid that bathes the brain and spinal cord

Spirillus   Any of a number of bacteria that have a curved or spiral shape

Spontaneous generation   The development of life from nonliving materials without the assistance of living life forms

Sporadic   An infrequent or irregular occurrence of an event

Spore   The asexual reproductive cells produced by fungi

Sporulation   The process of spore formation

Sterile   Without life or free from life

Streaking   The process of inoculation of solid media by sweeping a wire loop through the inoculum and across the agar

Subclinical   The occurrence of an infection wherein the symptoms of the disease are not manifest

Substrate   The compound acted on by an enzyme, resulting in a product

Sulfonamide   A sulfa drug. Antimicrobials containing the sulfanilamide group

Suppuration   Pertaining to the production of pus

Svedberg   A unit of sedimentation coefficient, equivalent to 10^{-13} seconds

Synovial fluid   A thick, transparent fluid found in association with synovial membranes and often occupying bone joint spaces

Systemic   Relating to the entire organism and not its separate parts

T cell   A thymus-derived lymphocyte primarily involved in cellular-type immunity

Taxonomy   The organization or classification of objects into logical relationships

Temperate phage   A bacterial virus that can become integrated into host cell DNA or replicate as a virulent virus

Tincture   A mixture containing alcohol as a solvent

Titer   The concentration of a substance in a solution as determined by measuring its presence in a series of increasing dilutions. The highest dilution containing the substance is the titer

Toxic   Poisonous

Toxin   A biologically produced poison

Toxoid   A toxin that has been modified in order to reduce toxicity without altering antigenicity. Used as a vaccine

Trachea   Windpipe

Transcription   The transfer of genetic information from DNA to messenger RNA

Transduction   The transfer of bacterial genetic information between bacteria by means of a bacterial virus

Transformation   The nonmediated transfer of bacterial DNA between bacterial cells

Translation   The transfer of genetic information from messenger RNA into a protein molecule

Transovarian passage   The transmission of infectious agents to offspring through the ovary by infection of the egg cell

Trichous   Hairlike

Triplet code   A set of three nucleotide bases that code for one amino acid

Trophozoite   The active, vegetative, form of a parasite as opposed to its cyst

Tubercle   A firm granulomatous lesion resulting from an infection with *Mycobacterium tuberculosis*

Turbid   Cloudy, a solution that is not clear

Ulcer   An area of inflammation where the epithelial layer has been lost

Ultraviolet   Area of the electromagnetic spectrum whose wavelength is between 4 and 400 nm

Urethritis   Infection of the urethra

Vaccination   The process of using a vaccine to immunize against disease

Vaccine   An antigen used in the process of vaccination

Vector   An insect, often an arthropod, that can transmit disease producing agents

Vehicle   An object that can serve to transmit an infectious agent

Venereal   Relating to or resulting from sexual intercourse

Virion   The complete viral particle, including both capsid and genome as well as envelope if present

Virulence   Relating to the capacity of an organism to overcome host resistance factors

Vitamin   An organic compound that is essential for health but that cannot be synthesized by the cells of the individual

Volutin   A polyphosphate complex found in some bacterial cells that stains with analine dyes

Zoonosis   Diseases of lower animals that can be transmitted to humans

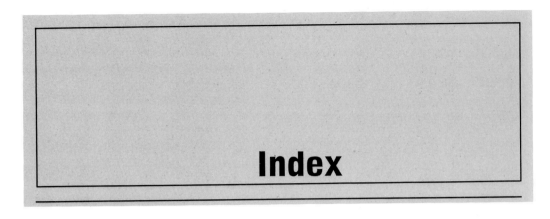

Index